Autism Spectrum Disorder: Understanding the Female Phenotype

Luigi Mazzone
Martina Siracusano • Kevin A. Pelphrey
Editors

Autism Spectrum Disorder: Understanding the Female Phenotype

Springer

Editors
Luigi Mazzone
Department of System Medicine
University of Rome Tor Vergata
Rome, Italy

Martina Siracusano
Department of Biomedicine and Prevention
University of Rome Tor Vergata
Rome, Italy

Kevin A. Pelphrey
Department of Neurology
University of Virginia
Charlottesville, VA, USA

ISBN 978-3-031-62071-3   ISBN 978-3-031-62072-0 (eBook)
https://doi.org/10.1007/978-3-031-62072-0

This Springer imprint is published by the registered company Springer Nature Switzerland AG
The registered company address is: Gewerbestrasse 11, 6330 Cham, Switzerland

Contents

Part I

Autistic Female Phenotype: Gender Differences from Infancy to Adulthood

Autism Spectrum Disorder: Prevalence and Symptoms' Onset

1

Martina Siracusano and Luigi Mazzone

1.1 Which Is the Sex/Gender Prevalence of ASD?

The Centers for Disease Control and Prevention's (CDC) Autism and Developmental Disabilities Monitoring (ADDM) Network estimated that about 1 in 36 children has been diagnosed with autism spectrum disorder (ASD) among children aged 8 years [1], reporting a 4.3:1 male-to-female ratio, resulting in a significant sex/gender difference in prevalence. The male-to-female ratio increases as the severity of intellectual disability decreases [2]. Thereafter, 42.1% of females diagnosed in the spectrum are characterized by intellectual disability (intelligence quotient [IQ] ≤70), which is a higher percentage in comparison to male individuals (36.9%) [1].

The sex/gender prevalence rate estimated has been considered as the objective of a "male bias" [3, 4]. Among the factors contemplated as responsible for this male prevalence, there are methodological issues (the use of sex/gender-biased diagnostic tools and the population samples included in the studies) and questions related to developmental sex/gender differences [3, 5]. The whole book attempts to clarify (at different levels: clinical, genetic) the reason why ASD prevalence is actually reported to be higher in males; within this chapter, we introduce the topic.

M. Siracusano (✉)
Department of Biomedicine and Prevention, University of Rome Tor Vergata, Rome, Italy

Child Neurology and Psychiatry Unit, Department of Wellbeing of Mental and Neurological, Dental and Sensory Organ Health, Policlinico Tor Vergata Hospital, Rome, Italy
e-mail: martina.siracusano@uniroma2.it

L. Mazzone
Child Neurology and Psychiatry Unit, Department of Wellbeing of Mental and Neurological, Dental and Sensory Organ Health, Policlinico Tor Vergata Hospital, Rome, Italy

Systems Medicine Department, University of Rome Tor Vergata, Rome, Italy
e-mail: luigi.mazzone@uniroma2.it

L. Mazzone et al. (eds.), *Autism Spectrum Disorder: Understanding the Female Phenotype*, https://doi.org/10.1007/978-3-031-62072-0_1

1.2 Why ASD Is More Frequently Reported in Males?

Are there less females with an autism condition or girls less easily and later diagnosed in comparison to their male peers? Whether ASD is less represented in females or it is underestimated in this sex/gender remains an open question, being an objective of a growing body of research.

Misdiagnosis or later diagnosis? Nosological or diagnostic challenge [3, 5]?

Several can be the reasons why girls are exposed to these phenomena (Fig 1.1), and two are the main diagnostic conditions which frequently occur: females receiving later diagnosis (condition of "**later age of diagnosis**") and females diagnosed in early infancy (condition of "**more severe profile leading to earlier diagnosis**") [3].

Autistic females with higher cognitive skills (low level of support needs) may be under-recognized [6, 7] due to the better communicative skills (verbal and nonverbal) and good social motivation [8, 9]; the difficulties in friendships' maintenance [3] and the restricted and repetitive interests—due to the less atypical content (i.e., singers, celebrities) in comparison to their male peers [10]—may be hardly identified until late childhood, adolescence, and even adulthood (condition of "**later age of diagnosis**").

However, the presence of comorbid cognitive delay (high level of support needs) defines a "classical male-typical presentation," which implies a minor diagnostic challenge (condition of "**more severe profile leading to earlier diagnosis**") [3] (see Chap. 3).

Recent research discussed whether "[…] *our understanding of autism may have been substantially biased towards males* […]" identifying the so-called diagnostic challenge in females [3, 4].

First of all, a problem of diagnostic tools has been hypothesized: instruments employed for capturing symptoms of ASD (ADOS-2; ADI-R) may be male biased and therefore less sensitive in detecting autism features among females [6, 11–17]. Moreover, culture-related gender developmental differences may contribute masking social difficulties (females are culturally expected as being shy) and atypical behaviors in females. Thus, these symptoms are later identified as related to the condition of ASD [3, 18].

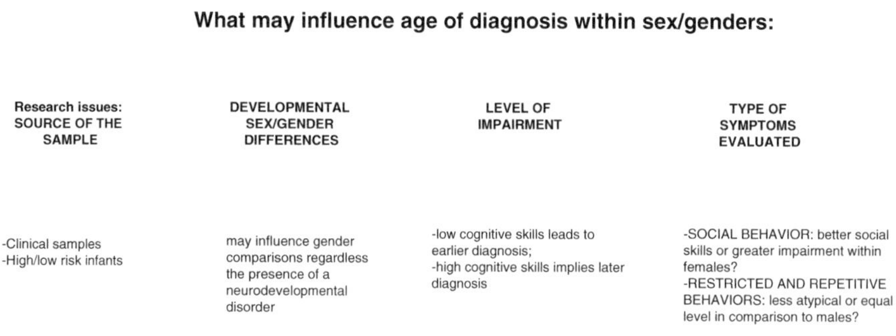

Fig. 1.1 Main factors with a possible influence on sex/gender difference in ASD onset

"*Setting the scene for future research*" is a critical issue as suggested by Lai et al. [3] trying to understand the implications from the actual research on sex/gender and ASD, in order to contribute to the design of future studies. In particular, the authors identified the need of using representative sample size of both sexes/genders as one of the main methodological concerns in gender research. Most of the studies, in fact, include a number of female participants according to the wide male–female ratio 4:1, leading to male-biased study [3]. In these terms, research may be in some ways responsible for the prevalence rate.

1.3 Is There Any Sex/Gender Difference in Autism Symptoms' Onset?

How ASD symptoms appear/arise/come out in early infancy is variable, and different clinical patterns have been identified as a possible way of ASD onset [19] (see Table 1.1). Even if ASD prevalence is significantly higher in males in comparison to females, this aspect may not reflect a sex/gender difference in the emergence of autism symptoms in early childhood [3]. However, despite the growing interest in defining an autism female phenotype, few researches have specifically investigated if there are evident sex/gender differences in early autism manifestations [20–24].

Some studies including infants and toddlers with ASD did not reveal significant sex/gender differences at these early stages of life [23, 25, 26]. In contrast, other researches identified better social communication skills and reduced RRBs as characteristics of young females with ASD in comparison to their male counterpart [24, 9]. Others found equal level of RRBs within sex/gender in early infancy but greater impairment of social skills [27].

These varied findings lead to a huge confusion, which has been attributed to clinical and research issues such as broad age ranges of the samples (6 months–5 years of age) with a possible influence of developmental issues on the autism manifestations rather than reflecting a specific gender phenotype [27]. For example, studies conducted on early infancy samples may hardly capture sex/gender differences in RRBs: Are children too young to show significant differences in the symptoms' manifestation [26]?

As a matter of fact, an important point is whether **developmental sex differences** may influence gender comparisons regardless of the presence of a neurodevelopmental disorder. In regard to this, a Baby Siblings Research Consortium study conducted on a sample of 1824 infants (including 1241 high-risk siblings, 583

Table 1.1 Based on Rogers [20], Pearson et al. [21] and Boterberg et al. [22]

	Congenital	Plateau	Regression	Mixed
ASD SYMTPOMS'ONSET	Emergence of atypical behaviors in the first year of life	Early milestone achievement followed by a developmental plateau	Attainment of developmental milestones followed by a regression/loss of skills	Pattern of early delays followed by later loss

low-risk)—evaluated at different age time (18, 24, 36 months)—examined sex differences in the development of ASD symptoms and in cognitive skills.

Interestingly, the authors found that, regardless of the condition of risk (high or low) and outcome (ASD/non-ASD), lower levels of cognitive functioning and higher levels of restrictive and repetitive behaviors emerged within males in comparison to females. Thus, this study suggests that "early sex differences are not autism specific" but mirror a sex-related variability not linked to the neurodevelopmental disorder [28].

Moreover, not only age—and subsequent developmental issues—but also **source of the sample** (clinical, high/low-risk individuals) may be responsible for the varied and inconsistent results actually characterizing sex/gender research. In fact, it is necessary to specify that most of the studies were conducted on clinical samples (infants and toddlers already diagnosed with ASD) [23, 24, 27] and few on cohorts including high-risk infant samples (i.e., siblings of ASD individuals) [29, 30]. In regard to studies conducted on clinical samples, Lawson et al. [27] examined (across time) sex/gender differences in early autism clinical manifestations and cognitive development in a very young community-ascertained sample of toddlers with ASD aged from 24 to 48 months. More social communication impairment emerged within females in comparison to the male counterpart.

When sex/gender differences were examined within high-risk infant cohorts, higher social skills better characterized females (i.e., increased attention to social stimuli) in comparison to male peers.

However, also results obtained from high-risk cohort studies—due to the fact that they include siblings—cannot reflect ASD as a whole but withstand underlying genetic mechanisms linked to ASD multiplex families.

Therefore, actual research on the topic does not clarify whether ASD symptoms differently emerge within sex/gender, but it has focused its attention on a possible female phenotype in early infancy characterized by less RRBs and better social skills (see Chap. 2). However, further studies are necessary in order to better investigate and understand this puzzling issue.

Specifically concerning **social behavior**, atypical attention to social stimuli is considered an important attentional and behavioral issue of ASD risk in early childhood [29, 31]. In this context, eye-tracking technology represents the main objective way to measure these abilities, in particular the attentional patterns [32].

What we have learned from eye-tracking studies is that toddlers with ASD or at risk for this condition present less attention to social targets and stimuli (faces of interactive people, objects attended by others, activities performed by interactive partners) [32].

Preliminary eye-tracking research shows that sex/gender differences may exist in ASD children specifically concerning social attention [33–35]. Of particular interest, an eye-tracker prospective research (experimental study of social attention) suggests that, in early infancy (6 and 12 months of age, period during which social cognitive skills are expected to develop), **females** at high risk for ASD (siblings of ASD children) are characterized by a "social advantage" consisting of increased attention to socially relevant targets such as faces, in comparison to males with the same risk of ASD and peers of both genders with lower risk [29]. Interestingly, high-risk females were characterized by a greater attention to social stimuli also in comparison to females at low risk of ASD. This neurobehavioral finding, even if preliminary, is in line with clinical researches reporting better clinical social skills in females later diagnosed with ASD (social camouflage theory).

Noteworthily, differences in social attention at early stages of life may be responsible for developmental trajectories, predicting later behavioral outcome [29, 36]. For example, less attention to social scenes in toddlers with ASD was related to poor cognitive and language outcome at 3 years [36].

In fact, given the relevant role of social attention in learning derived from experience—with subsequent effect on shaping the cognitive system—the existence of sex/gender differences in social attention in early infancy may influence developmental trajectories [37]. In this context, further research specifically investigating sex/gender differences in the development of social attention within population at risk for ASD is necessary in order to better understand if such female social advantage in early infancy corresponds to a different developmental trajectory in terms of ASD symptom severity and comorbid conditions.

Finally, as reported in previous paragraphs, different patterns of ASD onset may occur (Table 1.1), including "**regression**" (meant as a loss of acquired skills—not specifically defined in terms of onset time and type of ability) occurring in 32% of cases, which represent one of the main parental concerns. However, no sex/gender differences have been reported specifically concerning this way of onset, or this issue has not been deeply investigated yet [20].

Noteworthily, a study investigating if the **initial impression** (5-min observation of toddlers presenting for an ASD evaluation) of expert clinicians matched the final ASD diagnosis did not find sex/gender differences in its results (ASD diagnosis matched in 92% of cases) [19]. These findings highlight the fact that being female or male did not significantly influence the match between first impression and diagnosis of clinicians who are expert in the field. Thus, sex did not make more difficult "diagnosis at a glance in 5 min" within their very young sample. However, age and developmental aspects should be taken into account before going to conclusions. In fact, the study included toddlers referring for an ASD evaluation at very early age (part of a multicenter screening project), more likely affected by evident atypical features in comparison to children who later refer for mild socio-communicative difficulties, which could necessitate an evaluation longer than 5 min for a correct diagnosis.

1.4 Conclusion

We are still far away from understanding with certainty why the male prevalence of ASD is significantly higher in comparison to female and if a sex/gender pattern of ASD symptom onset—independently or not from developmental sex differences—exists indeed.

However, even if most of the questions addressed in this chapter remain unanswered, we can affirm that the greater awareness of a "female diagnostic challenge" is leading to a greater consciousness of families, teachers, researchers, and clinicians.

Key Points

- ASD prevalence is significantly higher in males in comparison to females.
- Main question is if females are later diagnosed or misdiagnosed.
- A more severe clinical profile with associated intellectual disability leads to earlier diagnosis.
- A sex difference in the emergence of autism symptoms in early childhood has not been concordantly reported.
- Developmental sex differences may influence gender comparisons regardless of the presence of a neurodevelopmental disorder.

References

1. Maenner MJ, Warren Z, Williams AR, et al. Prevalence and characteristics of autism spectrum disorder among children aged 8 years—autism and developmental disabilities monitoring network, 11 sites, United States, 2020. MMWR Surveill Summ. 2023;72(2):1–14. https://doi.org/10.15585/mmwr.ss7202a1.
2. Zeidan J, Fombonne E, Scorah J, et al. Global prevalence of autism: a systematic review update. Autism Res. 2022;15(5):778–90. https://doi.org/10.1002/aur.2696.
3. Lai MC, Lombardo MV, Auyeung B, Chakrabarti B, Baron-Cohen S. Sex/gender differences and autism: setting the scene for future research. J Am Acad Child Adolesc Psychiatry. 2015;54(1):11–24. https://doi.org/10.1016/j.jaac.2014.10.003.
4. Ochoa-Lubinoff C, Makol BA, Dillon EF. Autism in women. Neurol Clin. 2023;41(2):381–97. https://doi.org/10.1016/j.ncl.2022.10.006.
5. Di Vara S, Guerrera S, Menghini D, et al. Characterizing individual differences in children and adolescents with autism spectrum disorder: a descriptive study. Front Psychol. 2024;15:1323787. Published 2024 Feb 27. https://doi.org/10.3389/fpsyg.2024.1323787.
6. Lai MC, Lombardo MV, Pasco G, et al. A behavioral comparison of male and female adults with high functioning autism spectrum conditions. PLoS One. 2011;6(6):e20835. https://doi.org/10.1371/journal.pone.0020835.
7. Lai M-C, Lombardo MV, Ruigrok AN, Chakrabarti B, Auyeung B, Szatmari P, et al. Quantifying and exploring camouflaging in men and women with autism. Autism. 2017a;21:690–702. https://doi.org/10.1177/1362361316671012.
8. Napolitano A, Schiavi S, La Rosa P, Rossi-Espagnet MC, Petrillo S, Bottino F, et al. Sex differences in autism Spectrum disorder: diagnostic, neurobiological, and behavioral features. Front. Psych. 2022;13:889636. https://doi.org/10.3389/fpsyt.2022.889636.
9. Knutsen J, Crossman M, Perrin J, Shui A, Kuhlthau K. Sex differences in restricted repetitive behaviors and interests in children with autism spectrum disorder: an autism treatment network study. Autism. 2019;23:858–68. https://doi.org/10.1177/1362361318786490.
10. Saure E, Castrén M, Mikkola K, Salmi J. Intellectual disabilities moderate sex/gender differences in autism spectrum disorder: a systematic review and meta-analysis. J. Intellect. Disabil. Res. 2023;67:1–34. https://doi.org/10.1111/jir.12989.
11. Rutter M, Caspi A, Moffitt TE. Using sex differences in psychopathology to study causal mechanisms: unifying issues and research strategies. J Child Psychol Psychiatry. 2003;44(8):1092–115. https://doi.org/10.1111/1469-7610.00194.

12. Gould J, Ashton-Smith J. Missed diagnosis or misdiagnosis: girls and women on the autism spectrum. Good Autism Pract. 2011;12:34–41.
13. Constantino JN, Charman T. Gender bias, female resilience, and the sex ratio in autism. J Am Acad Child Adolesc Psychiatry. 2012;51(8):756–8. https://doi.org/10.1016/j.jaac.2012.05.017.
14. Lai MC, Lombardo MV, Chakrabarti B, Baron-Cohen S. Subgrouping the autism "spectrum": reflections on DSM-5. PLoS Biol. 2013;11(4):e1001544. https://doi.org/10.1371/journal.pbio.1001544.
15. Kreiser NL, White SW. ASD in females: are we overstating the gender difference in diagnosis? Clin Child Fam Psychol Rev. 2014;17(1):67–84. https://doi.org/10.1007/s10567-013-0148-9.
16. Tillmann J, Ashwood K, Absoud M, Bölte S, Bonnet-Brilhault F, Buitelaar JK, et al. Evaluating sex and age differences in ADI-R and ADOS scores in a large European multi-site sample of individuals with autism spectrum disorder. J. Autism Dev. Disord. 2018;48:2490–505. https://doi.org/10.1007/s10803-018-3510-4.
17. Navarro-Pardo E, López-Ramón F, Alonso-Esteban Y, Alcantud-Marín F. Diagnostic tools for autism Spectrum disorders by gender: analysis of current status and future lines. Children (Basel). 2021;8:262. https://doi.org/10.3390/children80402.
18. Lai M-C, Szatmari P. Sex and gender impacts on the behavioural presentation and recognition of autism. Curr. Opin. Psychiatry. 2020;33:117–23. https://doi.org/10.1097/YCO.0000000000000575.
19. Wieckowski AT, de Marchena A, Algur Y, et al. The first five minutes: initial impressions during autism spectrum disorder diagnostic evaluations in young children. Autism Res. 2021;14(9):1923–34. https://doi.org/10.1002/aur.2536.
20. Rogers SJ. Developmental regression in autism spectrum disorders. Ment Retard Dev Disabil Res Rev. 2004;10(2):139–43. https://doi.org/10.1002/mrdd.20027.
21. Pearson N, Charman T, Happé F, Bolton PF, McEwen FS. Regression in autism spectrum disorder: reconciling findings from retrospective and prospective research. Autism Res. 2018;11(12):1602–20. https://doi.org/10.1002/aur.2035.
22. Boterberg S, Charman T, Marschik PB, Bölte S, Roeyers H. Regression in autism spectrum disorder: a critical overview of retrospective findings and recommendations for future research. Neurosci Biobehav Rev. 2019;102:24–55. https://doi.org/10.1016/j.neubiorev.2019.03.013.
23. Postorino V, Fatta LM, De Peppo L, et al. Longitudinal comparison between male and female preschool children with autism spectrum disorder. J Autism Dev Disord. 2015;45(7):2046–55. https://doi.org/10.1007/s10803-015-2366-0.
24. Hartley SL, Sikora DM. Sex differences in autism spectrum disorder: an examination of developmental functioning, autistic symptoms, and coexisting behavior problems in toddlers. J Autism Dev Disord. 2009;39(12):1715–22. https://doi.org/10.1007/s10803-009-0810-8. Epub 2009 Jul 7. PMID: 19582563; PMCID: PMC3590797
25. Andersson GW, Gillberg C, Miniscalco C. Pre-school children with suspected autism spectrum disorders: do girls and boys have the same profiles? Res Dev Disabil. 2013;34(1):413–22. https://doi.org/10.1016/j.ridd.2012.08.025.
26. Van Wijngaarden-Cremers PJ, van Eeten E, Groen WB, Van Deurzen PA, Oosterling IJ, Van der Gaag RJ. Gender and age differences in the core triad of impairments in autism spectrum disorders: a systematic review and meta-analysis. J Autism Dev Disord. 2014;44(3):627–35. https://doi.org/10.1007/s10803-013-1913-9.
27. Lawson LP, Joshi R, Barbaro J, Dissanayake C. Gender differences during toddlerhood in autism spectrum disorder: a prospective community-based longitudinal follow-up study. J Autism Dev Disord. 2018;48(8):2619–28. https://doi.org/10.1007/s10803-018-3516-y.
28. Messinger DS, Young GS, Webb SJ, Ozonoff S, Bryson SE, Carter A, Carver L, Charman T, Chawarska K, Curtin S, Dobkins K, Hertz-Picciotto I, Hutman T, Iverson JM, Landa R, Nelson CA, Stone WL, Tager-Flusberg H, Zwaigenbaum L. Early sex differences are not autism-specific: A Baby Siblings Research Consortium (BSRC) study. Mol Autism. 2015;6:32. https://doi.org/10.1186/s13229-015-0027-y. PMID: 26045943; PMCID: PMC4455973.

29. Chawarska K, Macari S, Powell K, DiNicola L, Shic F. Enhanced social attention in female infant siblings at risk for autism. J Am Acad Child Adolesc Psychiatry. 2016;55(3):188–95.e1. https://doi.org/10.1016/j.jaac.2015.11.016.
30. Zwaigenbaum L, Bryson SE, Szatmari P, et al. Sex differences in children with autism spectrum disorder identified within a high-risk infant cohort. J Autism Dev Disord. 2012;42(12):2585–96. https://doi.org/10.1007/s10803-012-1515-y.
31. Di Giorgio E, Rosa-Salva O, Frasnelli E, et al. Abnormal visual attention to simple social stimuli in 4-month-old infants at high risk for Autism. Sci Rep. 2021;11(1):15785. Published 2021 Aug 4. https://doi.org/10.1038/s41598-021-95418-4.
32. Hamner T, Vivanti G. Eye-tracking research in autism spectrum disorder: what are we measuring and for what purposes? Curr Dev Disord Rep. 2019;6:37–44. https://doi.org/10.1007/s40474-019-00158-w.
33. Harrop C, Jones D, Zheng S, Nowell SW, Boyd BA, Sasson N. Sex differences in social attention in autism spectrum disorder. Autism Res. 2018;11(9):1264–75. https://doi.org/10.1002/aur.1997.
34. Kleberg JL, Nyström P, Bölte S, Falck-Ytter T. Sex differences in social attention in infants at risk for autism. J Autism Dev Disord. 2019;49(4):1342–51. https://doi.org/10.1007/s10803-018-3799-z.
35. Frazier TW, Strauss M, Klingemier EW, Zetzer EE, Hardan AY, Eng C, et al. A meta- analysis of gaze differences to social and nonsocial information between individuals with and without autism. J Am Acad Child Adolesc Psychiatry. 2017;56(7):546–55.
36. Campbell DJ, Shic F, Macari S, Chawarska K. Gaze response to dyadic bids at 2 years related to outcomes at 3 years in autism spectrum disorders: a subtyping analysis. J Autism Dev Disord. 2014;44(2):431–42. https://doi.org/10.1007/s10803-013-1885-9.
37. Chawarska K, Macari S, Shic F. Decreased spontaneous attention to social scenes in 6-month-old infants later diagnosed with autism spectrum disorders. Biol Psychiatry. 2013;74(3):195–203. https://doi.org/10.1016/j.biopsych.2012.11.022.

Female Autism Phenotype

2

Martina Siracusano, Claudia Marcovecchio, Elisa Carloni, Assia Riccioni, and Luigi Mazzone

2.1 Introduction

The existence of a specific "female phenotype of autism" has been proposed during the last few years, suggesting that the female diagnostic challenge may be mediated by two distinct factors contrasting but not mutually exclusive.

On the one hand, a *female protective effect* (FPE theory) has been hypothesized, which implies an innate protective factor in females, according to which they require a greater environmental and/or genetic load than males to express the same degree of autistic characteristics [1].

On the other hand, it has been proposed that diagnostic biases (employment of male-biased instruments; male-focused diagnostic criteria) contribute to delayed diagnosis or even missed diagnosis in females [2, 3].

M. Siracusano (✉)
Department of Biomedicine and Prevention, University of Rome Tor Vergata, Rome, Italy

Child Neurology and Psychiatry Unit, Department of Wellbeing of Mental and Neurological, Dental and Sensory Organ Health, Policlinico Tor Vergata Hospital, Rome, Italy
e-mail: martina.siracusano@uniroma2.it

C. Marcovecchio · E. Carloni · A. Riccioni
Child Neurology and Psychiatry Unit, Department of Wellbeing of Mental and Neurological, Dental and Sensory Organ Health, Policlinico Tor Vergata Hospital, Rome, Italy

L. Mazzone
Child Neurology and Psychiatry Unit, Department of Wellbeing of Mental and Neurological, Dental and Sensory Organ Health, Policlinico Tor Vergata Hospital, Rome, Italy

Systems Medicine Department, University of Rome Tor Vergata, Rome, Italy
e-mail: luigi.mazzone@uniroma2.it

L. Mazzone et al. (eds.), *Autism Spectrum Disorder: Understanding the Female Phenotype*, https://doi.org/10.1007/978-3-031-62072-0_2

Understanding and recognizing female autism phenotype are necessary to allow early identification and diagnosis of autistic females and to develop sex/gender-appropriate intervention for ASD.

In this chapter, we explore sex/gender differences in phenotypic presentation of ASD, focusing on the two core symptoms according to the DSM 5 TR [4, 5]: *social communication, social interaction abilities,* and *restricted and repetitive behaviors* (RRBs).

2.2 Social Communication and Social Interaction Skills

One of the main questions the research is attempting to answer within ASD is whether there are—and how are they influenced by—sex/gender differences in socio-communicative skills (Table 2.1).

Table 2.1 Persistent deficits in social communication and social interaction across multiple contexts (Autism Spectrum Disorder, Domain A, DSM 5 TR [5])

A1. ***Deficits in social-emotional reciprocity*** Ranging from abnormal social approach and failure of normal back-and-forth conversation through reduced sharing of interests, emotions, and affect and response to total lack of initiation of social interaction	• Unusual social initiations (intrusive touching, licking of others) • Use of others as tools • One-sided conversation/monologues • Impairment in join attention • Lack of showing or pointing out objects to other people • Failure to share enjoyment, excitement, or achievements with others • Indifference/aversion to physical contact and affection
A2. ***Deficits in nonverbal communicative behaviors used for social interaction*** Ranging from poorly integrated, verbal and nonverbal communication, through abnormalities in eye contact and body language, or deficits in understanding and use of nonverbal communication, to total lack of facial expression or gestures	• Abnormal prosody, rhythm, intonation, or volume in speech • Inability to coordinate eye contact or body language with words • Impairment in the use of facial expressions (limited or exaggerated) • Impairment in the use and understanding of gesture (i.e., nodding/shaking head, pointing, waving) or posture (i.e., facing away from a listener)
A3. ***Deficits in developing and maintaining relationships, appropriate to developmental level (beyond those with caregivers)*** Ranging from difficulties adjusting behavior to suit different social contexts through difficulties in sharing imaginative play and in making friends to an apparent absence of interest in people	• Inability to take another person's perspective • Unaware of social convention and appropriate social behavior (ask socially inappropriate questions) • Inappropriate expression of emotion (i.e., laughing or smiling out of context) • Withdrawn, lack interest in peers • Has an interest in friendship but lacks understanding of the convention of social interaction (i.e., extremely directive or rigid; overly passive)

2.2.1 Are There Sex/Gender Differences in Socio-Communicative Skills?

Females on the spectrum—even if displaying a social impairment in comparison to females with typical development—generally exhibit greater social skills when compared to autistic males such as greater desire and awareness of social interactions, tendency to imitate others, compensatory strategies masking difficulties in relationships, better language abilities, and greater imagination [6, 7]. Better social skills of females may contribute to the lower rate of ASD diagnosis in girls or at least they may be responsible for the masked behavioral difficulties [2, 8].

Currently, scientific evidence shows that among factors influencing sex/gender differences within ASD, there is mainly the level of impairment and subsequently the degree of support needed.

Age of first parental concern (early or late childhood and adolescence) may be linked to the level of their daughters' social impairment. As a matter of fact, girls who refer for a clinical assessment during *toddlerhood/early childhood* are characterized by a greater impairment in engaging social interaction and in reciprocal social communication [9]. On the other hand, females of same age with less social difficulties and showing higher levels of social motivation (i.e., greater desire to form friendship) may be missed during routine surveillance [9]. These girls will probably undergo psychiatric assessment during school age and/or adolescence [6, 8]. As a matter of fact, given that as age increases, the social demand rises, girls who have masked their difficulties until scholar age/adolescence might probably exhibit a social impairment—still less evident in comparison to autistic males—at this stage of life.

Specifically considering scholar age, females are more likely to show greater ability to engage in reciprocal conversation, to initiate friendship, and to share interests [6]. Furthermore, girls show greater abilities to adapt behaviors in public across different situations compared to boys including larger social setting and school environment (i.e., monitoring volume of voice, avoiding socially inappropriate comments) [2, 6, 10]. This sex/gender socio-communicative profile persists at older ages (adolescents and young adults), when female adolescents in the spectrum report a better friendship quality and empathy in comparison to autistic males [8] (Fig. 2.1).

Overall, these aspects may make cognitive-able females less likely to be identified at all stages of life, leading to late diagnosis, prejudicing them from receiving appropriately targeted health care, early intervention, and educational resources.

2.2.1.1 Sex/gender differences related to the level of support needs

Level of functioning (actually defined with the level of support needs) in autism spectrum disorder represents a crucial point on the definition of the autistic phenotype, influencing the determination of sex/gender differences between male and female [6].

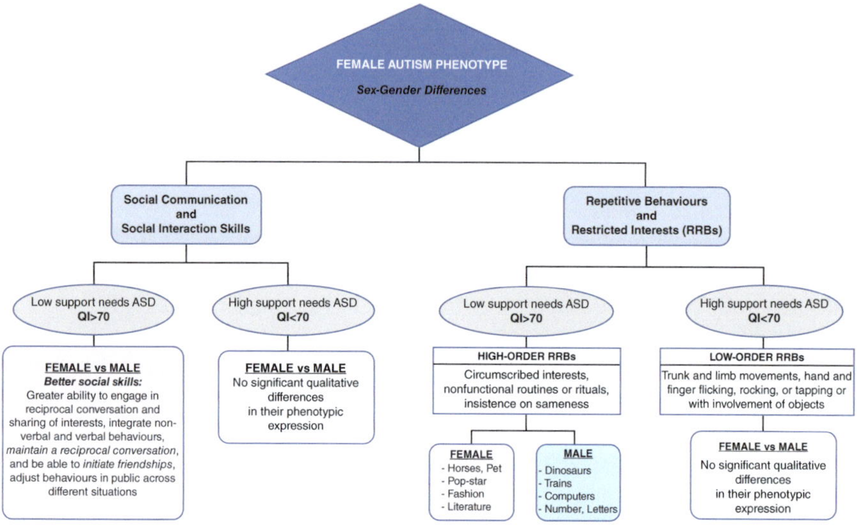

Fig. 2.1 Sex differences in symptom domains of ASD: Social Communication Skills and RRBs

Evidence of sex/gender differences in the social and communication domain may be related to different levels of support needs (Fig. 2.1). Indeed, during childhood and adolescence, both ASD males and females with high support needs did not show significant differences from each other in socio-communicative domain [11], reflecting overlapping profiles between males and females [12] (Fig. 2.1).

On the other hand, autistic females with low support needs, who possess strong social skills compared to males, require greater impairment of other core symptoms to obtain a diagnosis. Although it is currently estimated that four males are diagnosed with ASD for every one female [13], gender ratios have been seen to begin to decrease if individuals with intellectual disability are considered, making the differences between sexes/genders less apparent. These findings suggest that in individuals requiring a lower support, there may be a high portion of ASD females who go unnoticed, raising the added complexity of determining who should receive a diagnosis [2, 8].

The apparent better social functioning of autistic females compared to autistic males suggests that females may show a superficial understanding of appropriate social etiquette, and they may be able to mask their deficits through imitation and mimicry [14].

These findings could be explained by the "*camouflage hypothesis*" proposed by Wing [15] that refers to the use of conscious or unconscious strategies that allow females with ASD to develop social skills and coping mechanisms to blend in or camouflage themselves into society, obscuring a likely diagnosis of ASD, even though there may be other indications of the condition (see Box 2.1). Although camouflaging is an adaptive mechanism, it may enclose several negative implications, such as misdiagnosis, late diagnosis, or underdiagnosis that can prevent from adequate or timely intervention [16].

Therefore, the apparent advantage showed by autistic females over males may partly explain gender ratio (M:F = 4:1) within ASD. Understanding and recognizing the social female phenotype of ASD and the camouflage hypothesis may be useful to reconsider in a sex/gender prospective the social communication diagnostic criteria. This could allow to diagnose a larger number of females leading to a prompt and adequate intervention [8].

2.3 Repetitive Behaviors and Restricted Interests

Restricted and repetitive behaviors (RRBs) are core symptoms of autism spectrum disorder, but they are not unique to children with autism; indeed, they can be found in children with other neurodevelopmental disorders, such as intellectual disability and language disorders, and also in other psychiatric conditions (i.e., obsessive–compulsive disorder) [17]. RRBs are also common during early typical development, but what makes the RRBs of children with typical development different from those RRBs exhibited by autistic individuals is their intensity [18]. RRBs have been found to be one of the earliest signs exhibited by infants later diagnosed with ASD and early predictors of outcome [19].

In Table 2.2, restricted, repetitive patterns of behavior, typical of ASD—regardless of sex/gender differences—are reported as stated by the DSM 5 TR [5].

Table 2.2 Restricted, repetitive patterns of behavior, interests, or activities (Autism Spectrum Disorder, Domain B, DSM-5) with clinical examples

B1. ***Stereotyped or repetitive speech, motor movements, or use of objects*** Such as simple motor stereotypies, echolalia, repetitive use of objects, lining up toys or flipping objects, or idiosyncratic phrases	• Repetitive hand movements (i.e., flapping, clapping) • Toe walking • Unusually formal language (speaking like an adult) • Repetitive vocalization, words, phrases, or songs • Nonfunctional play with objects • Repetitively opens and closes doors or turns lights on–off
B2. ***Insistence on sameness, excessive adherence to routines, ritualized patterns of verbal or nonverbal behavior, or excessive resistance to change*** Such as motoric rituals, insistence on same route or food, rigid thinking patterns, repetitive questioning, or extreme distress at small changes	• Excessively rigid, inflexible in behavior and thought, and following specific unusual routines • Inability to understand nonliteral aspects of speech (i.e., irony, implied meaning) • Overreaction to trivial changes
B3. ***Highly restricted, fixated interests that are abnormal in intensity or focus*** Such as strong attachment to or preoccupation with unusual objects, excessively circumscribed or perseverative interests	• Attachment to unusual inanimate object (i.e., piece of string, wire, rubber band) • Excessive focus on nonrelevant or nonfunctional parts of objects (i.e., car wheels) • Focused on the same few objects, topics, or activities (i.e., planets, animals)

(continued)

Table 2.2 (continued)

B4. ***Hyper- or hypo-reactivity to sensory input or unusual interest in sensory aspects of environment*** Such as strong attachment to or preoccupation with unusual objects, excessively circumscribed or perseverative interests	• High tolerance for pain • Tactile defensiveness (i.e., does not like to be touched by certain objects or textures) • Significant aversion to having hair or toenails cut or teeth brushed • Looks at objects and people out of the corner of the eye • Extreme interest in watching movement of objects (i.e., spinning wheels of toys, spinning the washing machine) • Licking or sniffing objects

2.3.1 Do Restricted and Repetitive Behaviors Differ Between Sex/Gender Within ASD?

Little is known about RRBs' sex/gender differences in ASD: are RRBs less or more represented in females? Have RRBs a different qualitative expression in females leading to a specific clinical phenotype? In this paragraph, we attempt to examine sex/gender differences from both quantitative and qualitative points of view.

2.3.1.1 RRBs' Quantitative Sex/Gender Differences

Contradictory findings about quantitative sex/gender differences of RRBs are actually available [18]. Indeed, although most of the studies showed that autistic males had significantly more RRBs compared to autistic females [6, 20, 21], other researches found no significant evidence of such differences in RRBs in ASD [22, 23]. These contrasting findings may be in part due to different methodologies of the studies (i.e., small female sample, specific inclusion/exclusion criteria, wide age range, parent-reported measures, lack of cognitive information) [18].

Interestingly, the difference in RRBs' presentation among sex/gender may be related to *age*.

In this regard, results from a recent study, conducted with the aim to investigate sex differences in RRBs through the administration of the parent-reported questionnaire RBS-R (Repetitive Behavior Scale-Revised), showed similar scores among school-age male and female, while during preschool age, males were characterized by higher scores compared to females [24]. These data suggest that *females could later develop evident RRBs*; otherwise, at younger ages, these behaviors are less evident and more difficult to be detected by parent rating evaluation scales [24].

2.3.1.2 RRBs' Qualitative Sex/Gender Differences

If it is not clear whether females present less RRBs in comparison to males, even fewer is known about qualitative sex/gender differences of these interests and behaviors [25]. Interestingly, a study conducted by Antezana et al. [26] found sex/gender differences in a subset of RBS-R items (the scale most employed to measure RRBs): autistic girls exhibited higher scores on insistence on sameness, compulsive, and self-injurious behavior items and lower scores on stereotyped behavior and restricted interest items compared to affected boys. Noteworthily, emerging research pointed out a correlation between insistence on sameness, executive function deficits, and internalizing problems [22, 27–30]. Specifically, the link between executive function deficits and RRBs is explained as the greater is the executive function impairment (less behavioral inhibition, less cognitive flexibility), the higher is the level of RRBs (insistence on sameness). Thus, the positive relation between RRBs and internalizing problems (depression) could be mainly attributed to an alternative strategy for emotional regulation difficulties [31–33].

Specifically regarding the quality of circumscribed interests, females with ASD exhibit more engagement in gender and developmentally normative areas (horses, pets, literature, fashion, popstars), rather than objects/things (numbers, letters, dinosaurs, trains, computers) which characterize autistic boys [7]. These findings suggest that results obtained by available parent rating evaluation scales (i.e., RBS-R) [25] may be biased by the fact that these instruments do not include the full range of RRB types. As a matter of fact, these tools have been developed using samples including predominantly males [10]. This represents one of the main issues contributing to misdiagnosis in females.

2.3.1.3 Relationship Between RRBs, cognitive skills and Level of support needs

Different types of RRBs seem to be correlated with specific level of cognitive ability and support needs. In particular, individuals with ASD and **low cognitive abilities and high level of support needs** most frequently exhibit RRBs defined as low order (i.e., stereotypies such as hand and finger flicking, trunk and limb movements, manipulation of objects, self-injurious behavior, and sensory and motor repetitive behaviors) [34, 35], without significant qualitative differences between males and females in their phenotypic expression [11] (Fig. 2.1). However, in terms of quantitative sex/gender differences, few data suggest that among children with a high level of support needs (up to 8 years old), females show fewer impairments in RRBs than males [36].

On the other hand, individuals with ASD and **high cognitive abilities and low level of support needs** display RRBs defined as high order (i.e., insistence on sameness, unusual attachment to objects, repetitive language, and circumscribed interests) [34, 35] (Fig. 2.1). Therefore, greater cognitive skills seem to correspond to a reduced expression of RRBs, which is *independent from sex and age*, since autistic individuals with higher cognitive functioning can mask repetitive behaviors [34, 35]. However, this masking ability is even more evident in autistic females with low level of support needs, who tend to show pattern of RRBs hardly to identify as atypical (or as a sign of ASD)—especially at a younger age—and less likely to impair the daily functioning and, thus, less expressed by parents as a concern [6].

Consequently, within autistic females with good cognitive skills, RRBs may be masked and less identifiable leading to undiagnosis or misdiagnosis [24, 37, 38]. This reinforces the camouflage hypothesis, which accounts for the difficulty in the definition of a clear behavioral female autistic phenotype.

Given the importance of RRBs in influencing the long-term outcome of the autistic individual [24] and the relative difficulty in early recognizing RRBs in females with ASD, there is a need to further explore sex/gender differences using currently comprehensive RRB measures and improve them with female-specific assessments. Understanding and recognizing female-specific RRBs could help clinicians to create better targeted treatments oriented towards specific needs of girls with ASD [26].

2.4 Conclusion

Finally, the clear definition of a clinical female autistic phenotype is still hardly feasible in autistic females independently from the cognitive skills and level of support needs.

On the one hand, it seems to be "easier" to identify a specific sex/gender clinical phenotype among autistic individuals requiring a lower level of support in both autism core domains, socio-communicative skills and RRBs (Fig. 2.1). On the other hand, clinical symptoms of females with good cognitive skills are more frequently masked (leading to a delayed diagnosis) in comparison to ASD females with low cognitive skills where the clinical profile overlaps that of their male counterpart.

Box 2.1 Camouflaging

"Camouflage" refers to a process through which individuals with autism mask their autistic traits, using conscious or unconscious behavioral and cognitive strategies in order to minimize the visibility of their social difficulties [16, 39].

Three stages of camouflaging process:

1. **Motivation *(why?)*:** desire to fit in socially, to satisfy social expectations, and to limit peer rejection with the final aim to be included in social and work contexts, which could be less accessible in the presence of autism condition [8].
2. **Camouflaging (*how?*):** through several strategies which mask/camouflage their autistic traits:
   - **Assimilation:** adopting behaviors or developing new interests which help them fit in a social group (i.e., copying body language, clothing, or interests).
   - **Masking:** the use of coping strategies learned from real (social interactions) or virtual social life (TV, Web). These strategies include hiding, suppressing, and controlling inappropriate behaviors typical of ASD (i.e., use intentional eye contact, minimize their responses to sensory overstimulation, avoid talking about a particular topic).

- **Compensation:** strategies used by ASD individuals to compensate their atypical traits to meet others' expectations during a conversation (i.e., learning and rehearsing a social script or prompts)

3. **Consequences (*pros and cons*):**
   - **Pros:** camouflaging represents a strength of autistic individuals because it enhances their adaptive functioning, improving their quality of life in terms of independence and social integration (i.e., increase the ability to hide in with others, improve connections and relationships with others, improve employment opportunities) [8].
   - **Cons:** delayed diagnosis of ASD and subsequently delayed therapeutic intervention [8]. Given that camouflaging is a behavior mentally exhausting, it increases the risk of developing *internalizing symptoms* (depression, anxiety, loss of identity, self-injures, and/or suicidal thought) [39].

Gender Differences in Camouflaging

Camouflaging strategies are adopted by both autistic males and females, without co-occurring intellectual disability [39]. However, successful camouflaging techniques are more likely to be implemented by women probably due to culture-based sex/gender role expectations.

As a matter of fact, autistic females seem to suffer more social pressure, while autistic males experience their atypical behaviors as more accepted by society. As a whole, camouflaging, even if representing a "compensatory" strategy, contributes to delayed ASD diagnosis especially within females; thus, it may represent a potential explanation of the sex/gender prevalence rate [16].

The phenomenon of camouflage is summarized in this box; however, each chapter addresses this topic from the specific point of view of the subject discussed.

Key Points
Social Communication and Social Interaction Skills

- Females on the spectrum exhibit *more developed social skills* and *higher levels of social motivation* compared to males with ASD, contributing to the lower rate of ASD diagnosis in girls.
- Females who refer for a *clinical assessment during* ***toddlerhood*** *are those presenting with a* ***greater impairment*** in reciprocal social communication.
- Females who possess stronger social skills and low level of support needs compared to males, require greater impairment in other core symptoms to obtain a diagnosis.
- Females with low cognitive skills and high level of support needs did not show significant gender differences in socio-communicative domain.

Restricted and Repetitive Behaviors (RRBs)

- ***Females who possess stronger cognitive skills and low level of support needs*** most frequently exhibits low-order RRBs, *without significant gender differences* between males and females in their phenotypic expression.
- ASD females with low cognitive skills and high level of support needs displays significantly high-order RRBs, and in *females, RRBs may be masked* and less clinically identifiable.
- Females with ASD exhibit more circumscribed interests in gender and developmentally normative areas compared to affected boys, making it *difficult to identify a clear female autistic* phenotype.

References

1. Robinson EB, Lichtenstein P, Anckarsäter H, Happé F, Ronald A. Examining and interpreting the female protective effect against autistic behavior. Proc Natl Acad Sci USA. 2013;110(13):5258–62. https://doi.org/10.1073/pnas.1211070110.
2. Dworzynski K, Ronald A, Bolton P, Happé F. How different are girls and boys above and below the diagnostic threshold for autism spectrum disorders? J Am Acad Child Adolesc Psychiatry. 2012;51(8):788–97. https://doi.org/10.1016/j.jaac.2012.05.018.
3. Russell G, Steer C, Golding J. Social and demographic factors that influence the diagnosis of autistic spectrum disorders. Soc Psychiatry Psychiatr Epidemiol. 2011;46(12):1283–93. https://doi.org/10.1007/s00127-010-0294-z.
4. American Psychiatric Association. Diagnostic and statistical manual of mental Disorders-5. Washington, DC: American Psychiatric Association; 2013.
5. American Psychiatric Association. Diagnostic and statistical manual of mental disorders (5th ed., text rev.) 2022. https://doi.org/10.1176/appi.books.9780890425787.
6. Hiller RM, Young RL, Weber N. Sex differences in autism spectrum disorder based on DSM-5 criteria: evidence from clinician and teacher reporting. J Abnorm Child Psychol. 2014;42(8):1381–93. https://doi.org/10.1007/s10802-014-9881-x.
7. Lai MC, Lombardo MV, Auyeung B, Chakrabarti B, Baron-Cohen S. Sex/gender differences and autism: setting the scene for future research. J Am Acad Child Adolesc Psychiatry. 2015;54(1):11–24. https://doi.org/10.1016/j.jaac.2014.10.003.
8. Head AM, McGillivray JA, Stokes MA. Gender differences in emotionality and sociability in children with autism spectrum disorders. Mol Autism. 2014;5(1):19. https://doi.org/10.1186/2040-2392-5-19.
9. Lawson LP, Joshi R, Barbaro J, Dissanayake C. Gender differences during toddlerhood in autism spectrum disorder: a prospective community-based longitudinal follow-up study. J Autism Dev Disord. 2018;48(8):2619–28. https://doi.org/10.1007/s10803-018-3516-y.
10. Mandy W, Chilvers R, Chowdhury U, Salter G, Seigal A, Skuse D. Sex differences in autism spectrum disorder: evidence from a large sample of children and adolescents. J Autism Dev Disord. 2012;42(7):1304–13. https://doi.org/10.1007/s10803-011-1356-0.
11. Nguyen C, Ronald A. How do girls with low functioning autism compare to boys with autism and typically developing girls with regard to behavior, cognition, and psychopathology? Scand J Child Adolesc Psychiatry Psychol. 2014;2(2):55–65.
12. Rutter M, Bailey A, Lord C. The social communication questionnaire: manual. Western Psychological Services; 2003.
13. Maenner MJ, Warren Z, Williams AR, et al. Prevalence and characteristics of autism spectrum disorder among children aged 8 years—autism and developmental disabilities monitoring network, 11 sites, United States, 2020. MMWR Surveill Summ. 2023;72(2):1–14. https://doi.org/10.15585/mmwr.ss7202a1.

14. Attwood T, Grandin T, Bolick T, Faherty C, Iland L, Myers JM, Wroble M. Asperger's and girls. Texas: Future Horizons; 2006.
15. Wing L. Sex ratios in early childhood autism and related conditions. Psychiatry Res. 1981;5(2):129–37. https://doi.org/10.1016/0165-1781(81)90043-3.
16. Tubío-Fungueiriño M, Cruz S, Sampaio A, Carracedo A, Fernández-Prieto M. Social camouflaging in females with autism spectrum disorder: a systematic review. J Autism Dev Disord. 2021;51(7):2190–9. https://doi.org/10.1007/s10803-020-04695-x.
17. Muthugovindan D, Singer H. Motor stereotypy disorders. Curr Opin Neurol. 2009;22(2):131–6. https://doi.org/10.1097/WCO.0b013e328326f6c8.
18. Allely C. Exploring the female autism phenotype of repetitive behaviours and restricted interests (RBRIs): a systematic PRISMA review. Adv Autism. 2019;5(3):171–86. https://doi.org/10.1108/AIA-09-2018-0030.
19. Troyb E, Knoch K, Herlihy L, et al. Restricted and repetitive behaviors as predictors of outcome in autism spectrum disorders. J Autism Dev Disord. 2016;46(4):1282–96. https://doi.org/10.1007/s10803-015-2668-2.
20. Park S, Cho S-C, Cho IH, Kim B-N, Kim J-W, Shin M-S, et al. Sex differences in children with autism spectrum disorders compared with their unaffected siblings and typically developing children. Res Autism Spectr Disord. 2012;6(2):861–70.
21. Szatmari P, Chawarska K, Dawson G, et al. Prospective longitudinal studies of infant siblings of children with autism: lessons learned and future directions. J Am Acad Child Adolesc Psychiatry. 2016;55(3):179–87. https://doi.org/10.1016/j.jaac.2015.12.014.
22. Solomon M, Miller M, Taylor SL, Hinshaw SP, Carter CS. Autism symptoms and internalizing psychopathology in girls and boys with autism spectrum disorders. J Autism Dev Disord. 2012;42(1):48–59. https://doi.org/10.1007/s10803-011-1215-z.
23. Knutsen J, Crossman M, Perrin J, Shui A, Kuhlthau K. Sex differences in restricted repetitive behaviors and interests in children with autism spectrum disorder: an autism treatment network study. Autism. 2019;23(4):858–68. https://doi.org/10.1177/1362361318786490.
24. Siracusano M, Postorino V, Riccioni A, et al. Sex differences in autism spectrum disorder: repetitive behaviors and adaptive functioning. Children (Basel). 2021;8(5):325. https://doi.org/10.3390/children8050325.
25. Bodfish JW, Symons FJ, Parker DE, Lewis MH. Varieties of repetitive behavior in autism: comparisons to mental retardation. J Autism Dev Disord. 2000;30(3):237–43. https://doi.org/10.1023/a:1005596502855.
26. Antezana L, Factor RS, Condy EE, Strege MV, Scarpa A, Richey JA. Gender differences in restricted and repetitive behaviors and interests in youth with autism. Autism Res. 2019;12(2):274–83. https://doi.org/10.1002/aur.2049.
27. White EI, Wallace GL, Bascom J, et al. Sex differences in parent-reported executive functioning and adaptive behavior in children and young adults with autism spectrum disorder. Autism Res. 2017,10(10):1653–62. https://doi.org/10.1002/aur.1811.
28. Factor RS, Condy EE, Farley JP, Scarpa A. Brief report: insistence on sameness, anxiety, and social motivation in children with autism Spectrum disorder. J Autism Dev Disord. 2016;46(7):2548–54. https://doi.org/10.1007/s10803-016-2781-x.
29. Mosconi MW, Kay M, D'Cruz AM, et al. Impaired inhibitory control is associated with higher-order repetitive behaviors in autism spectrum disorders. Psychol Med. 2009;39(9):1559–66. https://doi.org/10.1017/S0033291708004984.
30. Wigham S, Rodgers J, South M, McConachie H, Freeston M. The interplay between sensory processing abnormalities, intolerance of uncertainty, anxiety and restricted and repetitive behaviours in autism spectrum disorder. J Autism Dev Disord. 2015;45(4):943–52. https://doi.org/10.1007/s10803-014-2248-x.
31. Baribeau DA, Vigod S, Pullenayegum E, et al. Co-occurring trajectories of anxiety and insistence on sameness behaviour in autism spectrum disorder. Br J Psychiatry. 2021;218(1):20–7. https://doi.org/10.1192/bjp.2020.127.
32. Schwartzman JM, Williams ZJ, Richards JK, Mattheiss SR, Gotham KO. Neuroticism drives associations between repetitive behaviors and depression in autistic adults. Front Psychiatry. 2022;13:803361. https://doi.org/10.3389/fpsyt.2022.803361.

33. Postorino V, Mazzone L, Reaven J. Editorial: Internalizing disorders in individuals with autism spectrum disorder. Front Psychiatry. 2023;13:1112633. https://doi.org/10.3389/fpsyt.2022.1112633.
34. Turner M. Annotation: repetitive behaviour in autism: a review of psychological research. J Child Psychol Psychiatry. 1999;40(6):839–49.
35. Militerni R, Bravaccio C, Falco C, Fico C, Palermo MT. Repetitive behaviors in autistic disorder. Eur Child Adolesc Psychiatry. 2002;11(5):210–8. https://doi.org/10.1007/s00787-002-0279-x.
36. Lord C, Schopler E, Revicki D. Sex differences in autism. J Autism Dev Disord. 1982;12(4):317–30. https://doi.org/10.1007/BF01538320.
37. Frazier TW, Georgiades S, Bishop SL, Hardan AY. Behavioral and cognitive characteristics of females and males with autism in the Simons simplex collection. J Am Acad Child Adolesc Psychiatry. 2014;53(3):329–40.e403. https://doi.org/10.1016/j.jaac.2013.12.004.
38. Postorino V, Fatta LM, De Peppo L, et al. Longitudinal comparison between male and female preschool children with autism spectrum disorder. J Autism Dev Disord. 2015;45(7):2046–55. https://doi.org/10.1007/s10803-015-2366-0.
39. Cook J, Hull L, Crane L, Mandy W. Camouflaging in autism: a systematic review. Clin Psychol Rev. 2021;89:102080. https://doi.org/10.1016/j.cpr.2021.102080.

Further Reading

Head AM, McGillivray JA, Stokes MA. Gender differences in emotionality and sociability in children with autism spectrum disorders. Mol Autism. 2014;5(1):19. https://doi.org/10.1186/2040-2392-5-19.

Hull L, Petrides KV, Allison C, et al. "Putting on my best normal": social camouflaging in adults with autism spectrum conditions. J Autism Dev Disord. 2017;47(8):2519–34. https://doi.org/10.1007/s10803-017-3166-5.

Jorgenson C, Lewis T, Rose C, Kanne S. Social camouflaging in autistic and neurotypical adolescents: a pilot study of differences by sex and diagnosis. J Autism Dev Disord. 2020;50(12):4344–55. https://doi.org/10.1007/s10803-020-04491-7.

Milner V, Mandy W, Happé F, Colvert E. Sex differences in predictors and outcomes of camouflaging: comparing diagnosed autistic, high autistic trait and low autistic trait young adults. Autism. 2023;27(2):402–14. https://doi.org/10.1177/13623613221098240.

Pearson A, Rose K. A conceptual analysis of autistic masking: understanding the narrative of stigma and the illusion of choice. Autism Adulthood. 2021;3(1):52–60. https://doi.org/10.1089/aut.2020.0043.

Tubío-Fungueiriño M, Cruz S, Sampaio A, Carracedo A, Fernández-Prieto M. Social camouflaging in females with autism spectrum disorder: a systematic review. J Autism Dev Disord. 2021;51(7):2190–9. https://doi.org/10.1007/s10803-020-04695-x.

3 Cognition and Neuropsychological Profiles

Martina Siracusano, Lucrezia Arturi, Assia Riccioni, and Luigi Mazzone

3.1 Introduction

Understanding neuropsychological profiles in autism spectrum disorder (ASD) represents a clinical and research issue as important as challenging, because of the complexity of the construct itself and the heterogeneity of symptoms expressed within people in the spectrum.

To date, research interest regarding behavioural differences between sex/gender is growing. However, little is still known about cognition and neuropsychological phenotype of autistic females, with the exception of a small number of studies showing possible differences in executive function and visuospatial processing [1].

In neurotypical population, there are no sex/gender differences in intelligence quotient (IQ) levels, but differences in specific cognitive skills have been described. Although most of the differences in typical population are due to life experiences and environmental stimulations to which people have been exposed, animal studies have suggested the presence of a biological substrate underlying these differences.

M. Siracusano
Department of Biomedicine and Prevention, University of Rome Tor Vergata, Rome, Italy

Child Neurology and Psychiatry Unit, Department of Wellbeing of Mental and Neurological, Dental and Sensory Organ Health, Policlinico Tor Vergata Hospital, Rome, Italy

L. Arturi · A. Riccioni
Child Neurology and Psychiatry Unit, Department of Wellbeing of Mental and Neurological, Dental and Sensory Organ Health, Policlinico Tor Vergata Hospital, Rome, Italy

L. Mazzone (✉)
Child Neurology and Psychiatry Unit, Department of Wellbeing of Mental and Neurological, Dental and Sensory Organ Health, Policlinico Tor Vergata Hospital, Rome, Italy

Systems Medicine Department, University of Rome Tor Vergata, Rome, Italy
e-mail: luigi.mazzone@uniroma2.it

L. Mazzone et al. (eds.), *Autism Spectrum Disorder: Understanding the Female Phenotype*, https://doi.org/10.1007/978-3-031-62072-0_3

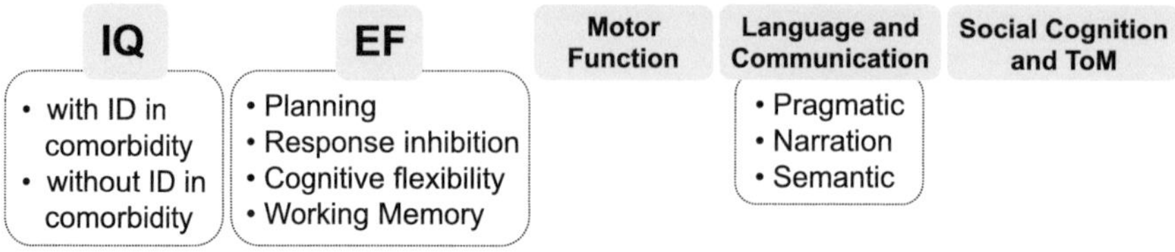

Fig. 3.1 Outline of the cognitive domains discussed in the following paragraphs. *IQ* intelligence quotient, *ID* intellectual disability, *EF* executive functions, *ToM* theory of mind

For example, males perform better in spatial navigation, map reading and mathematical problems [2, 3], while females perform better in social sensitivity, emotion recognition and language abilities [4–6].

In this framework—where the "systemizing functioning" of males with typical development is emphasized—fits the Baron-Cohen [7] *Extreme Male Brain (EMB)* theory, which conceptualizes the ASD phenotype as the result of an extreme male brain functioning. Specifically, systemizing style of functioning represents the capacity to analyse and infer rules governing mechanistic systems, and peculiar restricted interests of ASD individuals may be an expression of this cognitive tendency to focus on systems (and not on other people's emotions or thoughts) [8]. The use of systemizing strategies (e.g. insistence on sameness, obsession, restricted interest, islets of peculiar abilities) also determines difficulties in predicting other people's mental states, leading to the characteristic social deficits of ASD.

Even though the "extreme male brain" [9] provided an important contribution in understanding the cognitive functioning of ASD individuals [10], this theory did not give a full explanation of gender differences in ASD population.

In this context and for these reasons, a better comprehension of sex/gender differences in cognitive skills, language abilities, mechanism of perceptual processing of environmental and social stimuli [11]—and their interaction with autism symptoms and quality of life—represents an essential topic in order to better define the female ASD clinical phenotype and to drive sex/gender-oriented treatment.

Thus, in the following paragraphs are highlighted the main differences in cognitive and neuropsychological functioning of females with ASD, in comparison to autistic males and typical development in female peers (Fig. 3.1).

3.2 Intelligence Quotient (IQ)

The cognitive profile includes different intellectual skills essential for managing everyday tasks.

Planning and *performing* tasks, *memory*, *language*, *attention*, *reasoning* and *mental states encoding* are specific domains which together build the overall intelligence, measured by intelligence quotient (IQ).

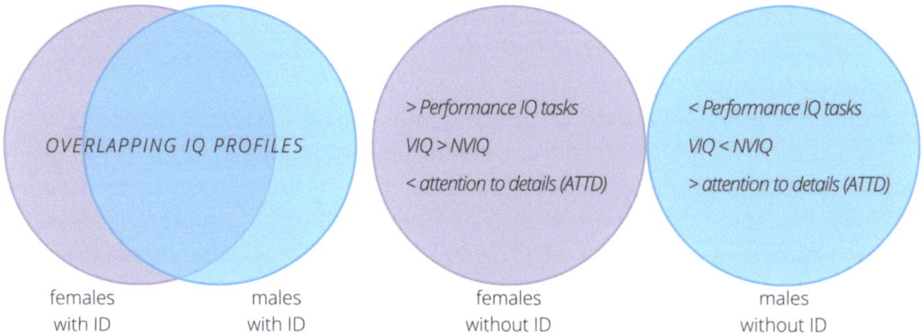

Fig. 3.2 Differences in IQ profiles between sex/genders in ASD with and without comorbid ID

Within ASD population, a specific endophenotype has been described characterized by impairment of intellectual abilities, including production and comprehension language skills, with better visual-spatial and non-verbal reasoning skills [12–15].

Intellectual functioning is a powerful outcome predictor of autistic symptoms in adulthood, and from a clinical point of view, IQ assessment is useful to guide clinician in the choice of the more appropriate treatment [16, 17].

Within ASD population, it is possible to distinguish two different cognitive profiles in terms of IQ: *low intellectual abilities (IQ <70)* or *average/high intellectual abilities (IQ >85).*

The relationship between autism phenotype and sex/gender is still controversial and unclear, especially since ASD is more diagnosed in males [18], with a 4:1 ratio, that decreases in the presence of comorbid intellectual disability (ID) [19].

In this chapter, we will discuss female IQ domains in presence or absence of limitations in cognitive functioning, which correspond to a different need of support from the environment (family, school, therapy, job) (Fig. 3.2).

3.2.1 Autistic Females with Intellectual Disability and High Level of Support Need

ASD individuals whose cognitive functioning is below average IQ levels (<70) generally, require high level of support and are characterized by increased dysfunctional behaviours, reduced adaptive skills and language impairment (DSM-5-TR, [20]).

Estimates of intellectual disability (ID) (IQ <70) within autistic population indicate higher prevalence of cognitive deficit in females (39%), compared to males (32%) [21].

Most of the studies have placed females at the lower ends of the IQ distribution, delineating a worse intellectual impairment in this sex/gender [22]. In fact, after controlling for diagnosis, females perform worse than males in standardized cognitive scales requiring language abilities (e.g. Wechsler Intelligence Scales) or not (e.g. Leiter International Performance Scales) [23].

Instead, a study conducted by Nguyen and Ronald [24] on a sample of individuals with ASD and comorbid ID, found no differences in cognitive abilities between males and females, reflecting overlapping profiles among sexes/genders. The only exception was found on block design (BD) tasks—a subtest of Wechsler Scales which measures attention to details (ATTD) [25]—where males outperformed autistic females. However, it is important to take into account that BD tasks require the ability to focus on pictures' details, which probably represents a peculiar skill of autistic males [26]. Indeed, no differences were found in BD performance between autistic and neurotypical females matched for mental age [24].

In conclusion, the reduction of male/female ASD ratio in the presence of comorbid ID [19] suggests that higher level of ID severity plays a role in the decrease of phenotypical differences between males/females, making autistic symptomatology more easily to detect through clinicians, also in female population [27].

Noteworthily, to the best of our knowledge, no research gave an exhaustive clinical description—specifically depicting a female phenotype—of the skills directly linked to the level of IQ among genders.

3.2.2 Autistic Females without Intellectual Disability and Low Level of Support Need

Generally, individuals with ASD without comorbid ID requires a low level of support (DSM-5-TR, [20]).

From both clinical and statistical points of view, females without ID are underrepresented, due to their abilities to mask atypical behaviours and social difficulties [28]. In fact, commonly, the verbal and social abilities exhibited by ASD females with higher levels of IQ lead to misdiagnosis given that the autistic symptoms remain below the clinical thresholds [29, 30].

With regard to ASD individuals who do not exhibit ID, sex/gender differences have been described specifically depending on the cognitive *task* proposed and on the basis of the cognitive index evaluated: *verbal (VIQ)* or *non-verbal (NVIQ)* [26, 31].

Higher scores in specific task included in the "performance IQ" index and in "processing speed index" of Wechsler Intelligence Scale for Children-III were described among females with ASD without comorbid ID [26]. In particular, results at the Coding and Symbol Search (processing speed index subtests) reflect female higher skills in attention and speed, while less tendency to circumstantiality and perfectionism in comparison to males.

Interestingly, the worse performances on block design task previously seen in individuals with ASD and comorbid ID are also confirmed in females without intellectual impairment [26, 31], highlighting sex/gender differences in cognitive style (ASD females characterized by less attention to details than males).

For what concerns the discrepancy between verbal and non-verbal IQ levels, a mild discrepancy was found in favour of VIQ in females in comparison to males (NVIQ > VIQ) [32]. This discrepancy decreases in females with ASD at the highest levels of the IQ distribution, where the NVIQ and VIQ domains are essentially overlapping [32, 33].

The fact that individuals with adequate intellectual abilities are characterized by higher verbal cognitive skills (no discrepancy between VIQ and NVIQ) may contribute to misdiagnosis or late diagnosis within this clinical population.

3.3 Executive Functions (EF)

The term *executive functions (EF)* is used to define interconnected cognitive processes necessary to plan, organize, regulate and implement functional actions to achieve goals [34].

Their organization in ASD is complex, due to the atypical functioning of brain structures involved in cognitive flexibility and information processing mechanisms, such as the prefrontal cortex, the caudate nucleus and the nucleus accumbens [35, 36]. Because of these abnormalities, ASD has also been defined as an "*executive disorder*" [37] linked to alterations in the ability to direct attention and implement appropriate behaviours [38].

Impaired capacities in *planning*, *inhibition*, *set-shifting* and *cognitive flexibility* are frequently associated with ASD condition [39], and the link between the executive dysfunction, behavioural atypia, lack in theory of mind (ToM) and social interaction difficulties is observed [40]. A study [31] comparing cognition between ASD males and females without intellectual disability (IQ >70) found that females outperformed males into higher order EF domains, such as conceptual abilities, and found an association with lower restricted interest and repetitive behaviours.

Since the study of specific EF deficits has been useful for understanding psychological basis of ASD symptomatology and given the inconsistent scientific evidences, defining a female developmental, behavioural and neuropsychological profile represents a priority for clinical practice.

In this chapter, the executive profile—*planning*, *inhibition*, *cognitive flexibility* and *working memory*—characteristics of females with ASD are described.

3.3.1 Planning

Planning abilities represent the capacity to identify alternatives, make choices, organize behaviours and predict consequences [39]. ASD individuals perform worse than neurotypical peers on standardized tests assessing these abilities (Tower of London or Tower of Hanoi), reflecting several difficulties in this area [39]. However, there is no consensus in literature with respect to sex/gender differences in planning performance, as some studies report greater difficulties in ASD females [41], while others show no sex/gender differences [42].

Discrepancy among studies may be related to methodological limitations. In particular, given that instruments assessing EF often involve visual-spatial skills in completing tasks—and knowing that females are more deficient in that cognitive areas—this issue could negatively affect female performance. Furthermore, it is important to take into consideration the significant influence of IQ levels on EF evaluation (higher IQ is generally related with a better performance). Therefore, sex/gender differences in EF could represent the effect of several vulnerability factors (including IQ), rather than being expression of a real gender difference.

3.3.2 Response Inhibition

Neurobehavioural profile overlapping was observed in males and females with high cognitive-functioning ASD and low level of support need, even when comparing them to neurotypical individuals. In particular, Lemon et al. [43] examining sex/gender differences in response inhibition skills within ASD individuals without intellectual disability (IQ >70) demonstrated worse performances in ASD females, compared with both neurotypical peers and autistic males. Specifically, stop-task revealed reduced speed ability in the stopping process, which is reflected in poorer behavioural inhibition performance, while ASD males performed equally as neurotypical peers. Despite this, difficulties in other inhibition process abilities (such as stopping automatic behaviours) have not been observed [43]. Furthermore, the speed impairment in response inhibition might negatively impact social interaction skills, particularly during high states of arousal (such as significant anxiety and/or cognitive load) with several consequences in daily-life organization.

3.3.3 Cognitive Flexibility

Cognitive flexibility is the ability to initiate adaptive and functional behaviours, in order to perform daily activities and regulate social life [40]. Regardless of sex/gender, evidences report considerable difficulties in this domain for ASD people [44]. Impairment of cognitive flexibility and related problem-solving difficulties represent two main issues for people with ASD, contributing to behavioural repetitiveness [39].

Some authors describe no significant sex/gender differences in specific tasks related to this domain [31, 45], while others report a worse performance among ASD females [40]. Outperformance of females with ASD without intellectual disability, in terms of cognitive flexibility, was found [42]: in particular, although in the presence of a greater number of perseveration errors, more strategic skills characterize this sex/gender.

Mental flexibility, together with IQ levels, plays a mediating role in adaptive skills and daily-life activities [46].

3.3.4 Working Memory (WM)

Differences in working memory (WM) are observed between sex and genders in typical population [47], with an advantage of males over females. This finding is consistent with results obtained within ASD population [42].

ASD individuals perform worse than neurotypical people on WM tasks; impairment in this area is associated with the presence of repetitive behaviours and lower adaptive skills [48]. In particular, it was found that females, in comparison to males with ASD, exhibit overall WM impairment, with a discrete superior proficiency on digit span task (a neuropsychological test used to assess verbal and number memory).

Results obtained by females with ASD in digit span tasks reflect greater abilities in recalling longer sequences of numbers [42]. WM domain is also strongly influenced by IQ, and it is possible that a fewer impairment in this area is related to compensation by cognitive system.

In conclusion, evidences revealed sex/gender differences in EF in both neurotypical and ASD populations. However, it is still difficult to delineate a female-specific profile of executive functioning, because of the heterogeneity and the lack of clarity about the EF organization in ASD.

3.4 Motor Function

Taking into account that motor functions are supported by cognitive skills [49] and are closely related to EF [1], the analysis of this domain is important in order to delineate an exhaustive profile of neuropsychological function within ASD females.

Although motor clumsiness is not considered a diagnostic feature of ASD, dyspraxic condition is often associated with autism. In fact, movement abnormalities, such as difficulties in gross and fine motor skills or coordination, are frequently found in ASD individuals [1].

The relationship between neurological comorbidities, IQ and behavioural impairments is close, and motor clumsiness aspects are associated with more compromised behavioural and IQ profiles [50]. An overlap between males and females with ASD regarding motor skills has been described, even if some authors report worse gross motor function in females [32, 51]. Thus, trivial tasks—such as throwing or catching a ball or running—are more challenging for ASD female in comparison to their male peers, whereas ASD males have more difficulty in tasks requiring complex motor skills (e.g. assembly tasks) such as coordination, planning, inhibition and speed. In fact, although females with ASD report difficulties in gross motor skills, they better perform in fine motor skills [52]. From a clinical point of view, it might be useful to considerate the in-depth and sex/gender-specific assessment of motor and executive functions, in order to facilitate clinicians in designing personalized rehabilitation programmes.

3.5 Language and Communication

Language abilities represent a pivotal factor for socialization and are crucial to establish interpersonal relationships [53]. Difficulties in socio-communication and narrative skills are characteristic features of ASD individuals. In ASD population, the impairment of both language production and comprehension emerges in early childhood and appears associated with difficulties in decoding and using non-verbal communicative signals (such as gestures, eye contact, facial expressions).

Several variables (such as IQ and social motivation) may influence language abilities leading to wide heterogeneity of communicative skills within ASD individuals (from absence/limited communication skills to fluent and functional language) [51].

However, impairment of communicative pragmatic skills is homogeneously distributed in this clinical population, with important impact on their quality of life and school success [54].

Sex/gender differences in communication skills are also known in neurotypical individuals [55]: first words' production appears earlier in females; girls are characterized by a better integration of non-verbal skills (such as gestures) [56, 57]; female communication style is more complex, focused on emotional details and incline to collaboration/negotiation with others [55, 58].

However, to date, little is known about language aspects based on sex/gender differences in ASD population. In fact, research studies predominantly include male samples, not being representative of female autistic population [59].

The following paragraphs will analyse from a sex/gender point of view the main language domains within ASD individuals exhibiting fluent verbal skills: *pragmatics*, *narration* and *semantic*.

3.5.1 Pragmatic

Within ASD, difficulties in pragmatic and inferential aspects of language have been widely investigated [60]. In particular, the use of causal and temporal connectors is impaired within both sexes/genders [54].

The development of pragmatic skills requires social interaction and conversation; therefore, the aetiology of its alteration might be ascribable to social cognition deficits characteristic of ASD [61]. The greater social awareness and motivation observed in autistic females make them more prone in modulating gestures, facial expressions and prosody and in respecting the conversational timing. Hiller et al. [62] study demonstrated better proficiency in pragmatic skills and social reciprocity in autistic females (when compared to autistic males), although worse than neurotypical females. In their sample, one-third of girls did not present impairment of verbal and non-verbal integration, in comparison to boys, who demonstrated greater difficulties in this area and in other communicative behaviours (e.g. less use of social gestures).

Taking together, all these characteristics contribute to the effectiveness (in terms of both quality and quantity) of ASD females' communicative exchange [63].

The underlying communication difficulties could not be easily captured by standardized tests commonly used in clinical evaluation settings; a qualitative analysis of socio-relational and communicative skills should be necessary [55]. Normal IQ and good language abilities contribute to misdiagnosis and/or delay in ASD diagnosis within girls.

For these reasons and from a therapeutic point of view, the identification of communicative and language domain peculiarities of females with ASD is essential in preventing emotional sphere problems, which are strongly associated with language and social interaction difficulties.

3.5.2 Narration

Among ASD individuals with fluent verbal abilities, deficit in narrative skills is shared between males and females [55]. In particular, the use of a concrete language and an object-oriented storytelling (e.g. frequent use/production of nouns; high labelling specificity in naming objects and characters) is a trait common to both sexes/genders; however, girls generally present an additional distinctive language profile defined as "*blended phenotype*" [59] characterized by good speaking abilities in describing and providing details, together with a frequent use of expressions related to cognitive and emotional domains, judgements and perceptions [49, 54, 64]. On the one hand, this better proficiency in narrative skills—characterizing females with autism—is likely attributable and may be strictly linked to their greater social motivation [65, 66]; nonetheless, on the other hand, female lower communicative impairment may contribute to misdiagnosis or later diagnosis in this gender.

3.5.3 Semantic

The impairment of this language domain is commonly observed across the lifespan within ASD individuals, with limited *priming effect* (words' semantic association: a psychological mechanism in which the exposure to one stimulus influences the response to subsequent stimuli) and persistent difficulties in *categorization* [67, 68]. The aetiology of this impairment is attributable to difficulties in linking words with their meanings, leading to impaired access to mental representations of categories [68].

To date, knowledge on this language topic is still limited specifically concerning gender differences [69].

3.6 Social Cognition and Theory of Mind (ToM)

Social cognition is the ability to encode, process and use social information in order to initiate appropriate social behaviours and manage interpersonal relationships [70].

This psychological construct consists of different subdomains responsible for self-other interface: understanding of other people (ToM, empathy) and self-understanding/control (agency, self-recognition, impulse control) [71].

Social cognition impairment represents one of the core symptoms of ASD condition: the *social-emotional* reciprocity deficit [70].

Sex/gender differences in social-cognition have been widely investigated within both neurotypical and ASD individuals [9]. According to the "empathizing-systemizing theory" (E-S) proposed by Baron-Cohen, neurotypical females are generally characterized by *empathizing* abilities, whereas males present greater *systemizing skills* [72].

The term "*systemizing*" refers to a logical rule-based tendency to interpret contexts, while "*empathizing*" refers to the ability of understanding other people's mental states (emotions, intention, beliefs) and to respond in an emotionally appropriate manner.

In this theoretical framework, ASD social functioning (of both genders) has been described by Baron-Cohen as a *systematizing functioning,* subsequently impairing *theory of mind (ToM) abilities*—a social cognition subdomain involved in the understanding of other people's emotions and mental states [73]. Deficits in ToM are linked to mind-reading skills, leading to low proficiency in managing social situations [74].

Although in ASD condition ToM performance appears sex/gender independent [1, 75], females with low level of support need exhibit more effective social skills (making friends and maintaining relationships) [66] and social strategies than males [76], camouflaging their difficulties in the social domain [75, 77]. Interestingly, the evolutive trajectory of socialization-empathization competences appears stable during adulthood, with ASD women showing persisting less socio-communicative impairment in comparison to adult males [74].

Noteworthily, cognitive abilities have a role in social skill development and according to previous literature, lower IQ levels are associated with greater overall social impairment [32, 78].

In sum, the less severe female social phenotype, together with symptomatic camouflage in other domains (greater verbal and non-verbal communicative skills; restricted interests similar to typical-development females), contributes to misdiagnosis or late diagnosis within this gender.

Key Points

- **IQ**
  - Overlapping IQ profiles between sexes and genders in ASD individuals with lower levels of IQ.
  - Higher VIQ, performance IQ and processing speed exhibited by ASD females with IQ levels in/above the average.
  - Less attention to detail on block design tasks regardless the level of IQ.
- **EF**
  - A specific EF profile of ASD females has not yet been outlined.

- **Motor function**
  - ASD females present gross motor difficulties, while fine motor abilities are not impaired.
- **Language and communication**
  - ASD females exhibiting fluent verbal abilities present better pragmatic skills, social reciprocity and proficiency (good verbal and non-verbal integration, better use of social gestures).
  - A "*blinded phenotype*" characterizes verbal fluent ASD females' narrative skills.
- **Social cognition and ToM**
  - Presence of ToM impairment in both sexes and genders and within both type of cognitive functioning.
  - Females with low level of support need present moderate social cognition skills, despite impaired ToM system.
  - High level of social motivation and social reciprocity characterizing females without intellectual and language impairments, may contribute to masking ToM impairment.

References

1. Lai MC, Lombardo MV, Ruigrok ANV, Chakrabarti B, Wheelwright SJ, et al. Cognition in males and females with autism: similarities and differences. PLoS One. 2012;7(10):e47198. https://doi.org/10.1371/journal.pone.0047198.
2. Kimura D. Sex and cognition. Cambridge: Massachusetts Institute of Technology (MIT) Press; 1999.
3. Lawson S, Baron-Cohen S, Wheelwright J. Empathising and systemising in adults with and without Asperger syndrome. Autism Dev Disord. 2004;34:301–10.
4. Baron-Cohen S, O'Riordan M, Jones R, Stone V, Plaisted K. J Autism Dev Disord. 1999;29:407.
5. McClure EB. A meta-analytic review of sex differences in facial expression processing and their development in infants, children, and adolescents. Psychol Bull. 2000;126:424–53. https://doi.org/10.1037/0033-2909.126.3.424.
6. Hyde JS, Linn MC. Gender differences in verbal ability: a meta-analysis. Psychol Bull. 1988;104:53–69. https://doi.org/10.1037/0033-2909.104.1.53.
7. Baron-Cohen S. The extreme male brain theory of autism. Trends Cogn Sci. 2002;1(6):248–54. https://doi.org/10.1016/s1364-6613(02)01904-6.
8. Baron-Cohen S, Wheelwright S. 'Obsessions' in children with autism or Asperger syndrome content analysis in terms of core domains of cognition. Br J Psychiatry. 1999;175:484–90. https://doi.org/10.1192/bjp.175.5.484.
9. Baron-Cohen S, Knickmeyer RC, Belmonte MK. Sex differences in the brain: implications for explaining autism. Science. 2005;310(5749):819–23. https://doi.org/10.1126/science.1115455.
10. Kimura D. Sex differences in the brain. Sci Am. 1992;267(3):118–25. https://doi.org/10.1038/scientificamerican0992-118.
11. Volkmar FR, Lord C, Bailey A, Schultz RT, Klin A. Autism and pervasive developmental disorders. J Child Psychol Psychiatry. 2004;45(1):135–70. https://doi.org/10.1046/j.0021-9630.2003.00317.x.

12. Allen MH, Lincoln AJ, Kaufman AS. Sequential and simultaneous processing abilities of high-functioning autistic and language-impaired children. J Autism Dev Disord. 1991;21:483–502.
13. Lincoln A, Courchesne E, Kilman B, Elmasian R, Allen M. A study of intellectual abilities in high-functioning people with autism. J Autism Dev Disord. 1988;18:505–24.
14. Ohta M. Cognitive disorders of infantile autism: a study employing the WISC, spatial relationships, conceptualization, and gestural imitation. J Autism Dev Dis. 1987;17:45–62.
15. Shah A, Frith U. Why do autistic individuals show superior performance on the block design task? J Child Psychol Psychiatry. 1993;34:1351–64.
16. Begovac I, Begovac B, Majić G, Vidović V. Longitudinal studies of IQ stability in children with childhood autism—literature survey. Psychiatr Danub. 2009;21(3):310–9.
17. Volkmar FR, Pauls D. Autism. Lancet. 2003;362(9390):1133–41.
18. Ankenman K, Elgin J, Sullivan K, Vincent L, Bernier R. Nonverbal and verbal cognitive discrepancy profiles in autism spectrum disorders: influence of age and gender. Am J Intellect Dev Dis. 2014;119(1):84–99. https://doi.org/10.1352/1944-7558-119.1.84.
19. Hartley SL, Sikora DM. Sex differences in autism spectrum disorder: an examination of developmental functioning, autistic symptoms, and coexisting behavior problems in toddlers. J Autism Dev Disord. 2009;39:175–1722. https://doi.org/10.1007/s10803-009-0810-8.
20. American Psychiatric Association. Diagnostic and statistical manual of mental Disorders, Fifth Edition, text revision (DSM-5-TR). Washington, DC: American Psychiatric Association; 2022.
21. Maenner KJ, Shaw KA, Baio J, et al. Prevalence of autism spectrum disorder among children aged 8 years-autism and developmental disabilities monitoring network, 11 sites, United States, 2016. MMWR Surveill Summ. 2009;69(4):1–12. https://doi.org/10.15585/mmwr.ss6904a1.
22. Halladay AK, et al. Sex and gender differences in autism spectrum disorder: summarizing evidence gaps and identifying emerging areas of priority. Mol Autism. 2015;6:36. https://doi.org/10.1186/s13229-015-0019-y.
23. Volkmar F, Szatmari P, Sparrow S. Sex differences in pervasive developmental disorders. J Autism Dev Dis. 1993;23:579–91.
24. Nguyen C, Ronald A. How do girls with low functioning autism compare to boys with autism and typically developing girls with regard to behavior, cognition, and psychopathology? Scand J Child Adolesc Psychiatry Psychol. 2014;2(2):55–65. https://doi.org/10.21307/sjcapp-2014-009.
25. Happè F, Frith U. The weak coherence account: detail-focused cognitive style in autism spectrum disorders. Autism Dev Disord. 2006;36(1):5–25. https://doi.org/10.1007/s10803-005-0039-0.
26. Koyama T, Kamio Y, Inada N, Kurita H. Sex differences in WISC-III profiles of children with high-functioning pervasive developmental disorders. J Autism Dev Disord. 2009;39:135–41.
27. Yeargin-Allsopp M, Rice C, Karapurkar T, Doernberg N, Boyle C, Murphy C. Prevalence of autism in a US metropolitan area. JAMA. 2003;289(1):49–55. https://doi.org/10.1001/jama.289.1.49.
28. Cage E, Troxell-Whitman Z. Understanding the reasons, contexts and costs of camouflaging for autistic adults. J Autism Dev Disord. 2019;49(5):1899–911. https://doi.org/10.1007/s10803-018-03878-x.
29. Head AM, McGillivray JA, Stokes MA. Gender differences in emotionality and sociability in children with autism spectrum disorders. Mol Autism. 2014;5:19. https://doi.org/10.1186/2040-2392-5-19.
30. Lai MC, Lombardo MV, Pasco G, Ruigrok AN, Wheelwright SJ, Sadek SA, et al. A behavioral comparison of male and female adults with high functioning autism spectrum conditions. PLoS One. 2011;6(6):e20835. https://doi.org/10.1371/journal.pone.0020835.
31. Bölte S, Duketis E, Poustka F, Holtmann M. Sex differences in cognitive domains and their clinical correlates in higher-functioning autism spectrum disorders. Autism. 2011;15(4):497–511. https://doi.org/10.1177/1362361310391116.
32. Frazier TW, Georgiades S, Bishop SL, Hardan AY. Behavioral and cognitive characteristics of females and males with autism in the Simons simplex collection. J Am Acad Child Adolesc Psychiatry. 2014;53(3):329–40. https://doi.org/10.1016/j.jaac.2013.12.004.

33. Doi H, Kanai C, Ohta H. Transdiagnostic and sex differences in cognitive profiles of autism spectrum disorder and attention-deficit/hyperactivity disorder. Autism Research. 2022;15:1130–1141. https://doi.org/10.1002/aur.2712.
34. Stuss DT, Benson DF. The frontal lobes. New York: Raven Press; 1986.
35. Ozonoff S, Cook I, Coon H, et al. Performance on Cambridge neuropsychological test automated battery subtests sensitive to frontal lobe function in people with autistic disorder: evidence from the collaborative programs of excellence in autism network. J Autism Dev Disord. 2004;34(2):139–50.
36. Alvarez JA, Emory E. Executive function and the frontal lobes: a meta-analytic review. Neuropsychol Rev. 2006;16:17–42.
37. Russell J. Autism as an executive disorder. New York: Oxford University Press; 1997.
38. Ridley RM. The psychology of perserverative and stereotyped behaviour. Prog Neurobiol. 1994;44:221–31.
39. Hill EL. Evaluating the theory of executive dysfunction in autism. Dev Rev. 2004;24:189–233.
40. Memari AH, Ziaee V, Shayestehfar M, Ghanouni P, Mansournia MA, Moshayedi P. Cognitive flexibility impairments in children with autism spectrum disorders: links to age, gender and child outcomes. Res Dev Disabil. 2013;34:3218–25. https://doi.org/10.1016/j.ridd.2013.06.033.
41. Nydén A, Hjelmquist E, Gillberg C. Autism spectrum and attention-deficit disorders in girls. Some neuropsychological aspects. Eur Child Adolesc Psychiatry. 2000;9:180–5.
42. Kiep M, Spek AA. Executive functioning in men and women with an autism spectrum disorder. International Society for Autism Research INSAR; 2016.
43. Lemon JM, Gargaro B, Enticott PG, Rinehart NJ. Brief report: Executive functioning in autism spectrum disorders: a gender comparison of response inhibition. J Autism Dev Disord. 2011;41:352–6. https://doi.org/10.1007/s10803-010-1039-2.
44. Verté S, Geurts HM, Roeyers H, Oosterlaan J, Sergeant JA. Executive functioning in children with autism and Tourette syndrome. Dev Psychopathol. 2005;17:415–45.
45. Demetriou EA, Pepper KL, Park SH, Pellicano L, Song YJC, Naismith SL, Hickie IB, Thomas EE, Guastella AJ. Autism spectrum disorder: an examination of sex differences in neuropsychological and self report measures of executive and non-executive cognitive function. Autism. 2021;25:2223. https://doi.org/10.1177/13623613211014991.
46. White EI, Wallace GL, Bascom J, Armour AC, Register Brown K, Popal HS, Ratto AB, Martina A, Kenworthy L. Sex differences in parent-reported executive functioning and adaptive behavior in children and young adults with autism spectrum disorder, vol. 10. INSAR, Wiley Periodicals, Inc.; 2017. p. 1653. https://doi.org/10.1002/aur.1811.
47. Hill AC, Laird AR, Robinson JL. Gender differences in working memory networks: a BrainMap meta-analysis. Biol Psychol. 2014;102:18–29.
48. Kercood S, Grskovic JA, Banda D, Begeske J. Working memory and autism: a review of literature. Res Autism Spectr Disord. 2014;8(10):1316–32.
49. Haaland KY, Harrington DL. Neuropsychological assessment of motor skills. In: Goldstein G, Nussbaum PD, Beers SR, editors. Neuropsychology. Human brain function (assessment and rehabilitation). Boston: Springer; 1998. https://doi.org/10.1007/978-1-4899-1950-2_19.
50. Fournier KA, Hass CJ, Naik SK, Lodha N, Cauraugh JH. Motor coordination in autism spectrum disorders: a synthesis and meta-analysis. J Autism Dev Disord. 2010;40:1227–40.
51. Saure E, Castrén M, Mikkola K, Salmi J. Intellectual disabilities moderate sex/gender differences in autism spectrum disorder: a systematic review and meta-analysis. J Intellect Disabil Res. 2023;67(1):1–34. https://doi.org/10.1111/jir.12989.
52. Mandy W, Chilvers R, Chowdhury U, et al. Sex differences in autism spectrum disorder: evidence from a large sample of children and adolescents. J Autism Dev Disord. 2012;42:1304–13.
53. Siller M, Swanson MR, Serlin G, Teachworth AG. Internal state language in the storybook narratives of children with and without autism spectrum disorder: investigating relations to theory of mind abilities. Res Autism Spectr Disord. 2014;8(5):589–96. https://doi.org/10.1016/j.rasd.2014.02.002.

54. Kauschke C, van der Beek B, Kamp-Becker I. Narratives of girls and boys with autism spectrum disorder: gender differences in narrative competence and internal state language. J Autism Dev Disord. 2016;46:840–52. https://doi.org/10.1007/s10803-015-2620-5.
55. Sturrock A, Adams C, Freed J. A subtle profile with a significant impact: language and communication difficulties for autistic females without intellectual disability. Front Psychol. 2021;12:621742. https://doi.org/10.3389/fpsyg.2021.621742.
56. Bleses D, Vach W, Slott M, et al. The Danish communicative developmental inventories: validity and main developmental trends. J Child Lang. 2008;35:651–69. https://doi.org/10.1017/s0305000907008574.
57. Eriksson M, Marschik PB, Tulviste T, et al. Differences between girls and boys in emerging language skills: evidence from 10 language communities. Br J Dev Psychol. 2012;30:326–43. https://doi.org/10.1111/j.2044-835x.2011.02042.x.
58. Bouchard C, Trudeau N, Sutton A, Boudreault MC, Deneault J. Gender differences in language development in French Canadian children between 8 and 30 months of age. Appl Psycholinguist. 2009;30:685–707. https://doi.org/10.1017/s0142716409990075.
59. Boorse J, Cola M, Plate S, Yankowitz L, Pandey J, Schultz RT, Parish-Morris J. Linguistic markers of autism in girls: evidence of a "blended phenotype" during storytelling. Mol Autism. 2019;10:14. https://doi.org/10.1186/s13229-019-0268-2.
60. Loukusa S, Moilanen I. Pragmatic inference abilities in individuals with Asperger syndrome or high-functioning autism. A review. Res Autism Spectr Disord. 2009;3:890–904. https://doi.org/10.1016/j.rasd.2009.05.002.
61. Volden J, Dodd E, Engel K, et al. Beyond sentences: using the expression, reception, and recall of narratives instrument to assess communication in school-aged children with autism spectrum disorder. J Speech Lang Hear Res. 2017;60:2228–40. https://doi.org/10.1044/2017_jslhr-l-16-0168.
62. Hiller RM, Young RL, Weber N. Sex differences in autism spectrum disorder based on DSM-5 criteria: evidence from clinician and teacher reporting. J Abnorm Child Psychol. 2014;42:1381–93. https://doi.org/10.1007/s10802-014-9881-x.
63. Cola ML, Plate S, Yankowitz L, et al. Sex differences in the first impressions made by girls and boys with autism. Mol Autism. 2020;11:49. https://doi.org/10.1186/s13229-020-00336-3.
64. Cola M, et al. Friend matters: sex differences in social language during autism diagnostic interviews. Molecular Autism. 2022;13:5. https://doi.org/10.1186/s13229-021-00483-1.
65. Harrop C, Jones D, Zheng S, Nowell SW, Boyd BA, Sasson N. Sex differences in social attention in autism spectrum disorder. Autism Res. 2018;11:1264–75. https://doi.org/10.1002/aur.1997.
66. Sedgewick F, Hill V, Yates R, Pickering L, Pellicano E. Gender differences in the social motivation and friendship experiences of autistic and non-autistic adolescents. J Autism Dev Dis. 2016;46:1297–306. https://doi.org/10.1007/s10803-015-2669-1.
67. Kamio Y, Robins D, Kelley E, Swainson B, Fein D. Atypical lexical/semantic processing in high-functioning autism spectrum disorders without early language delay. J Autism Dev Disord. 2007;37:1116–22.
68. Naigles LR, Kelley E, Troyb E, Fein D. Residual difficulties with categorical induction in children with a history of autism. J Autism Dev Disord. 2013;43:2048–61.
69. Groen WB, Zwiers MP, van der Gaag RJ, Buitelaar JK. The phenotype and neural correlates of language in autism: an integrative review. Neurosci Biobehav Rev. 2008;32:1416–25. https://doi.org/10.1016/j.neubiorev.2008.05.008.
70. Sasson NJ, Pinkham AE, Carpenter KL, Belger A. The benefit of directly comparing autism and schizophrenia for revealing mechanisms of social cognitive impairment. J Neurodev Disord. 2011;3:87–100. https://doi.org/10.1007/s11689-010-9068-x.
71. Martins-Junior FE, Sanvincente Vieira B, Grassi Oliveira R, Brietzke E. Social cognition and theory of mind: controversies and promises for understanding major psychiatric disorders. Psychol Neurosci. 2011;4(3):347–51. https://doi.org/10.3922/j.psns.2011.3.008.

72. Baron-Cohen S. The essential difference: men, women and the extreme male brain. London: Penguin; 2003.
73. Fernyhough C, Jones SR, Whittle C, Waterhouse J, Bentall RP. Theory of mind, schizotypy, and persecutory ideation in young adults. Cogn Neuropsychiatry. 2008;13(3):233–49.
74. Baron-Cohen S, Wheelwright J. The empathy quotient: an investigation of adults with Asperger syndrome or high functioning autism, and normal sex differences. Autism Dev Disord. 2004;34:163–75. https://doi.org/10.1023/B:JADD.0000022607.19833.00.
75. Wood-Downie H, Wong B, Kovshoff H, Mandy W, Hull L, Hadwin JA. Sex/gender differences in camouflaging in children and adolescents with autism. J Autism Dev Disord. 2021;51:1353–64. https://doi.org/10.1007/s10803-020-04615-z.
76. van Ommeren TB, Koot HM, Scheeren AM, Begeer S. Sex differences in the reciprocal behaviour of children with autism. Autism. 2016;21:795. https://doi.org/10.1177/1362361316669622.
77. Lacroix A, Dutheil F, Logemann A, Cserjesi R, Peyrin C, Biro B, Gomot M, Mermillod M. Flexibility in autism during unpredictable shifts of socio-emotional stimuli: investigation of group and sex differences. Autism. 2022;26(7):1681–97. https://doi.org/10.1177/13623613211062776.
78. Livingston LA, Colvert E, Bolton P, Happé F. Good social skills despite poor theory of mind: exploring compensation in autism spectrum disorder. J Child Psychol Psychiatry. 2018;60(1):102–10. https://doi.org/10.1111/jcpp.12886.

4 Adulthood: Do the Sex/Gender Differences in Autistic Phenotype Persist in Adult Life?

Roberto Keller, Domenica Leone, Angela Aresi, Luana Salerno, Elisa Carloni, Martina Siracusano, and Luigi Mazzone

4.1 Evolution of Autism Symptoms in Adulthood

Doubtlessly, autism is a lifelong condition, extending from early childhood and adolescence into adulthood [1]. However, the expression of autistic phenotype evolves in the transition from young to adult age. Outcomes appear highly variable, but most individuals with autism tend to show improvements during this transition [2].

Globally, the severity of autism core symptoms tends to reduce over time, with improvements in several aspects. Indeed, regarding language and communication abilities, a reduction of anomalies in speech is observed (such as lowering of

R. Keller (✉) · D. Leone · A. Aresi
Adult Autism Center, Mental Health Department, Local Health Unit, ASL Città di Torino, Turin, Italy
e-mail: roberto.keller@aslcittaditorino.it

L. Salerno
Institute of Neuroscience INS, Florence, Italy

E. Carloni
Child Neurology and Psychiatry Unit, Department of Wellbeing of Mental and Neurological, Dental and Sensory Organ Health, Policlinico Tor Vergata Hospital, Rome, Italy

M. Siracusano
Child Neurology and Psychiatry Unit, Department of Wellbeing of Mental and Neurological, Dental and Sensory Organ Health, Policlinico Tor Vergata Hospital, Rome, Italy

Department of Biomedicine and Prevention, University of Rome Tor Vergata, Rome, Italy

L. Mazzone
Child Neurology and Psychiatry Unit, Department of Wellbeing of Mental and Neurological, Dental and Sensory Organ Health, Policlinico Tor Vergata Hospital, Rome, Italy

Systems Medicine Department, University of Rome Tor Vergata, Rome, Italy

L. Mazzone et al. (eds.), *Autism Spectrum Disorder: Understanding the Female Phenotype*, https://doi.org/10.1007/978-3-031-62072-0_4

repetitive language use), and nonverbal individuals tend to acquire some useful verbal communication skills [3]. Moreover, improvements in social-relational abilities are reported, with increased communicative intentionality and more strategies of interacting with other people [2]. A reduction in ritualistic behaviors and sensory seekness is also noticed, making these aspects less impairing as the individual gets older [3]. However, significant difficulties in communication and socio-relational abilities tend to persist during time, particularly regarding pragmatic language abilities and eye contact modulation [3].

A fundamental aspect for the individual's quality of life is represented by adaptive skills, meaning the abilities needed to adapt to the surrounding environment and to face daily challenges. Although intellectual quotient is known to remain stable in time, adaptive skills can be implemented through specific intervention [4]; indeed, in individuals with autism who pass from adolescence to adulthood, adaptive skills appear to improve over time [5].

However, although improvements in adaptive abilities are frequently observed, many autistic individuals continue to present significant disadvantages in adulthood [6]. In fact, several researches in the last decades demonstrated poor outcomes in terms of employment, social relationships, and independence in daily-life activities, in this population [7]. Overall, around a fifth of adult individuals with autism could be considered as well integrated within the society, while almost half of them seem to show poor or very poor quality of life [4] (Fig. 4.1).

Several factors (both individual and environmental) may have a significant impact on the outcome of autism spectrum disorder in adulthood. Among individual factors, two main aspects were demonstrated to be associated with better outcomes in the long term: intellectual quotient and language abilities [5]. Individuals who do not present intellectual disability and who develop effective verbal communication

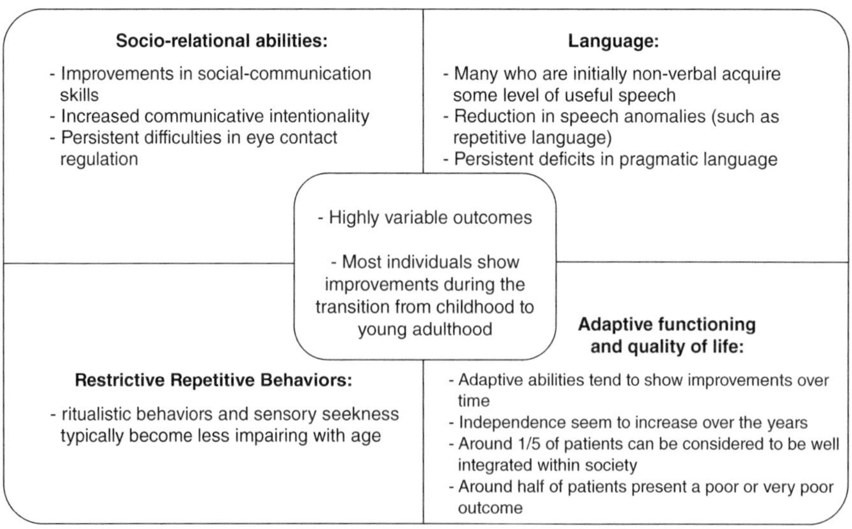

Fig. 4.1 Evolution of ASD core symptoms in adulthood

skills show higher levels of independence and significant better quality of life, compared to nonverbal autistic people with cognitive impairment [4]. On the contrary, a negative correlation between favorable outcome and psychiatric/physical comorbidities was demonstrated in different researches. Specifically, co-occurring mental health conditions are frequently described in individuals with autism (around 70% of them present at least one comorbid mental disorder, while around 50% show multiple co-occurring psychiatric conditions) with increased risk of worse long-term outcome and mortality [8, 9]. For example, individuals with autism frequently show co-occurring attention-deficit hyperactivity disorder (with greater impairment in adaptive and executive functions), anxiety disorders (with increased social difficulties, repetitive behaviors, and sensory seeking), depressive disorders (with increased risk of suicide), or psychosis [10–12], with negative effect on the outcome and quality of life. Among physical conditions associated with worsening clinical pictures, there are immune diseases, gastrointestinal problems and obesity, sleep disorders, seizures, and, finally, side effects of medications [13, 14].

Furthermore, different environmental features can modify the course of autism spectrum disorder during time, such as support in several contexts of life (family, school, post-school) and positive/adverse experiences. Family factors can both have positive and negative influences: a supportive family environment, with parents who have learned how to manage their child's difficulties and support him in daily activities, plays a crucial role in improving the individual's quality of life, while parental mental health difficulties, socio-economic issues, or conflictual relationships between parents may negatively impact the individual's well-being [15]. Negative experiences, such as bullying, social isolation and poor interaction with peers, or lack of adequate support, both in school and post-school periods, were described as associated with worse outcome in adult age [16] (Fig. 4.2).

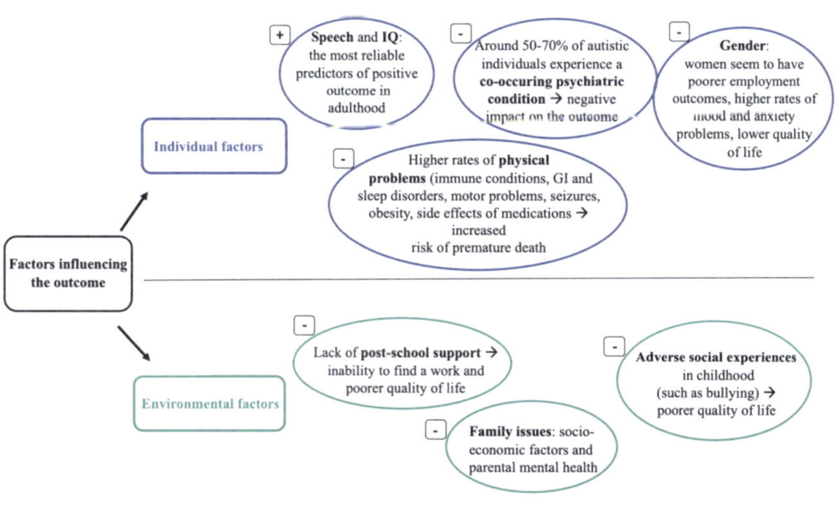

Fig. 4.2 Factors which may positively (+) or negatively (−) influence ASD outcome in adulthood

4.2 Evolution of Autism Symptoms in Adulthood: Differences Between Males and Females

Despite the relevant differences in clinical presentation of autism symptoms in males and females, with distinct profiles of strengths and difficulties, at the moment, only few studies have investigated the different evolution of autistic symptoms in adulthood, depending on the individual's sex/gender.

Most of the recent research has focused on the assessment of psychiatric comorbidities in adults with autism, both males and females. Particularly, evidence suggests that during the transition from adolescence to adulthood, females show higher risk of developing specific co-occurring conditions, such as anxiety and mood disorders, compared to males [2, 17].

Furthermore, when considering quality of life and outcomes in different life contexts, women seem to present poorer social and employment outcomes, with worse overall quality of life [2, 6], while men show specific strengths in physical quality of life [2]; this may be due to difficulties in the recognition of autism symptoms in female gender, with delayed diagnosis and lack of adequate support, with subsequent relevant impact on quality of life. Indeed, gender ratio between males and females in adults with autism varies from 2:1 to 9:1, depending on the different studies considered [18, 19], pointing out the prevalence of autism diagnosis in the male population in diagnostic services for adults (indicatively 3:1) [20].

To the best of our knowledge, there is only one study which evaluates, within adult individuals with autism, sex/gender differences in executive functions [21]. Lai et al. found no significant differences between men and women in terms of mentalizing skills, recognition of facial emotions, and inhibitory response control: these impairments are equally present in both sexes/genders. However, ASD adult males seem to be characterized by difficulties in details' perception, not found in autistic females [21] (Fig. 4.3).

	Men	Women
Mentalizing difficulties	✓	✓
Facial emotion recognition difficulties	✓	✓
Inhibitory control difficulties	✓	✓
Difficulties in attention to details	✓	✕
Higher social quality of life	✕	✓
Higher physical quality of life	✓	✕
Better employment outcome	✓	✕
Higher rates of mood and anxiety	✕	✓
Overall poorer quality of life	✕	✓

Legend
✓: presence
✕: absence

Fig. 4.3 Adults with ASD: differences between males and females

The lack of information regarding sex/gender profiles of adults with autism draws attention to the need of developing further research on this topic. As a matter of fact, the identification of strengths and weaknesses specifically related to sex/gender could help to define an effective intervention and to detect support strategies in adulthood, with the final aim of preventing long-term complications and comorbidities (Box 4.1).

Box 4.1 Camouflaging in Adulthood

What is it?

- Camouflaging strategies involve ***conscious or unconscious masking*** of autistic characteristics during interactions, allowing individuals with autism to mix themselves in social situations, reduce the sense of shame (related to victimization, bullying, or abusive relationships), and try to cope with the world through behaviors that follow social standards [22].
- Camouflaging has been documented in both genders, but it is doubtlessly more frequent in ***women*** with autism [23].

What does it lead to?

- Possible ***underestimation or misrecognition*** of autistic traits, with delayed specific diagnostic evaluation and ***late diagnosis*** in adulthood [22].
- Lack of access to specific ***support services*** [24].
- Experience of ***internal distress*** in individuals with autism, due to their desire to conform with society expectations and rules, beyond the intense effort required [23].
- Development of ***mental health problems*** [22].

Why is it important to identify it?

- To facilitate the ***assessment*** of autistic symptoms in adulthood, with implemented diagnostic abilities and ***access to specific support*** [25].
- To reduce ***distress*** linked to camouflaging and misdiagnosis, in order to prevent internalizing difficulties and psychiatric comorbidities [22].
- To improve ***outcomes*** in terms of well-being, mental health, education, employment, and independence [22].

References

1. Happé F, Frith U. Annual research review: looking back to look forward–changes in the concept of autism and implications for future research. J Child Psychol Psychiatry. 2020;61(3):218–32.
2. Howlin P. Adults with autism: changes in understanding since DSM-111. J Autism Dev Disord. 2021;51(12):4291–308.
3. Le Couteur A, Szatmari P, et al. Autism spectrum disorder. In: Thapar A, editor. Rutter's child and adolescent psychiatry; 2015. p. 665–72.
4. Pickles A, McCauley JB, Pepa LA, Huerta M, Lord C. The adult outcome of children referred for autism: typology and prediction from childhood. J Child Psychol Psychiatry. 2020a;61(7):760–7.
5. Gillespie-Lynch K, Sepeta L, Wang Y, Marshall S, Gomez L, Sigman M, Hutman T. Early childhood predictors of the social competence of adults with autism. J Autism Dev Disord. 2012;42(2):161–74.
6. Howlin P, Magiati I. Autism spectrum disorder: outcomes in adulthood. Curr Opin Psychiatry. 2017a;30(2):69–76. https://doi.org/10.1097/YCO.0000000000000308.
7. Mason D, Capp SJ, Stewart GR, Kempton MJ, Glaser K, Howlin P, Happé F. A meta-analysis of outcome studies of autistic adults: quantifying effect size, quality, and meta-regression. J Autism Dev Disord. 2021;51(9):3165–79. https://doi.org/10.1007/s10803-020-04763-2.
8. Lai MC, Kassee C, Besney R, Bonato S, Hull L, Mandy W, Szatmari P, Ameis SH. Prevalence of co-occurring mental health diagnoses in the autism population: a systematic review and meta-analysis. Lancet Psychiatry. 2019;6(10):819–29. https://doi.org/10.1016/S2215-0366(19)30289-5.
9. Schendel DE, Overgaard M, Christensen J, et al. Association of psychiatric and neurologic comorbidity with mortality among persons with autism spectrum disorder in a Danish population. JAMA Pediatr. 2016;170:243–50.
10. Sikora DM, Vora P, Coury DL, Rosenberg D. Attention-deficit/hyperactivity disorder symptoms, adaptive functioning, and quality of life in children with autism spectrum disorder. Pediatrics. 2012;130(suppl 2):S91–7.
11. Wood JJ, Drahota A, Sze K, Har K, Chiu A, Langer DA. Cognitive behavioral therapy for anxiety in children with autism spectrum disorders: a randomized, controlled trial. J Child Psychol Psychiatry. 2009;50:224–34.
12. Cassidy S, Bradley L, Shaw R, Baron-Cohen S. Risk markers for suicidality in autistic adults. Mol Autism. 2018;9:42.
13. Mason D, Ingham B, Urbanowicz A, Michael C, Birtles H, Woodbury-Smith M, et al. A systematic review of what barriers and facilitators prevent and enable physical healthcare services access for autistic adults. J Autism Dev Disord. 2019;49(8):3387–400.
14. Croen LA, Zerbo O, Qian Y, Massolo ML, Rich S, Sidney S, Kripke C. The health status of adults on the autism spectrum. Autism. 2015;19(7):814–23.
15. Woodman AC, Smith LE, Greenberg JS, Mailick MR. Change in autism symptoms and maladaptive behaviors in adolescence and adulthood: the role of positive family processes. J Autism Dev Disord. 2015;45(1):111–26.
16. Hong J, Bishop-Fitzpatrick L, Smith LE, Greenberg JS, Mailick MR. Factors associated with subjective quality of life of adults with autism spectrum disorder: self-report versus maternal reports. J Autism Dev Disord. 2016;46(4):1368–78. https://doi.org/10.1007/s10803-015-2678-0.
17. Fombonne E. Editorial: camouflage and autism. J Child Psychol Psychiatry. 2020;61(7):735–8. https://doi.org/10.1111/jcpp.13296.
18. Brugha T, McManus S, Meltzer H, et al. Autism spectrum disorders in adults living in households throughout England: Report from the adult psychiatric morbidity survey 2007. Leeds: NHS Information Centre for Health and Social Care; 2009.
19. Hofvander B, Delorme R, Chaste P, et al. Psychiatric and psychosocial problems in adults with normal-intelligence autism spectrum disorders. BMC Psychiatry. 2009;9(1):35.

20. Rutherford M, McKenzie K, Johnson T, Catchpole C, O'Hare A, McClure I, Murray A. Gender ratio in a clinical population sample, age of diagnosis and duration of assessment in children and adults with autism spectrum disorder. Autism. 2016;20:628–34.
21. Lai M, Lombardo MV, Auyeung B, Chakrabarti B, Baron-Cohen S. Sex/gender differences and autism: setting the scene for future research. J Am Acad Child Adolesc Psychiatry. 2015;54(1):11–24.
22. Rynkiewicz A, Janas-Kozik M, Slopien A. Girls and women with autism. Psychiatr Pol. 2019;53(4):737–52.
23. Green RM, Travers AM, Howe Y, McDougle CJ. Women and autism spectrum disorder: diagnosis and implications for treatment of adolescents and adults. Curr Psychiatry Rep. 2019;21(4):22. https://doi.org/10.1007/s11920-019-1006-3.
24. Hull L, Petrides KV, Allison C, Smith P, Baron-Cohen S, Lai MC, Mandy W. "Putting on my best normal": social camouflaging in adults with autism spectrum conditions. J Autism Dev Disord. 2017;47(8):2519–34. https://doi.org/10.1007/s10803-017-3166-5.
25. Lai M-C, Hull L, Mandy W, Chakrabarti B, Nordahl CW, Lombardo MV, Ameis SH, Szatmari P, Baron-Cohen S, Happè F, Livingston LA. Commentary: 'Camouflaging' in autistic people—reflection on Fombonne (2020). J Child Psychol Psychiatry. 2021;62(8):1037–41.

Part II

Neurogenetics of Female Autism

Neurogenetics of Autism Spectrum Conditions in Individuals Assigned Female at Birth

5

Allison Jack, Goldie A. McQuaid, and Abha R. Gupta

Study of the biological bases of autism spectrum conditions has long been limited by several major challenges, including heterogeneous phenotypes and etiologies, differences in the expression of endophenotypes across development, and difficulties obtaining samples of sufficient size and representativeness to model this variability [1]. Characteristics of autism in female individuals have been particularly understudied historically, with the sex ratio currently reported at four diagnoses of male individuals to every one diagnosis for a female individual [2] in the United States; this skewed diagnostic ratio has often translated into research samples that underrepresent female autistic people. From a public health perspective, this is a crucial problem, as female autistic people appear more likely to experience missed or late diagnosis than male individuals [3–5], and this may be due in part to gender-based ascertainment biases. For example, studies that use active (vs. passive) case ascertainment suggest a ~3:1, not ~4:1, male-to-female prevalence estimate [6], indicating that typical referral practice in the community may regularly overlook female individuals and/or those assigned female at birth (AFAB; see Table 5.1 for the list of all abbreviations used in this chapter). The fact that autism diagnostic criteria are exclusively based on observed behavior, as are gold-standard diagnostic confirmation measures, likely contributes to this problem (e.g., D'Mello et al. [7]). Identifying objective biomarkers relevant to autism in AFAB individuals would help

A. Jack (✉) · G. A. McQuaid
Department of Psychology, George Mason University, Fairfax, VA, USA
e-mail: ajack@gmu.edu; gmcquaid@gmu.edu

A. R. Gupta
Department of Pediatrics, Child Study Center, Yale School of Medicine, New Haven, CT, USA

Department of Neuroscience, Yale School of Medicine, New Haven, CT, USA
e-mail: abha.gupta@yale.edu

L. Mazzone et al. (eds.), *Autism Spectrum Disorder: Understanding the Female Phenotype*, https://doi.org/10.1007/978-3-031-62072-0_5

Table 5.1 Abbreviations used in this chapter

Abbreviation	Definition
AFAB	Assigned female at birth
AMAB	Assigned male at birth
CNV	Copy number variant
fMRI	Functional magnetic resonance imaging
FPE	Female protective effect (hypothesis)
mPFC	Medial prefrontal cortex
NAcc	Nucleus accumbens
OT	Oxytocin
OXTR/*OXTR*	Oxytocin receptor/oxytocin receptor gene
PFC	Prefrontal cortex
PRS	Polygenic risk score(s)
RAP	Region-aligned prediction
sMRI	Structural magnetic resonance imaging
SNc	Substantia nigra pars compacta
SNP	Single nucleotide polymorphism
TD	Typically developing
TH	Tyrosine hydroxylase

address this issue. Combining information from genetic and brain-based assays is one promising means of narrowing the available search space and thus advancing progress in the characterization of autism biology generally and autism in AFAB persons specifically.

5.1 Organization and Scope of this Chapter

In this chapter, we first briefly review major relevant findings regarding the neural and genetic bases of autism broadly speaking, as well as a leading theory related to the etiology of autism, specifically in AFAB persons (the "female protective effect" hypothesis). Thereafter, we review and comment on the existing literature addressing the intersection of genetic and neural factors in the emergence and expression of autism (here called "neurogenetic" studies) in AFAB individuals. To conclude, we briefly review ethical considerations related to autism neurogenetic work, particularly with regard to concerns raised within the autism community.

We focus specifically on the neurogenetic characteristics of autistic individuals based on their sex assigned at birth, rather than their gender identity. Given that gender diversity is more prevalent in the autistic than non-autistic population [8–10] and similarly autistic traits are overrepresented in the transgender versus cisgender population [11], considering both sex- and gender-related factors in autism research is crucial [12]. Precision when describing the samples under consideration is similarly important; in much of the extant literature, samples are described regarding the representation of "male" versus "female" participants, but it is unclear whether this refers to sex assigned at birth or current gender identity. We focus here on AFAB individuals to the extent possible, because regardless of gender, this population is likely to share (at least some) common biological factors in terms of their prenatal and infant brain development (that is, during the period of greatest etiological relevance), as well as common early-life socialization experiences that adults typically direct toward infants and children whom they perceive as female (e.g., Aznar and Tenenbaum [13].

Finally, a note on language: Conventional terms used in the field of autism brain and genetic research presuppose that autism is pathological—for example, genetic variants associated with greater autism likelihood are typically called "risk variants," and factors associated with the reduction of autism likelihood are termed "protective." As we discuss further in our closing section on ethical considerations, many autistic people consider their autism an intrinsic part of their identity (similar to members of Deaf culture [14, 15]) and consequently find such language dehumanizing and offensive. While some use of these terms in this chapter is unavoidable, we use nonevaluative language whenever possible.

5.2 Genetic and Neural Bases of Autism

5.2.1 Genetic Bases of Autism

Autism is highly heritable [16]; many genes have been identified as associated with the condition [17], with rare and common gene variants implicated, as well as both inherited and de novo variants [16]. Studies have revealed a highly heterogeneous and complex picture of the genetic etiologies for autism, concordant with the condition's heterogeneous and complex phenotypical presentations [16]. Most individual cases of autism are thought to be likely polygenic in nature, involving one or more rare genetic variants in combination with common variants [18]. Additionally, studies have demonstrated substantial pleiotropy, where genes associated with autism are also associated with attention-deficit/hyperactivity disorder, Tourette's syndrome, depression, and intellectual disability, all conditions that commonly co-occur with autism [16].

5.2.2 Neural Features Associated with Autism

As with the genetic picture of autism, many neural features have been identified as potentially associated with autism diagnosis. Neuroimaging studies reveal structural differences from non-autistic controls in superior temporal cortex [19–21], striatum [22], amygdala [19, 22, 23], prefrontal cortex [21, 22, 24, 25], cerebellum [21, 24, 26, 27], corpus callosum [25, 27–29], and cerebrospinal fluid and ventricular systems [22, 27, 30–32]; for review, see McPartland et al. [33]. Postmortem brain tissue analyses also implicate a number of these structures, especially the cerebellum and prefrontal cortex, and suggest that synaptic, immune, apoptotic, metabolic, and proliferation-related processes (among others) may contribute to autism etiology [34].

The multiplicity of implicated processes and systems is likely related to heterogeneity in underlying genotypes and etiologies (see, e.g., Ellegood et al. [35]) and variability in sample size, composition, and developmental period. Thus, as previously suggested [33], traditional case-control analytic designs aimed at detecting features that distinguish autistic from non-autistic groups are unlikely to advance the field substantially. For example, while functional connectivity differences from neurotypicals are frequently observed in autistic samples using such case-control designs (e.g., Di Martino et al. [36]), identification of consistent *patterns* (both in terms of networks affected and in terms of the direction of the effects, e.g., elevated or reduced connectivity) of connectivity differences has proved elusive [37, 38]. One important approach to untangling diverse and often contradictory findings regarding the biology of autism is to focus attention on particular subpopulations within the spectrum (such as AFAB individuals); another key approach involves combining information from multiple modalities, as described below.

5.2.3 Why Neurogenetic Approaches?

A study takes a *neurogenetic* approach when endophenotypic information about subjects' brains is combined with genetic information from those same subjects and/or when brain (or genetic) data from one subject cohort (or repository) is used to guide genetic (or brain) analyses from another cohort (or repository). Typically, imaging genetic [39] studies and postmortem brain tissue analyses constitute neurogenetic reports. Such approaches help address the problem of widely distributed brain differences and heterogeneous etiologies in autism biology by potentially allowing brain and genetic data to inform each other reciprocally. For example, guidance from imaging or histological findings can define boundaries within the vast genetic search space; genetic information may suggest which aspects of imaging results could be etiological in origin; and imaging or neuropathological findings may speak to the potential endophenotypic outcomes of genomic variation.

5.3 Neural and Genetic Features Associated with Female Autism

Work focused on identifying biological features associated with female autism has historically been limited. In recent years, an upswing in interest in this domain has occurred, with notable developments including collection of larger samples of female and/or AFAB autistic participants in major research cohorts such as ABIDE [36, 40], GENDAAR [41] (NIH Data Archive Collection #2021), EU-AIMS LEAP [42, 43], SPARK [44], and ENIGMA-ASD [22]. However, while such work is advancing, literature on the genetics and particularly the neuroscience of female autism is still relatively thin. A recent systematic review [45] summarizes the extant neuroimaging literature on sex/gender in autism as thin, typically underpowered, and prone to bias; moreover, of the three well-powered studies available in the literature at the time of review, no results converged upon a common network or region. While this report may seem grim, in testament to the rapid movement of the field, three out of four of the neuroimaging studies in autistic cohorts that we review in this chapter were published in the year since Mo and colleague's review.

5.3.1 The Female Protective Effect Hypothesis and Genetic Findings

The existence of a *female protective effect* (FPE; [46, 47]) is a common model, originating in the genetic literature, that is used to help explain the skewed sex ratio in autism. In models consistent with the hypothesis, greater etiologic load is posited to be necessary for the expression of autism in individuals of female versus male biological sex due to female-specific factors that reduce or offset the impact of other factors that increase autism likelihood. Evidence supporting the existence of such an effect comes from work including genetic analyses indicating that de novo mutations in female versus male probands are more frequent, larger in size, and more deleterious [48–50]. Of note, while genetic evidence supports the existence of female sex-specific mechanism(s) that reduce the likelihood that an autistic phenotype will emerge from a given etiological profile, it is as of yet unclear what these mechanism(s) may be. Neurogenetic approaches may be one way of addressing this question.

5.4 Neurogenetic Studies of Autism in Female Individuals

We conducted a systematic database search to identify reports that included human participants (either autistic participants or participants from whom a measure of autistic traits had been obtained), integrated neural and genetic levels of analysis (largely reports featuring imaging genetics or postmortem brain tissue analyses), and either conducted tests of sex differences or reported results of tests conducted on exclusively female samples. While we sought to focus on sex assigned at birth, in many cases, studies did not clarify the definition of "female" as referring to donors or participants in the study (in other words, it was often unclear if "female" represented gender, sex assigned at birth, chromosomal sex, gonadal sex, etc.). In the text that follows, we use "male" and "female" when discussing participants or donors within studies for which it is not known/confirmed whether these terms when used in the original reports refer to sex assigned at birth; otherwise, "AFAB" or assigned male at birth ("AMAB") is used. The inclusion and exclusion criteria for our search are found in Table 5.2; the search and review process details are provided in Fig. 5.1. Ultimately, 14 reports were identified as meeting the criteria for inclusion in this review. Summary characteristics of included reports are found in Table 5.3.

Table 5.2 Inclusion and exclusion criteria for the literature review

Inclusion criteria	Exclusion criteria
Includes at least one of the following: • Autistic participants or brain tissue donors • Participants or brain tissue donors for whom a measure of autistic traits is collected or available	Includes only male[a] individuals or organisms
Includes analysis/analyses of at least one of the following: • Sex differences • Gender differences • Female[a] individuals or tissue from female donors	Includes only analyses combined across sexes or genders
Integrates information from neural and genetic levels of analysis	Animal model studies

[a]"Female" and "male" are used here in reflection of the relatively imprecise terminology used by most reports screened. While our original intent was to focus on sex assigned at birth in our review, it was not possible to conclude participant sex assigned at birth based on information provided by many reports. Consequently, here we use the broad "male" and "female" language used in the reports reviewed and clarify in text where further details regarding sex and/or gender are available for a given sample

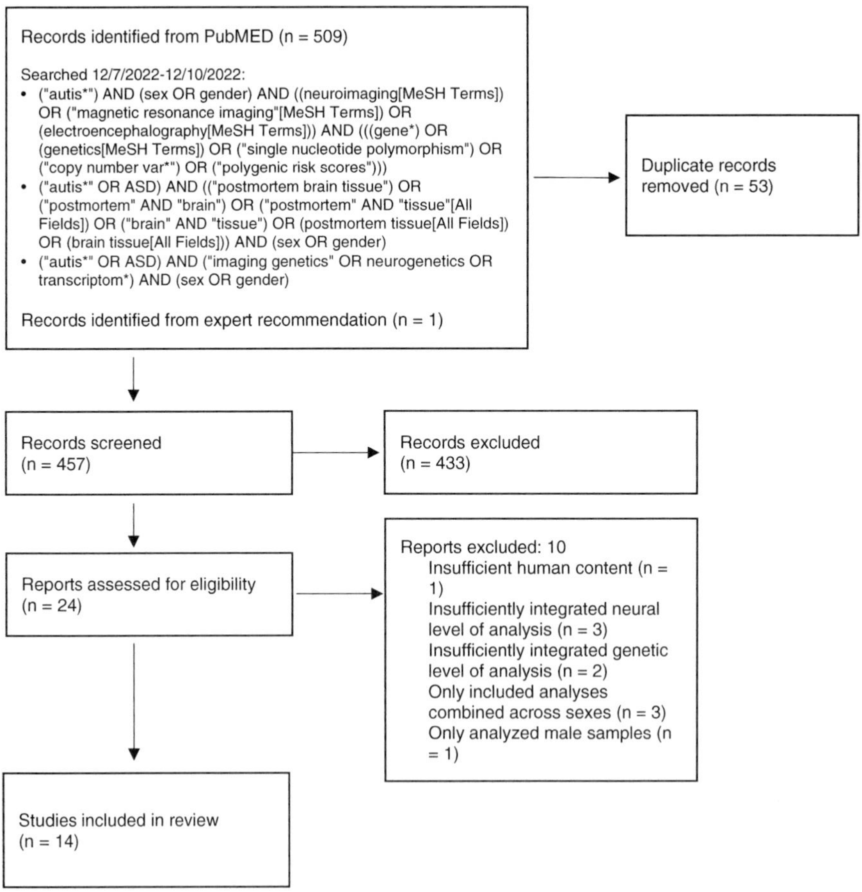

Fig. 5.1 Search, screening, and review process for articles included and excluded in this review

Table 5.3 Studies included in the review

First author (year)	Method	Subject type	SAB?	Total autistic *N* (*n* autistic female[a])	Non-autistic *ns* (*n* female)	System/site(s) potentially implicated	Cohort(s) or repository
Jack et al. [41]	Decoding imaging maps: task-based fMRI + BrainSpan atlas	Autistic participants (8–17 years)	Yes	92 (45) fMRI 127 (6[illegible]) genetics 2075 (291) replication genetics	TD 92 (45) fMRI genetics	Striatum including putamen	GENDAAR; SPARK
Floris et al. [51]	Decoding imaging maps: sMRI + Allen human brain atlas	Autistic participants (transfer/validation 5–56 years; testing 6–30 years)		Transfer/ validation: 641 (115) Testing: 395 (109)	Training: NT 14,503 (7584) Transfer/ validation: NT 771 (239) Testing: 286 (98)	Estrogen-downregulated genes; genes for prenatal excitatory neurons; posterior auditory cortex; fronto-temporal/fronto-occipital white matter	UK biobank; ABIDE I + II; EU-AIMS LEAP
Saito et al. [52]	sMRI + SNP	General population adults with AQ scores (21–40 years)		N/A	135 (56)	*OXTR* rs2254298; insula	N/A
Hernandez et al. [53]	Rs-fMRI + SNP	Autistic participants (8–17 years)	Yes	87 (50)	86 (52)	*OXTR* rs1042778, rs2254298, rs53576, and rs237887; NAcc connectivity with dorsal striatum (caudate and putamen), thalamus, PFC	GENDAAR
Sha et al. [54]	sMRI + PRS	General population adults		N/A	32,256 (16,968)	Null findings for sex-related analyses	UK biobank
Lawrence et al. [55]	Rs-fMRI + PRS	Autistic participants (8–17 years)	Yes	61 (31)	66 (28)	Salience network FC with sensorimotor processing regions (e.g., precentral gyrus, insula)	GENDAAR
Gui et al. [56]	s/fMRI + PRS	General population youth 9.91 years (±0.62); adults 63.84 years (±7.47)		N/A	ABCD: 4722 (2198) UK biobank s/ fMRI genetics: 21,523 (11,180)	Null findings	ABCD, UK biobank

(continued)

Table 5.3 (continued)

First author (year)	Method	Subject type	SAB?	Total autistic *N* (*n* autistic female[a])	Non-autistic *ns* (*n* female)	System/site(s) potentially implicated	Cohort(s) or repository
Plummer et al. [57]	Postmortem brain tissue	Autistic tissue donors	Yes	15 ASD (5) 5 RTT (5)	18 (8)	Superior temporal gyrus	Harvard brain tissue resource center, UMB BTB
Khan et al. [58]	Postmortem tissue	Autistic tissue donors (4–15 years)	Yes	10 (3)	11 (4)	Cortical regions, putamen	UMB BTB
Werling et al. [59]	Postmortem tissue	Neurotypical tissue donors (13–56 years)		N/A	28 (14)	Astrocytes and microglia	BrainSpan
Schumann et al. [60]	Postmortem tissue	Autistic tissue donors (5–50 years)	Yes	10 (5)	8 (2)	Superior temporal sulcus, primary auditory cortex	Harvard brain tissue resource center
Lee et al. [61]	Postmortem tissue + blood-based microarray	Autistic tissue donors (4–67 years)		13 (3)	39 (9)	Dorsolateral prefrontal cortex	NIMH neuropathology, UMB BTB, Stanley Medical Research Institute
Frehner et al. [62]	Postmortem tissue: Receptor binding and mRNA expression	Autistic tissue donors (4–27 years)	Yes	15 (7)	TD 15 (7)	OXTR in SNc	UMB BTB
Chen et al. [63]	Postmortem tissue	Autistic tissue donors		103	88	Neuroimmune system	Multiple studies

SAB? confirmation in report or from original description of cohort/repository that "female" refers to female sex assigned at birth, *AQ* Autism Spectrum Quotient, *FC* functional connectivity, *fMRI* functional magnetic resonance imaging, *NT* neurotypical, OXTR/*OXTR* oxytocin receptor/oxytocin receptor gene, *PFC* prefrontal cortex, *PRS* Polygenic Risk Score, *rs-fMRI* resting-state functional magnetic resonance imaging, *sMRI* structural magnetic resonance imaging, *SNc* substantia nigra pars compacta, *SNP* single nucleotide polymorphism, *TD* typically developing, *UMB BTB* University of Maryland Brain and Tissue Bank

[a]See note in Table 5.1

5.4.1 Studies Investigating the Oxytocinergic System

Within the limited literature on the neurogenetics of autism sex differences, three reports evaluate potential differences in the oxytocinergic system. Oxytocin (OT) is a neuropeptide that is sexually dimorphic in its effects [64, 65]; in addition to its contributions to childbirth and lactation, it also plays an important role in human social cognition and behavior, including processes related to social perception, social salience, affiliation, bonding, trust, and reward/motivation [66–68]. OT's ability to impact these diverse functions is thought to derive in part from its interactions with the mesocorticolimbic dopaminergic pathway of the brain [69]; this pathway is crucial for motivated behavior via dopamine's influence on reward drive [70–72]. OT projects to limbic regions in this pathway, including the ventral tegmental area, nucleus accumbens (NAcc), and amygdala, where it may modulate dopaminergic activity [69, 71]. The prefrontal cortex (PFC) constitutes the "cortical" aspect of the mesocorticolimbic dopaminergic pathway and, via its dense interconnections with other cortical regions, serves as a hub through which motivational factors (potentially modulated by OT) can shape attentional, perceptual, and cognitive processes [69, 71]. The social functions of OT and its sex-differential effects have led to ongoing interest in the potential role this system may play in autism etiologies (e.g., Carter [73]). Behavioral and imaging genetic studies investigating the association between common variation in the oxytocin receptor gene (*OXTR*) and autism have produced mixed results, particularly for any given single nucleotide polymorphism (SNP), but when taken together are overall suggestive of greater representation of so-called risk alleles in autism cases versus controls, and association between common variants and autism phenotypes and neuroendophenotypes [74].

Two SNP-focused imaging genetic studies, Saito et al. [52] and Hernandez et al. [53], suggest that certain *OXTR* alleles may contribute to sex-differential patterns of brain structure and function in ways related to autistic phenotype expression. Focusing on *OXTR* rs2254298, Saito et al. [52] examined associations among genotype, brain structure (assessed via voxel-based morphometry of MRI data), and autistic trait expression (assessed via a translation [75] of the Autism Spectrum Quotient [76]) in a general population sample of ethnically Japanese participants. Allele frequency for rs2254298 differs across populations based on ancestry, as does the association of particular alleles with a greater likelihood of autistic phenotypes [77]; in Chinese Han and Japanese ethnic samples, rs2254298A has been associated with greater autism likelihood [78, 79]. Consequently, in Saito et al. [52], the number of rs2254298A alleles (0, 1, or 2, corresponding to G/G, A/G, or A/A genotypes, respectively) carried was the genetic variable of interest. First, the team conducted whole-brain analyses of grey matter volume to determine regions where volume correlated with autistic trait scores; then, they examined whether the rs2254298A number was associated with volume in identified brain regions. Male, but not female, participants showed an association between what the authors termed a "prosociality" factor extracted from (primarily social communication) items on the Autism Spectrum Quotient and a region of right anterior insula; male participants with higher autistic trait levels had lower grey matter volume. Follow-up analysis indicated that lower grey matter volume of this insula region was significantly associated with higher rs2254298A number in male but not female individuals. This study is suggestive but has notable limitations. Autistic traits are indeed thought to vary on a continuum throughout the human population, and using general population samples is a particularly appropriate means to examine how common genetic variation relates to dimensional phenotypic variability. However, the degree to which the neurogenetic patterns described in this study might apply to people with autism diagnoses, including AFAB individuals, is unclear. More importantly, the examination of associations between brain structure and genotype conducted for this report must be framed as, at best, exploratory; if autistic trait levels are thought to relate to allele number, then limiting genetic analyses to brain regions already selected on the basis of association with autistic traits is likely to inflate estimation of effects.

Hernandez et al. [53] also examined common variations in *OXTR* but did so via a multi-SNP dosage approach in a sample that included youth with confirmed autism diagnoses (as well as matched neurotypical youth). SNPs considered were *OXTR* rs1042778, rs2254298, rs53576, and rs237887; each participant was assigned a cumulative score based on the number of autism-associated alleles they carried across the four SNPs. This genetic score was then used as a regressor in functional connectivity analyses of resting-state fMRI data. These analyses used a seed-based approach, examining the connectivity of the nucleus accumbens (NAcc) with the whole brain. Among AFAB autistic youth, a higher number of autism-associated alleles across *OXTR* SNPs was related to greater functional connectivity between the NAcc seed and dorsal striatum (caudate and putamen) and thalamus, and weaker connectivity between this seed and regions of inferior and superior lateral occipital cortex. A significant three-way interaction among allele dosage, sex, and group was also detected, such that sex assigned at birth predicted a differential relationship between allele dosage and NAcc connectivity in the autistic group only. Specifically, NAcc functional connectivity with prefrontal, dorsal striatal, and thalamic regions increased with greater allele number among AFAB autistic youth but decreased with greater allele number among AMAB autistic youth. Prefrontal areas implicated included a region of left medial prefrontal cortex (mPFC) highlighted by previous work on NAcc functional connectivity in a largely ($n = 71$ of 82) male sample [80]; in that report, consistent with the pattern demonstrated by AMAB youth in Hernandez et al. [53], autistic youth showed decreased NAcc-left mPFC resting-state functional connectivity as a function of increasing number of autism-associated alleles at *OXTR* rs1042778, rs2254298, rs53576, and rs237887, relative to increased NAcc-left mPFC connectivity with increased number among neurotypical youth. Hernandez and colleagues argue that these results indicate relative similarity between AFAB autistic and male neurotypical youth in terms of the endophenotypic and phenotypic profiles associated with common genetic variation in *OXTR*, with both AFAB autistic and male neurotypical youth showing greater NAcc-left mPFC functional connectivity with greater allele dosage and greater NAcc-left mPFC connectivity also associated with lower Social Responsiveness Scale scores (indicative of lower levels of autistic traits) for both groups [53, 80]. The authors suggest that NAcc-left mPFC connectivity may represent a compensatory mechanism involving increased linking of reward functions to prefrontal processes related to social cognition and inhibitory control. Further, they argue that the finding supports the FPE hypothesis in that this presumed compensatory modulation of functional connectivity in the presence of autism-associated genetic variation was found in AFAB but not AMAB autistic youth.

Frehner et al. [62] evaluated postmortem tissue from the substantia nigra pars compacta (SNc) of autistic and typically developing (TD) donors to test whether oxytocin receptor (OXTR) density (assessed via competitive binding receptor autoradiography) and gene expression (assessed via in situ hybridization to visualize OXTR mRNA) differed by sex (assigned at birth) and/or autism status. The project was partly motivated by the team's hypothesis that sex-differential OT regulation of dopaminergic activity in SNc might help explain features of the autistic phenotype that have been found to vary between male and female individuals. Consequently, the team also evaluated mRNA expression of tyrosine hydroxylase (TH), the rate-limiting enzyme in dopamine synthesis, in donor tissue samples, as condensed TH is indicative of the presence of dopaminergic neurons [81]. OXTR density results indicated significant effects for sex and for the interaction between sex and diagnosis, with AFAB autistic donors demonstrating less OXTR binding in SNc than any other group (AMAB autistic donors or TD donors of either sex). However, contrary to the team's predictions, neither OXTR nor TH mRNA differed by sex, group, or the interaction thereof. Thus, these results suggest that AFAB autistic donors in this sample had fewer mature OXTR on the cell surface in SNc, without differences in gene expression. Frehner and colleagues suggest several possible mechanisms for this pattern of results: delayed recycling of OXTR to the cell surface after agonist binding; enhanced OXTR desensitization; desensitization and internalization of OXTR in consequence of extensive agonist activity; or disruptions in the broader endocytotic pathway, not necessarily specific to the action of OT and its receptors. These findings may be compared to those of another case-control postmortem tissue study, which exclusively examined OXTR binding [82]. This study included tissue from five AFAB autistic donors and found higher oxytocin receptor (OXTR) binding in nucleus basalis and lower in ventral pallidum, among autistic versus control donors (with null results in global pallidus, superior colliculus, and periaqueductal grey), but no effects of sex or sex × diagnosis interaction effects for any region. (Of note, given the paucity of AFAB autistic brain tissue donors [n = 16 in NIH Biobank as of Dec 15, 2022; https://neurobiobank.nih.gov/subjects/], overlap between subjects across these two studies is likely.) Thus, it seems that sex differences in OXTR density among autistic individuals may be regionally specific, with no current evidence for sex differences in OXTR binding within various other regions relevant to OT action in the human brain.

5.4.2 Studies Using Polygenic Risk Scores (PRS)

In conditions with complex etiologies, examination of a specific genetic variant associated with an increased likelihood of a condition, typically called a "risk variant," may not yield adequate information to understand associations between genetic variation and other biological factors [83]. In contrast, polygenic risk scores (PRSs) are based not on a single variant but on composites of many variants. PRS thus quantifies genetic loading for a condition, and this quantification has utility, for example, in characterizing associations of genetic variation with brain structure and/or function.

To date, three studies have examined PRS as these scores relate to sex differences in autism. Lawrence et al. [55] investigated a potential neurogenetic basis for the female protective effect in autism. The authors examined associations between autism PRS and salience network functional connectivity in a sex-balanced sample of autistic and TD youth. PRSs were associated with increased functional connectivity between a salience network seed (right orbital frontoinsula) and somatosensory processing regions for AMAB autistic youth and with the primary motor cortex (precentral gyrus) for TD AMAB youth. In contrast, in both autistic and TD AFAB youth, no significant associations were found between PRS and salience network connectivity. Within autistic and TD youth, PRS associations with functional connectivity were modulated by sex. Among AMAB autistic youth with higher genetic load, greater connectivity was observed between salience network and sensorimotor processing regions. Within the TD group, AMAB youth with higher genetic load showed greater connectivity between salience network and primary motor cortex. The findings suggest a general sex-based association between functional connectivity and autism PRS, observed across autistic and non-autistic youth. The authors interpret the sex-differential effect of PRS on salience network functional connectivity with sensorimotor processing regions as a potential neurogenetic mechanism for the FPE in autism. Specifically, they argue that while AMAB youth with higher PRS showed potential impacts on sensorimotor regions, AFAB youth with higher PRS showed no such impacts, suggesting that this neural circuitry is "protected" in girls.

Two studies have examined autism PRSs as these relate to structural and functional brain metrics in general population cohorts. Sha et al. [54] investigated potential associations between autism PRS and multivariate indices of brain asymmetry, specifically examining whether PRS scores for autism were associated with "masculinized" or "more male-like" patterns of brain asymmetry. Forty-two structural asymmetry indices in the UK Biobank brain imaging genetic dataset were examined, including surface area, cortical thickness, and subcortical volume metrics. Autism PRS was associated with eight asymmetry indices in the temporal, frontal, and medial cortex and in the caudate nucleus. However, patterns of associations between PRS and these asymmetry indices did not provide evidence for a more male-like (or more female-like) pattern of brain asymmetry.

Gui et al. [56] investigated sex differences in the effect of autism PRS (along with PRS for five neuropsychiatric conditions) on brain function and structure in general population youth (ABCD) and adult (UK Biobank) cohorts. Neuroimaging metrics in two cohorts included resting-state fMRI, diffusion tensor imaging-based metrics, and morphometrics (e.g., sulcal depth, surface area, cortical thickness, and cortical and subcortical volume). No sex differences were found in the effect of autism PRS on brain function or structure in either cohort.

5.4.3 Studies Decoding Imaging Maps

Two recent studies (one our own) used imaging maps as a starting point for subsequent genetic analyses. Such approaches are relatively novel, but similar methods have begun to gain traction in the broader literature (e.g., [84–88]).

In the study of Jack et al. [41], we (AJ; ARG) used imaging and genetic data collected from Wave 1 of the GENDAAR cohort, which was also the cohort used in the reports by Lawrence et al. [55] and Hernandez et al. [53] that are reviewed in this chapter. Wave 1 of this cohort consisted of a sample of autistic youth (8–17 years) without intellectual disability who were balanced in terms of sex assigned at birth and a sample of TD comparison youth matched to the autistic group in terms of age, sex assigned at birth, and IQ. Our analyses used task-based fMRI to assess brain response to socially relevant stimuli (point-light displays of coherent biological or scrambled whole-body human motion [89, 90]) in these youth. Among our neuroimaging analyses, we chiefly sought to characterize how functional brain response among AFAB autistic youth differed from AFAB comparison youth within the experimental contrast (biological > scrambled). We found that autistic AFAB youth showed reduced response to human motion, relative to TD AFAB youth, in striatal, parietal, and posterior frontal regions, with largest effect sizes right-lateralized in motor and premotor areas, dorsolateral PFC, and putamen region of the striatum.

Subsequently, to explore whether any aspect of the fMRI-derived profile that differentiated autistic and TD AFAB youth (hereafter, the *autistic AFAB fMRI profile*) might relate to etiological (versus experiential) factors, we looked at evidence related to how the size of rare genetic copy number variants (CNVs) might vary between AFAB and AMAB. We expected that we would find that rare CNVs containing genes expressed in brain regions represented in autistic AFAB fMRI profiles, specifically during prenatal and early infant brain development, would be larger in size for autistic AFAB than AMAB youth. While previous work (described above) has demonstrated greater genetic "load" in autistic AFAB versus AMAB probands [48, 50], we tested the hypothesis that potential impacts to the specific brain regions implicated in the autistic AFAB fMRI profile would contribute to this load differential more so than mutational burden broadly defined. First, we categorized rare CNVs in our sample based on the pattern of spatiotemporal expression of gene(s) they contained using the BrainSpan exon-array transcriptome dataset [91]. CNVs of interest were those which were rare and contained gene(s) that were (1) expressed during early development (10 post-conceptual weeks to 24 months) and (2) expressed within 11 brain regions that were represented in the autistic AFAB fMRI profile and for which BrainSpan transcriptome data were available. For all 11 brain regions of interest combined, the autistic AFAB minus autistic AMAB difference in median CNV size was significant, and further exploratory analyses indicated that the difference appeared to be driven by the striatal regions of interest, with right and left striatal regions combined yielding a median size difference of 89,999 base pairs. By contrast, the median size difference between AFAB and AMAB autistic youth for rare CNVs *not* containing genes expressed in early striatal development was not significant (1002 base pairs). These genetic findings held under various permutation-based control tests and replicated in an independent cohort, the Simons Simplex Collection [92, 93]. One critique of our approach focused on our evaluation of rare genetic CNVs containing *any* gene(s), rather than just those with known associations to autism [94]. However, since the complete genetic contribution to autism is not yet known, examining only CNVs containing known autism genes would exclude those containing novel genes with potentially important associations with autism as well. Together, these results support the FPE hypothesis and suggest that the expression of an autistic phenotype in some AFAB individuals may relate to rare genetic variation potentially associated with the early development and later function of the striatum.

Floris et al. [51] also used a strategy that involved decoding imaging maps, on a larger sample of structural MRI (sMRI) data. Analyses in this project were designed to test the hypothesis that autism is associated with more typically "male-like" neuroanatomy (a prediction of what was originally termed the "Extreme Male Brain Theory" of autism [95, 96]). Additionally, the team sought to determine whether autistic brain features associated with a shift toward "maleness" were linked to autism-associated and/or sex-differential gene expression. As a first step, the authors trained a sex-prediction machine learning classifier on a very large sample of sMRI brain data from neurotypical adults (44–80 years [y]) in the UK Biobank; thereafter, this classifier was transferred and validated using ABIDE I + II sMRI data from neurotypical and autistic children, adolescents, and adults (5–56 years); finally, tuned models were applied to sMRI data from the EU-AIMS LEAP cohort of neurotypical and autistic children, adolescents, and adults (6–30 years). Region-aligned prediction (RAP; [20]) maps were generated for each participant, which provided a predicted probability of male sex for each individual brain region; these individual maps were then used to create group-level RAP maps that could be used to conduct group difference analyses (e.g., to examine regionally specific maleness predictions across the brain for autistic versus neurotypical female participants). Neurotypical male participants were most differentiated from neurotypical female participants by features of the posterior auditory cortex and frontotemporal/fronto-occipital white matter pathways. Autistic female participants similarly showed a greater likelihood (versus neurotypical female participants) of neurotypical male predictions in posterior auditory cortex and frontotemporal/fronto-occipital white matter, as well as corpus callosum and occipital fusiform gyrus. Autistic male participants, contrasted to neurotypical male participants, showed greater likelihood of neurotypical male prediction in the amygdala, pallidum, thalamus, cerebellum, medial frontal cortex, supplementary motor cortex, and superior fronto-occipital fasciculus.

Subsequently, Neurosynth [97] and Neurovault [98] gene expression decoding tools were used to identify genes whose patterns of expression were topologically similar to group difference RAP maps of interest: those for autistic versus neurotypical female participants, and autistic versus neurotypical male participants. Unlike Jack et al. [41], decoding was based on the Allen Human Brain gene expression atlas and thus was not specific to early brain development; this atlas instead focuses on gene expression as characterized from adult postmortem brain tissue [99, 100]. Candidate genes were retained if similarity analysis indicated that they had high expression in regions that were significantly associated with higher male probability in the RAP maps. The candidate gene list was then analyzed to examine enrichment for autism-associated genes, genes from prenatal cell types, and sex-differentially regulated genes.

The set of candidate genes whose expression patterns were similar to the patterns from the autistic female > neurotypical female RAP and autistic male > neurotypical male RAP difference maps was enriched for transcriptionally upregulated autism-associated genes; the set of candidate genes with expression patterns similar to those of the neurotypical male > neurotypical female RAP difference map was enriched for transcriptionally downregulated autism-associated genes. Candidate genes with expression patterns similar to the autistic female > neurotypical female RAP difference map showed enrichment for prenatal excitatory cell types, X-chromosomal male differentially expressed genes, estrogen-downregulated genes, and autosomal female differentially expressed genes. Candidate genes with expression patterns similar to the autistic male > neurotypical male RAP difference map demonstrated enrichment for dihydrotestosterone- and estrogen-upregulated genes and several prenatal cell types (microglial, progenitor, and radial glial). Overall, the authors interpret their results as supporting the hypothesis that autism is associated with a shift toward neurobiological features characteristic of neurotypical male individuals. In particular, they point to the relative similarity between the regions identified using the autistic female > neurotypical female and neurotypical male > neurotypical female RAP maps and the candidate genes associated with these maps. As the authors note, a limitation of this study is the focus only on neurobiological features associated with a "shift" toward a typically male neuroendophenotype; they acknowledge that any given human brain (including any autistic brain) typically demonstrates a composite of "male-like" and "female-like" features and indicate that future work should examine neurobiological features associated with a "female shift" as well.

5.4.4 Postmortem Human Brain Studies

Postmortem human brain tissue studies have provided valuable insights into how differences in gene expression might contribute to sex differences in autism. Werling et al. [59] presented one of the first studies investigating sex-differential gene expression in autism. The authors determined that sexually dimorphic processes, specifically involving neuronal-glial interactions, may account for the skewed sex prevalence of autism. They accomplished this by characterizing sex differences in gene expression in postmortem human neocortical tissue from neurotypical adults [total 10 subjects (5 female)] and fetuses [total 8 subjects (4 female)] from the BrainSpan dataset [91]. They then compared these patterns to gene expression modules derived from postmortem human cortical data from neurotypical [total 57 subjects (10 female)] and autistic donors [total 48 subjects (12 female)] [101, 102]. This analysis revealed that there was no enrichment of known autism-associated genes among genes expressed differentially between male and female neurotypical cortex. In other words, autism-associated genes, themselves, do not show sex-differential expression. However, the analysis did make the novel discovery that the set of genes found to be expressed at higher levels in neurotypical male versus female cortex is significantly enriched for genes that are also expressed at higher levels in postmortem autism cortex. The genes upregulated in autism cortex are associated with astrocyte and microglia markers. This provided the intriguing insight that neuronal–glial interactions and immune system function contribute to sex differences in autism. Furthermore, genes downregulated in autism cortex are enriched for genes differentially expressed in neurotypical female cortex and are associated with neuronal and synaptic function. The authors suggest that biological pathways downstream of autism-associated genes that intersect with naturally occurring sexually dimorphic processes influence sex differences in autism, rather than sex-differential expression of autism-associated genes.

Chen et al. [63] also investigated gene expression in postmortem brain tissue from autistic individuals and five other major psychiatric or neurological conditions (schizophrenia, bipolar disorder, depression, Alzheimer's disease, and Parkinson's disease). They focused on immune-related genes due to the implication of neuroinflammation in the pathophysiology of multiple brain disorders. Their analysis uncovered significant sex differences in immune-related dysregulation in autism and depression but not the other disorders. Immune-related genes showed greater differential expression in male versus female autism brains relative to control brains. In contrast, the brains of females with depression showed larger changes than males. This report provided further evidence that the neuroimmune system contributes to sex differences in autism.

Two other studies also focused on sex-differential gene expression of specific systems. Plummer et al. [57] analyzed transcriptional regulation of the *MET* receptor tyrosine kinase gene by MeCP2. *MET* is a gene associated with elevated autism likelihood; *MeCP2* mutations cause Rett syndrome, a neurodevelopmental disorder with autistic features that affects mostly female individuals. MeCP2 binds to the *MET* promoter, and *MET* gene expression is significantly reduced in postmortem female temporal cortex affected by Rett syndrome. The authors discovered reduced *MET* gene expression in autistic AMAB but not AFAB donors compared to controls. The authors suggest that distinct, but as of yet unclear, mechanisms lead to the reduction of *MET* in AFAB individuals affected by Rett syndrome and in autistic AMAB individuals. Khan et al. [58] based their postmortem human brain tissue examination on the hypothesis of brain thyroid hormone deficiency in autism. They found sex-differential expression of genes regulated by thyroid hormone. Many of these changes were detected in the putamen, with decreased gene expression in postmortem AMAB autistic putamen and increased gene expression in postmortem AFAB autistic putamen. The putamen, primarily involved in regulating movement, has also been implicated in language and social functions [103]. Intriguingly, our work found that the striatum, which contains the putamen, is a key component of the AFAB autistic neural profile through the imaging-genomics analysis discussed above [41].

Schumann et al. [60] extended the analysis of sex-differential expression of genes to small noncoding RNAs such as microRNAs, which themselves regulate gene expression. In postmortem temporal cortex from autistic donors, they found sex-differential expression of microRNAs involved in neuronal and oligodendrocyte differentiation and implicated in anxiety. The potential microRNA targets are significantly enriched in immune and nervous system pathways. Also, they found more dysregulated small noncoding RNAs, microRNA target genes, and pathways in brain tissue from autistic AFAB compared to AMAB donors. The authors suggest that this supports the observation of a greater genetic "burden" in autistic female individuals and is also relevant to the FPE as a possible reflection of a greater "protective" molecular response.

Finally, Lee et al. [61] identified sex-dependent biomarkers of autism by analyzing RNA-seq data from postmortem human brain tissue and conducting a meta-analysis of six blood-based microarray datasets. Rather than treating sex as a simple covariate, as often done in previous studies, the authors modeled the interaction of sex and autism directly. RNA-seq data analysis revealed that the top five transcripts showing the most sex-dependent dysregulation encode the proteins SLC13A4, DSP, OGN, PTGDS, and AEBP1, although these results were not statistically significant. Blood-based microarray data analysis identified four genes with significant sex-dependent dysregulation: *TTF2*, *UTY*, *KCNJ8*, and *NCS1*. Interestingly, the top hit, *TTF2*, is involved in thyroid development. As described above, Khan et al. [58] linked sex-differential expression of thyroid hormone target genes to autism.

5.5 Common Themes and Future Directions

While the extant neurogenetic literature on female autism is slim, some studies do converge upon common sites or systems. As discussed above, three studies directly investigated sex differences in the *oxytocinergic* system and found evidence for sex differences in autistic and autistic-like neuroendophenotypes associated with common variation in *OXTR* [52, 53], as well as OXTR density (but not OXTR mRNA expression) in SNc tissue [62]. In addition, the *striatum* and *neuroimmune* processes emerged as themes from studies included in this review.

5.5.1 Striatum

The striatum, comprised of caudate and putamen (dorsal striatum) and NAcc (ventral striatum), emerged as a potential system of interest in the work of Hernandez et al. [53], Jack et al. [41], and Khan et al. [58]. In particular, putamen emerged as a potential structure of interest in all three studies. This brain region is thought to serve as an interface for information about motivational value and voluntary behavior by virtue of the projections it receives from the motor, premotor, and prefrontal cortex [104, 105]; it appears likely to play a role in diverse functions including language, social behavior, and sensorimotor processes [103, 104]. Previously, striatal [22] and more specifically putaminal (e.g., [106, 107]) differences from neurotypicals have been documented within autistic samples broadly speaking (although typically in male-predominant samples). Thus, as we have previously suggested [41], these findings likely do not suggest that striatal (or putaminal) involvement is a unique component of the AFAB neurobiological profile. Rather, while not sex-*specific*, such results suggest that striatal involvement may have a particularly important role in AFAB etiologies. As Hernandez et al. [53] and Jack et al. [41] both analyzed the same GENDAAR cohort, further replication of such effects in independent samples will be required; however, the replication of striatal-related genetic findings from Jack et al. [41] in the SPARK cohort is suggestive. We could speculate that this might be related to what some might term "FPE" processes (e.g., that mechanisms involving striatum may reduce likelihood of expression of certain aspects of the autistic phenotype particularly in AFAB individuals); however, as of yet, extant data is insufficient to speak to such hypotheses.

5.5.2 Neuroimmune Processes

Sex differences potentially relevant to neuroimmune function were noted in the works of Werling et al. [59], Chen et al. [63], Floris et al. [51], and Schumann et al. [60]. Overall, results of these studies suggested that sex-differential variation in neuroimmune system may help partially explain the male bias in autism prevalence; autism-associated genes appear to be enriched for neuroimmune-relevant genes that have typically sex-differential expression (with upregulation in male individuals). These findings are in line with accumulating evidence suggesting that neuroimmune processes may be associated with autism etiology generally speaking [108, 109] and the theory that sexual dimorphism in these processes may be relevant to sex differences observed in autism prevalence and expression [110].

5.6 Ethical Considerations

Some within the autism community (which includes autistic self-advocates, autistic researchers, parents of autistic persons, as well as allies who are autism clinicians and researchers) express concerns regarding genetic and brain-based studies of autism. Themes are closely interlinked and include concerns regarding researchers' perception and study of autism from a strictly *medical model* standpoint; degree of *respect for autistic people as persons* (rather than simply as research subjects); and misgivings regarding the *potential uses* to which neurogenetic data could be applied (e.g., eugenics). Many of these concerns articulated within the autism community are also voiced within the broader disability rights communities (e.g., [111, 112]). These concerns necessitate attention and particularly careful consideration from researchers given that many autistic individuals consider their autism an intrinsic and inextricable aspect of their identity. Acknowledging, understanding, and respecting these concerns are a prerequisite for non-autistic researchers to reflect critically on their research goals and practices.

The *medical model* of autism conceptualizes autism as a disorder of atypical neurodevelopment. Under this conceptualization, autistic social and communication behaviors are viewed as medical symptoms requiring treatment. This has been the conventional lens through which the majority of autism-related research, educational, and clinical practice (and training) has been conducted, particularly neurogenetic research. By contrast, many, though not all (e.g., [113]; see also [114], for a discussion of common critiques), members of the autism community subscribe to a *neurodiversity* [115, 116] model of autism (and/or a broader *social model of disability* [117]). While the definition of neurodiversity can vary, broadly speaking, this model conceptualizes neurodevelopmental differences, including conditions such as autism, attention-deficit/hyperactivity disorder, and Tourette's (and their related traits and/or subclinical manifestations), as part of the spectrum of human diversity. Within the neurodiversity model, autistic differences in and of themselves (such as sensory differences; intense, focused interests; reduced eye contact; or "stimming" behaviors) are not considered pathological, but can be disabling due to a misfit between autistic needs and the expectations and affordances of a neurotypical-majority society [116]. Typically, co-occurring medical, genetic, psychiatric, or social conditions (e.g., depression, Ehlers-Danlos syndrome, poverty, trauma), rather than core autistic traits themselves, are highlighted by advocates as their chief sources of distress [118–120]. Thus, both language conventionally used in autism-related reports, textbooks, and assessment instruments and, more importantly, many key goals driving the last several decades of autism biomedical research, are antithetical to the principles and goals of the neurodiversity movement. Indeed, the conventional biomedical (and more broadly, neurotypical) view of autism strictly as pathology (and thus presumably separable from an underlying "healthy" individual identity that could be uncovered with treatment) was a major driving factor in the development of the neurodiversity movement (e.g., [121, 122]).

Neurogenetic researchers should be aware that intrinsic differences between the medical and neurodiversity models of autism serve as a major source of conflict within autism communities at the moment, particularly between parent/caregivers and autistic self-advocates. These parents/caregivers argue that autistic individuals with high support needs and co-occurring intellectual disability, particularly those who are minimally verbal (i.e., *nonrepresenting* autistic individuals), are not well represented by self-advocates (i.e., *representing* autistic individuals) [123–126]; typically, these voices endorse a medical model view of autism and argue that the neurodiversity model harms nonrepresenting individuals by reducing research, funding, and intervention efforts that would address their needs. By contrast, representing autistic individuals argue that they are best positioned to advocate on behalf of nonrepresenting autistic individuals, by virtue of their shared autism, and that non-autistic voices, such as those of non-autistic parents, have too long been centered in conversations regarding autism research and funding priorities.

The tendency within the biomedical literature to describe autism and autistic people through the lens of pathology also raises concerns about *respect for autistic people as persons* (rather than simply as research subjects). Concerns regarding respect for participants as persons within biomedical research are expressed particularly clearly in an opinion piece by Cos Michael, in which she describes a history of enthusiastic engagement in participatory research related to autism, and the factors that have since led her to opt out (2021).[1] She questions the attitudes of non-autistic researchers toward autistic participants, describing experiences of feeling tokenized and used primarily as a means to advance researchers' careers. Of particular importance for those engaged in neurogenetic research is her statement about her experiences participating in neuroscience studies: "Too many scientists research the brain as if it is a dissected specimen. Often, it really is just that, but even if it arrives complete with the messy detritus of our bodies, mucked up with imagination and opinions, it will always remain, to them, as this is an autistic adult brain. Not a person" [127]. Others have similarly expressed a sense that autism research treats autistic people merely as "objects of inspection," dismissing unique expertise that autistic people possess about autism [128, 129]. In the words of Becca Lory, who discusses her experiences as an autistic research participant and the priorities of autism research, autism science has disregarded "… a wealth of untapped, unarticulated information that could have been collected if we were not so keen on throwing money at genetics and zebra fish" [130]. Thus, some autistic people report feeling objectified, othered, ignored, and exploited in the context of autism research, including and perhaps especially biomedical research.

A different perspective has been expressed by other autistic people, who have detailed positive experiences with biomedical research, including participation in studies examining genetics and autism. For some autistic people, participation in research has provided a source of self-illumination for their personal histories. Amy Gravino, an autism advocate, details her participation in SPARK [44] and how this participation provided for a "new understanding and context" for her lived experiences [131]. Gravino writes that she hopes genetic findings from the study "will show that autism is less of a puzzle to be solved and more of a story to be told" and "open a discussion on how we can improve the quality of life" for autistic people, both now and in the future (2021). Autism researcher Zachary Williams discusses why he participates in autism research studies (including SPARK) and why he encourages other autistic people to participate in biomedical research as well (2022). Williams speaks generally about the benefits of genetic research and ways in which, armed with information from genetic testing, autistic people and their families are able to better understand and test for medical conditions that co-occur with autism. He also speaks of his personal experiences and ways in which participation in autism research has helped him to better understand himself and his autism [132].

Although there are autistic people and autistic researchers who identify positive experiences in and beneficial aspects of biomedical research, some within the autism community have expressed concerns regarding the *potential uses* to which neurogenetic data could be applied (e.g., eugenics). For example, efforts to determine genetic causes of autism prompt concerns related to the development of

[1] We cite and summarize here articles that detail autistic people's first-person experiences within autism research (either as research participants, autistic researchers, or both). We encourage all non-autistic persons engaged in autism research to read these articles in full.

prenatal tests that would allow for selective termination of pregnancies likely to produce an autistic child. As an illustration of the gravity that these concerns hold for the autistic community, Spectrum 10K, a research study aiming to collect genetic information from 10,000 autistic people and their biological family members, was quickly paused after its launch in 2021 [133] after autistic people and non-autistic allies delineated a variety of concerns related to the project, including the aims of the study and the ultimate uses of the genetic data collected [134]. In particular, the Boycott Spectrum 10K movement emphasized that public-facing information about the study (including study recruitment materials) substantively differed from scientific materials that were part of the funding application for the project. Public-facing materials announced that the study sought to improve well-being and quality of life for autistic people, which rank high among research priorities within the autism community [118, 135, 136]. However, the scientific materials for the study did not reference well-being or quality of life; rather, the study's stated aims were to identify the genetic causes of autism. This incident illustrates the gulf that exists between (largely non-autistic) biomedical researchers, especially those involved in neurogenetic work, and the autism community. As autism researcher Sue Fletcher-Watson has pointed out, the backlash against Spectrum 10K was not unforeseeable and could have been prevented by "more groundwork to engage with the community … and to design a study that would serve the community's needs" [133].

Considerations for neurogenetic researchers. Closing the gap between non-autistic researchers of autism and members of the autism community will require researchers to educate themselves regarding the needs, feelings, and priorities of autistic individuals and autistic communities. Researchers conducting neurogenetic work should consider how they interpret and communicate about their findings and the underlying biases that may undergird their choices.

Biomedical research, with its emphasis on symptoms, treatment, and prevention, typically frames autistic differences as indicative of "deficits" or "dysfunctions"; indeed, even superior task performance by autistic versus neurotypical persons may be framed as reflective of autistic deficits [137]. As an example, the observed behaviors of autistic people have frequently been interpreted as demonstrating that autistic people are not socially motivated or that they lack empathy [138, 139], and neuroimaging studies have claimed to have identified neural underpinnings of these putative deficits [140, 141]. Yet critical challenges have been presented to research making such claims [142–146]. Importantly, given the societal importance of human connection, (mis)characterizations of autistic people as aloof and unempathetic contribute to excess social stressors [147] and harm autistic people's mental health [148]. Brain-based and genetic research, in particular, can act as a powerful legitimizing force, providing "evidence" for stereotypes about autistic people. As such, non-autistic geneticists and neuroimaging investigators, at all stages of their research—study design, data collection, data analysis, data interpretation, and dissemination of results—have a responsibility to ensure that their research does not perpetuate harms or create a basis that society uses for marginalizing autistic people.

Fulfilling this responsibility will take work. It will mean shifts in how researchers ask scientific questions, design their studies, and carry out and interpret their research. Neurodiversity approaches offer alternatives to the medical model of autism that can help to guide these shifts (see [149], particularly Table 5.2). Neurodiversity approaches recognize that autistic people demonstrate strengths while also facing challenges and that challenges are not simply internally located within the autistic person but rather reflect transactions within an environment that has been optimized for neurotypical people. In particular, senior non-autistic investigators should regularly challenge their own assumptions and biases about autistic people and how they are interpreting differences between autistic and neurotypical people in their own datasets, and encourage and support non-autistic students and trainees to do the same.

The autism community provides resources for researchers, including toolkits developed by the Academic Autistic Spectrum Partnership in Research and Education (https://aaspire.org/). Publications centering autistic perspectives provide guidelines for non-autistic autism researchers [150], including guidelines for identifying and avoiding ableist language [151] and for conducting community-based participatory research and implementing inclusive research practices [150, 152]. Neurogenetic researchers can also learn from and model research studies that have advanced autism knowledge by successfully implementing community-based participatory research approaches [153, 154].

Above all, the inclusion of autistic researchers in neurogenetic research is key. This means that non-autistic principal investigators (and their institutions and funders) must create an environment that allows for the recruitment and retention of autistic researchers. Autistic people need to be meaningfully included, and the team should routinely examine whether this inclusion is indeed meaningful or instead reflects tokenism. This likely means engaging with ideas and perspectives that non-autistic investigators may find challenging, particularly when they call into question standard practices, theories, and ways of conducting research. However, these practices, if implemented consistently and critically, could bring about a paradigm shift in neurogenetics research in autism and transform how autistic people—who have the most to gain (and lose)—are involved in and are impacted by this research.

References

1. Lord C, Brugha TS, Charman T, Cusack J, Dumas G, Frazier T, Jones EJH, Jones RM, Pickles A, State MW, Taylor JL, Veenstra-VanderWeele J. Autism spectrum disorder. Nat Rev Dis Prim. 2020;6(1):5. https://doi.org/10.1038/s41572-019-0138-4.
2. Maenner MJ, Shaw KA, Baio J, Washington A, Patrick M, DiRienzo M, Christensen DL, Wiggins LD, Pettygrove S, Andrews JG, Lopez M, Hudson A, Baroud T, Schwenk Y, White T, Rosenberg CR, Lee LC, Harrington RA, Huston M, Dietz PM. Prevalence of autism spectrum disorder among children aged 8 years—autism and developmental disabilities monitoring network, 11 Sites, United States, 2016. MMWR Surveill Summ. 2020;69(4):1–12. https://doi.org/10.15585/MMWR.SS6904A1.
3. Atherton G, Edisbury E, Piovesan A, Cross L. Autism through the ages: a mixed methods approach to understanding how age and age of diagnosis affect quality of life. J Autism Dev Disord. 2022;52(8):3639–54. https://doi.org/10.1007/s10803-021-05235-x.

4. Huang Y, Arnold SRC, Foley K-R, Lawson LP, Richdale AL, Trollor JN. Factors associated with age at autism diagnosis in a community sample of Australian adults. Autism Res. 2021;14(12):2677–87. https://doi.org/10.1002/aur.2610.
5. Kavanaugh BC, Schremp CA, Jones RN, Best CR, Sheinkopf SJ, Morrow EM. Moderators of age of diagnosis in >20,000 females with autism in two large US studies. J Autism Dev Disord. 2021;53:864–9. https://doi.org/10.1007/s10803-021-05026-4.
6. Loomes R, Hull L, Mandy WPL. What is the male-to-female ratio in autism spectrum disorder? A systematic review and meta-analysis. J Am Acad Child Adolesc Psychiatry. 2017;56(6):466–74. https://doi.org/10.1016/j.jaac.2017.03.013.
7. D'Mello AM, Frosch IR, Li CE, Cardinaux AL, Gabrieli JDE. Exclusion of females in autism research: empirical evidence for a "leaky" recruitment-to-research pipeline. Autism Res. 2022;15(10):1929–40. https://doi.org/10.1002/aur.2795.
8. Corbett BA, Muscatello RA, Klemencic ME, West M, Kim A, Strang JF. Greater gender diversity among autistic children by self-report and parent-report. Autism Int J Res Pract. 2022;27:158–72. https://doi.org/10.1177/13623613221085337.
9. Strang JF, Janssen A, Tishelman A, Leibowitz SF, Kenworthy L, McGuire JK, Edwards-Leeper L, Mazefsky CA, Rofey D, Bascom J, Caplan R, Gomez-Lobo V, Berg D, Zaks Z, Wallace GL, Wimms H, Pine-Twaddell E, Shumer D, Register-Brown K, Anthony LG. Revisiting the link: evidence of the rates of autism in studies of gender diverse individuals. J Am Acad Child Adolesc Psychiatry. 2018;57(11):885–7. https://doi.org/10.1016/j.jaac.2018.04.023.
10. Strang JF, Kenworthy L, Dominska A, Sokoloff J, Kenealy LE, Berl M, Walsh K, Menvielle E, Slesaransky-Poe G, Kim K-E, Luong-Tran C, Meagher H, Wallace GL. Increased gender variance in autism spectrum disorders and attention deficit hyperactivity disorder. Arch Sex Behav. 2014;43(8):1525–33. https://doi.org/10.1007/s10508-014-0285-3.
11. Warrier V, Greenberg DM, Weir E, Buckingham C, Smith P, Lai M-C, Allison C, Baron-Cohen S. Elevated rates of autism, other neurodevelopmental and psychiatric diagnoses, and autistic traits in transgender and gender-diverse individuals. Nat Commun. 2020;11(1):3959. https://doi.org/10.1038/s41467-020-17,794-1.
12. Strang JF, van der Miesen AI, Caplan R, Hughes C, daVanport S, Lai M-C. Both sex- and gender-related factors should be considered in autism research and clinical practice. Autism. 2020;24(3):539–43. https://doi.org/10.1177/1362361320913192.
13. Aznar A, Tenenbaum HR. Gender and age differences in parent-child emotion talk. Br J Dev Psychol. 2015;33(1):148–55. https://doi.org/10.1111/bjdp.12069.
14. Jones M. Deafness as culture: a psychosocial perspective. Disabil Stud Q. 2002;22(2):2. https://doi.org/10.18061/dsq.v22i2.344.
15. Richardson KJ. Deaf culture: competencies and best practices. Nurse Pract. 2014;39(5):20. https://doi.org/10.1097/01.NPR.0000445956.21045.c4.
16. Thapar A, Rutter M. Genetic advances in autism. J Autism Dev Disord. 2021;51(12):4321–32. https://doi.org/10.1007/s10803-020-04685-z.
17. Qiu S, Qiu Y, Li Y, Cong X. Genetics of autism spectrum disorder: an umbrella review of systematic reviews and meta-analyses. Transl Psychiatry. 2022;12(1):249. https://doi.org/10.1038/s41398-022-02009-6.
18. Berg JM, Geschwind DH. Autism genetics: searching for specificity and convergence. Genome Biol. 2012;13(7):247. https://doi.org/10.1186/gb4034.
19. Patriquin MA, DeRamus T, Libero LE, Laird A, Kana RK. Neuroanatomical and neurofunctional markers of social cognition in autism spectrum disorder. Hum Brain Mapp. 2016;37(11):3957–78. https://doi.org/10.1002/hbm.23288.
20. Peng H, Beckmann C, Smith S, Vedaldi. Deep net region-aligned prediction (RAP) localises life factors affecting brain aging in UK Biobank. In: 26th Annual meeting of the organization for human brain mapping. 2020a.
21. Yang X, Si T, Gong Q, Qiu L, Jia Z, Zhou M, Zhao Y, Hu X, Wu M, Zhu H. Brain gray matter alterations and associated demographic profiles in adults with autism spectrum disorder: a meta-analysis of voxel-based morphometry studies. Aust N Z J Psychiatry. 2016;50(8):741–53. https://doi.org/10.1177/0004867415623858.

22. van Rooij D, Anagnostou E, Arango C, Auzias G, Behrmann M, Busatto GF, Calderoni S, Daly E, Deruelle C, Di Martino A, Dinstein I, Duran FLS, Durston S, Ecker C, Fair D, Fedor J, Fitzgerald J, Freitag CM, Gallagher L, Buitelaar JK. Cortical and subcortical brain morphometry differences between patients with autism spectrum disorder and healthy individuals across the lifespan: results from the ENIGMA ASD working group. Am J Psychiatry. 2018;175(4):359–69. https://doi.org/10.1176/appi.ajp.2017.17010100.
23. Peng Z, Chen J, Jin L, Han H, Dong C, Guo Y, Kong X, Wan G, Wei Z. Social brain dysfunctionality in individuals with autism spectrum disorder and their first-degree relatives: an activation likelihood estimation meta-analysis. Psychiatry Res Neuroimaging. 2020b;298:111063. https://doi.org/10.1016/j.pscychresns.2020.111063.
24. Liu J, Yao L, Zhang W, Xiao Y, Liu L, Gao X, Shah C, Li S, Tao B, Gong Q, Lui S. Gray matter abnormalities in pediatric autism spectrum disorder: a meta-analysis with signed differential mapping. Eur Child Adolesc Psychiatry. 2017;26:933–45. https://doi.org/10.1007/s00787-017-0964-4.
25. Rane P, Cochran D, Hodge SM, Haselgrove C, Kennedy DN, Frazier JA. Connectivity in autism: a review of MRI connectivity studies. Harv Rev Psychiatry. 2015;23(4):223–44. https://doi.org/10.1097/HRP.0000000000000072.
26. D'Mello AM, Crocetti D, Mostofsky SH, Stoodley CJ. Cerebellar gray matter and lobular volumes correlate with core autism symptoms. NeuroImage Clin. 2015;7:631–9. https://doi.org/10.1016/j.nicl.2015.02.007.
27. Pagnozzi AM, Conti E, Calderoni S, Fripp J, Rose SE. A systematic review of structural MRI biomarkers in autism spectrum disorder: a machine learning perspective. Int J Dev Neurosci. 2018;71:68–82. https://doi.org/10.1016/j.ijdevneu.2018.08.010.
28. Di X, Azeez A, Li X, Haque E, Biswal BB. Disrupted focal white matter integrity in autism spectrum disorder: a voxel-based meta-analysis of diffusion tensor imaging studies. Progr Neuro-Psychopharmacol Biol Psychiatry. 2018;82:242–8. https://doi.org/10.1016/j.pnpbp.2017.11.007.
29. Lefebvre A, Beggiato A, Bourgeron T, Toro R. Neuroanatomical diversity of corpus callosum and brain volume in autism: meta-analysis, analysis of the autism brain imaging data exchange project, and simulation. Biol Psychiatry. 2015;78(2):126–34. https://doi.org/10.1016/j.biopsych.2015.02.010.
30. Lange N, Travers BG, Bigler ED, Prigge MBD, Froehlich AL, Nielsen JA, Cariello AN, Zielinski BA, Anderson JS, Fletcher PT, Alexander AA, Lainhart JE. Longitudinal volumetric brain changes in autism spectrum disorder ages 6–35 years. Autism Res. 2015;8(1):82–93. https://doi.org/10.1002/aur.1427.
31. Shen MD. Cerebrospinal fluid and the early brain development of autism. J Neurodev Disord. 2018;10(1):39. https://doi.org/10.1186/s11689-018-9256-7.
32. Turner AH, Greenspan KS, van Erp TGM. Pallidum and lateral ventricle volume enlargement in autism spectrum disorder. Psychiatry Res Neuroimaging. 2016;252:40–5. https://doi.org/10.1016/j.pscychresns.2016.04.003.
33. McPartland JC, Lerner MD, Bhat A, Clarkson T, Jack A, Koohsari S, Matuskey D, McQuaid GA, Su W-C, Trevisan DA. Looking back at the next 40 years of ASD neuroscience research. J Autism Dev Disord. 2021;51(12):4333–53. https://doi.org/10.1007/s10803-021-05095-5.
34. Fetit R, Hillary RF, Price DJ, Lawrie SM. The neuropathology of autism: a systematic review of post-mortem studies of autism and related disorders. Neurosci Biobehav Rev. 2021;129:35–62. https://doi.org/10.1016/j.neubiorev.2021.07.014.
35. Ellegood J, Anagnostou E, Babineau BA, Crawley JN, Lin L, Genestine M, DiCicco-Bloom E, Lai JKY, Foster JA, Peñagarikano O, Geschwind DH, Pacey LK, Hampson DR, Laliberté CL, Mills AA, Tam E, Osborne LR, Kouser M, Espinosa-Becerra F, Lerch JP. Clustering autism: using neuroanatomical differences in 26 mouse models to gain insight into the heterogeneity. Mol Psychiatry. 2015;20(1):118–25. https://doi.org/10.1038/mp.2014.98.
36. Di Martino A, Yan C-G, Li Q, Denio E, Castellanos FX, Alaerts K, Anderson JS, Assaf M, Bookheimer SY, Dapretto M, Deen B, Delmonte S, Dinstein I, Ertl-Wagner B, Fair DA, Gallagher L, Kennedy DP, Keown CL, Keysers C, Milham MP. The autism brain imaging

data exchange: towards a large-scale evaluation of the intrinsic brain architecture in autism. Mol Psychiatry. 2014;19(6):659–67. https://doi.org/10.1038/mp.2013.78.
37. Hull JV, Jacokes ZJ, Torgerson CM, Irimia A, Van Horn JD, Aylward E, Bernier R, Bookheimer SY, Dapretto M, Gaab N, Geschwind D, Jack A, Nelson C, Pelphrey KA, State M, Ventola P, Webb SJ. Resting-state functional connectivity in autism spectrum disorders: a review. Front Psychiatry. 2017;7:205. https://doi.org/10.3389/fpsyt.2016.00205.
38. Picci G, Gotts SJ, Scherf KS. A theoretical rut: revisiting and critically evaluating the generalized under/over-connectivity hypothesis of autism. Dev Sci. 2016;19(4):524–49. https://doi.org/10.1111/desc.12467.
39. Bigos KL, Weinberger DR. Imaging genetics—days of future past. NeuroImage. 2010;53(3):804–9. https://doi.org/10.1016/j.neuroimage.2010.01.035.
40. Di Martino A, O'Connor D, Chen B, Alaerts K, Anderson JS, Assaf M, Balsters JH, Baxter L, Beggiato A, Bernaerts S, Blanken LME, Bookheimer SY, Braden BB, Byrge L, Castellanos FX, Dapretto M, Delorme R, Fair DA, Fishman I, Milham MP. Enhancing studies of the connectome in autism using the autism brain imaging data exchange II. Sci Data. 2017;4:170010. https://doi.org/10.1038/sdata.2017.10.
41. Jack A, Sullivan CAW, Aylward E, Bookheimer SY, Dapretto M, Gaab N, Van Horn JD, Eilbott JA, Jacokes ZJ, Torgerson CM, Bernier RA, Geschwind DH, McPartland JC, Nelson CA, Webb SJ, Pelphrey KA, Gupta AR, ACE GENDAAR Consortium. A neurogenetic analysis of female autism. Brain. 2021;144(6):1911–26. https://doi.org/10.1093/brain/awab064.
42. Charman T, Loth E, Tillmann J, Crawley D, Wooldridge C, Goyard D, Ahmad J, Auyeung B, Ambrosino S, Banaschewski T, Baron-Cohen S, Baumeister S, Beckmann C, Bölte S, Bourgeron T, Bours C, Brammer M, Brandeis D, Brogna C, Buitelaar JK. The EU-AIMS Longitudinal European Autism Project (LEAP): clinical characterisation. Mol Autism. 2017;8:27. https://doi.org/10.1186/s13229-017-0145-9.
43. Loth E, Charman T, Mason L, Tillmann J, Jones EJH, Wooldridge C, Ahmad J, Auyeung B, Brogna C, Ambrosino S, Banaschewski T, Baron-Cohen S, Baumeister S, Beckmann C, Brammer M, Brandeis D, Bölte S, Bourgeron T, Bours C, Buitelaar JK. The EU-AIMS Longitudinal European Autism Project (LEAP): design and methodologies to identify and validate stratification biomarkers for autism spectrum disorders. Mol Autism. 2017;8:24. https://doi.org/10.1186/s13229-017-0146-8.
44. SPARK Consortium. SPARK: a US cohort of 50,000 families to accelerate autism research. Neuron. 2018;97(3):488–93. https://doi.org/10.1016/j.neuron.2018.01.015.
45. Mo K, Sadoway T, Bonato S, Ameis SH, Anagnostou E, Lerch JP, Taylor MJ, Lai M C. Sex/gender differences in the human autistic brains: a systematic review of 20 years of neuroimaging research. NeuroImage Clin. 2021;32:102811. https://doi.org/10.1016/j.nicl.2021.102811.
46. Robinson EB, Lichtenstein P, Anckarsäter H, Happé F, Ronald A. Examining and interpreting the female protective effect against autistic behavior. Proc Natl Acad Sci U S A. 2013;110(13):5258–62. https://doi.org/10.1073/pnas.1211070110.
47. Werling DM, Geschwind DH. Sex differences in autism spectrum disorders. Curr Opin Neurol. 2013;26(2):146–53. https://doi.org/10.1097/WCO.0b013e32835ee548.
48. Gilman SR, Iossifov I, Levy D, Ronemus M, Wigler M, Vitkup D. Rare de novo variants associated with autism implicate a large functional network of genes involved in formation and function of synapses. Neuron. 2011;70(5):898–907. https://doi.org/10.1016/j.neuron.2011.05.021.
49. Jacquemont S, Coe BP, Hersch M, Duyzend MH, Krumm N, Bergmann S, Beckmann JS, Rosenfeld JA, Eichler EE. A higher mutational burden in females supports a "female protective model" in neurodevelopmental disorders. Am J Hum Genet. 2014;94(3):415–25. https://doi.org/10.1016/j.ajhg.2014.02.001.
50. Levy D, Ronemus M, Yamrom B, Lee Y, Leotta A, Kendall J, Marks S, Lakshmi B, Pai D, Ye K, Buja A, Krieger A, Yoon S, Troge J, Rodgers L, Iossifov I, Wigler M. Rare de novo and transmitted copy-number variation in autistic spectrum disorders. Neuron. 2011;70(5):886–97. https://doi.org/10.1016/j.neuron.2011.05.015.

51. Floris DL, Peng H, Warrier V, Lombardo MV, Pretzsch CM, Moreau C, Tsompanidis A, Gong W, Mennes M, Llera A, van Rooij D, Oldehinkel M, Forde NJ, Charman T, Tillmann J, Banaschewski T, Moessnang C, Durston S, Holt RJ, EU-AIMS LEAP Group. The link between autism and sex-related neuroanatomy, and associated cognition and gene expression. Am J Psychiatry. 2022;180:50–64. https://doi.org/10.1176/appi.ajp.20220194.
52. Saito Y, Suga M, Tochigi M, Abe O, Yahata N, Kawakubo Y, Liu X, Kawamura Y, Sasaki T, Kasai K, Yamasue H. Neural correlate of autistic-like traits and a common allele in the oxytocin receptor gene. Soc Cogn Affect Neurosci. 2014;9(10):1443–50. https://doi.org/10.1093/scan/nst136.
53. Hernandez LM, Lawrence KE, Padgaonkar NT, Inada M, Hoekstra JN, Lowe JK, Eilbott J, Jack A, Aylward E, Gaab N, Van Horn JD, Bernier RA, McPartland JC, Webb SJ, Pelphrey KA, Green SA, Geschwind DH, Bookheimer SY, Dapretto M. Imaging-genetics of sex differences in ASD: distinct effects of OXTR variants on brain connectivity. Transl Psychiatry. 2020;10(1):1. https://doi.org/10.1038/s41398-020-0750-9.
54. Sha Z, Schijven D, Francks C. Patterns of brain asymmetry associated with polygenic risks for autism and schizophrenia implicate language and executive functions but not brain masculinization. Mol Psychiatry. 2021;26(12):12. https://doi.org/10.1038/s41380-021-01204-z.
55. Lawrence KE, Hernandez LM, Fuster E, Padgaonkar NT, Patterson G, Jung J, Okada NJ, Lowe JK, Hoekstra JN, Jack A, Aylward E, Gaab N, Van Horn JD, Bernier RA, McPartland JC, Webb SJ, Pelphrey KA, Green SA, Bookheimer SY, GENDAAR Consortium. Impact of autism genetic risk on brain connectivity: a mechanism for the female protective effect. Brain. 2022;145(1):378–87. https://doi.org/10.1093/brain/awab204.
56. Gui Y, Zhou X, Wang Z, Zhang Y, Wang Z, Zhou G, Zhao Y, Liu M, Lu H, Zhao H. Sex-specific genetic association between psychiatric disorders and cognition, behavior and brain imaging in children and adults. Transl Psychiatry. 2022;12(1):347. https://doi.org/10.1038/s41398-022-02041-6.
57. Plummer JT, Evgrafov OV, Bergman MY, Friez M, Haiman CA, Levitt P, Aldinger KA. Transcriptional regulation of the MET receptor tyrosine kinase gene by MeCP2 and sex-specific expression in autism and Rett syndrome. Transl Psychiatry. 2013;3(10):e316. https://doi.org/10.1038/tp.2013.91.
58. Khan A, Harney JW, Zavacki AM, Sajdel-Sulkowska EM. Disrupted brain thyroid hormone homeostasis and altered thyroid hormone-dependent brain gene expression in autism spectrum disorders. J Physiol Pharmacol. 2014;65(2):257–72.
59. Werling DM, Parikshak NN, Geschwind DH. Gene expression in human brain implicates sexually dimorphic pathways in autism spectrum disorders. Nat Commun. 2016;7(10):717. https://doi.org/10.1038/ncomms10717.
60. Schumann CM, Sharp FR, Ander BP, Stamova B. Possible sexually dimorphic role of miRNA and other sncRNA in ASD brain. Mol Autism. 2017;8:4. https://doi.org/10.1186/s13229-017-0117-0.
61. Lee SC, Quinn TP, Lai J, Kong SW, Hertz-Picciotto I, Glatt SJ, Crowley TM, Venkatesh S, Nguyen T. Solving for X: evidence for sex-specific autism biomarkers across multiple transcriptomic studies. Am J Med Genet Part B Neuropsychiatr Genet. 2019;180(6):377–89. https://doi.org/10.1002/ajmg.b.32701.
62. Frehner SS, Dooley KT, Palumbo MC, Smith AL, Goodman MM, Bales KL, Freeman SM. Effect of sex and autism spectrum disorder on oxytocin receptor binding and mRNA expression in the dopaminergic pars compacta of the human substantia nigra. Philos Trans R Soc Lond Ser B Biol Sci. 2022;377(1858):20210118. https://doi.org/10.1098/rstb.2021.0118.
63. Chen Y, Dai J, Tang L, Mikhailova T, Liang Q, Li M, Zhou J, Kopp RF, Weickert C, Chen C, Liu C. Neuroimmune transcriptome changes in patient brains of psychiatric and neurological disorders. Mol Psychiatry. 2022;28:710–21. https://doi.org/10.1038/s41380-022-01854-7.
64. Bredewold R, Veenema AH. Sex differences in the regulation of social and anxiety-related behaviors: insights from vasopressin and oxytocin brain systems. Curr Opin Neurobiol. 2018;49:132–40. https://doi.org/10.1016/j.conb.2018.02.011.

65. Dumais KM, Veenema AH. Vasopressin and oxytocin receptor systems in the brain: sex differences and sex-specific regulation of social behavior. Front Neuroendocrinol. 2016;40:1–23. https://doi.org/10.1016/j.yfrne.2015.04.003.
66. Feldman R. The neurobiology of human attachments. Trends Cogn Sci. 2017;21(2):80–99. https://doi.org/10.1016/j.tics.2016.11.007.
67. Froemke RC, Young LJ. Oxytocin, neural plasticity, and social behavior. Annu Rev Neurosci. 2021;44:359–81. https://doi.org/10.1146/annurev-neuro-102320-102847.
68. Gordon I, Martin C, Feldman R, Leckman JF. Oxytocin and social motivation. Dev Cogn Neurosci. 2011;1(4):471–93. https://doi.org/10.1016/j.dcn.2011.07.007.
69. Gordon I, Jack A, Pretzsch CMCM, Vander Wyk BC, Leckman JFJF, Feldman R, Pelphrey KA. Intranasal oxytocin enhances connectivity in the neural circuitry supporting social motivation and social perception in children with autism. Sci Rep. 2016;6:35054. https://doi.org/10.1038/srep35054.
70. Berke JD. What does dopamine mean? Nat Neurosci. 2018;21(6):787–93. https://doi.org/10.1038/s41593-018-0152-y.
71. Love TM. Oxytocin, motivation and the role of dopamine. Pharmacol Biochem Behav. 2014;119:49–60. https://doi.org/10.1016/j.pbb.2013.06.011.
72. Wise RA. Dopamine, learning and motivation. Nat Rev Neurosci. 2004;5(6):6. https://doi.org/10.1038/nrn1406.
73. Carter CS. Sex differences in oxytocin and vasopressin: implications for autism spectrum disorders? Behav Brain Res. 2007;176(1):170–86. https://doi.org/10.1016/j.bbr.2006.08.025.
74. Kohlhoff J, Cibralic S, Hawes DJ, Eapen V. Oxytocin receptor gene (*OXTR*) polymorphisms and social, emotional and behavioral functioning in children and adolescents: a systematic narrative review. Neurosci Biobehav Rev. 2022;135:104573. https://doi.org/10.1016/j.neubiorev.2022.104573.
75. Wakabayashi A, Baron-Cohen S, Wheelwright S, Tojo Y. The Autism-Spectrum Quotient (AQ) in Japan: a cross-cultural comparison. J Autism Dev Disord. 2006;36(2):263–70. https://doi.org/10.1007/s10803-005-0061-2.
76. Baron-Cohen S, Wheelwright S, Skinner R, Martin J, Clubley E. The Autism-Spectrum Quotient (AQ): evidence from Asperger syndrome/high-functioning autism, males and females, scientists and mathematicians. J Autism Dev Disord. 2001;31(1):5–17. https://doi.org/10.1023/A:1005653411471.
77. Brüne M. Does the oxytocin receptor polymorphism (rs2254298) confer "vulnerability" for psychopathology or "differential susceptibility"? Insights from evolution. BMC Med. 2012;10(1):38. https://doi.org/10.1186/1741-7015-10-38.
78. Liu X, Kawamura Y, Shimada T, Otowa T, Koishi S, Sugiyama T, Nishida H, Hashimoto O, Nakagami R, Tochigi M, Umekage T, Kano Y, Miyagawa T, Kato N, Tokunaga K, Sasaki T. Association of the oxytocin receptor (OXTR) gene polymorphisms with autism spectrum disorder (ASD) in the Japanese population. J Hum Genet. 2010;55(3):137–41. https://doi.org/10.1038/jhg.2009.140.
79. Wu S, Jia M, Ruan Y, Liu J, Guo Y, Shuang M, Gong X, Zhang Y, Yang X, Zhang D. Positive association of the oxytocin receptor gene (OXTR) with autism in the Chinese Han population. Biol Psychiatry. 2005;58(1):74–7. https://doi.org/10.1016/j.biopsych.2005.03.013.
80. Hernandez LM, Krasileva K, Green SA, Sherman LE, Ponting C, McCarron R, Lowe JK, Geschwind DH, Bookheimer SY, Dapretto M. Additive effects of oxytocin receptor gene polymorphisms on reward circuitry in youth with autism. Mol Psychiatry. 2017;22(8):1134–9. https://doi.org/10.1038/mp.2016.209.
81. Pickel VM, Joh TH, Field PM, Becker CG, Reis DJ. Cellular localization of tyrosine hydroxylase by immunohistochemistry. J Histochem Cytochem. 1975;23(1):1–12. https://doi.org/10.1177/23.1.234988.
82. Freeman SM, Palumbo MC, Lawrence RH, Smith AL, Goodman MM, Bales KL. Effect of age and autism spectrum disorder on oxytocin receptor density in the human basal forebrain and midbrain. Transl Psychiatry. 2018;8(1):257. https://doi.org/10.1038/s41398-018-0315-3.

83. Plomin R, Simpson MA. The future of genomics for developmentalists. Dev Psychopathol. 2013;25(4 pt 2):1263–78. https://doi.org/10.1017/S0954579413000606.
84. Ecker C, Pretzsch CM, Bletsch A, Mann C, Schaefer T, Ambrosino S, Tillmann J, Yousaf A, Chiocchetti A, Lombardo MV, Warrier V, Bast N, Moessnang C, Baumeister S, Dell'Acqua F, Floris DL, Zabihi M, Marquand A, Cliquet F, Murphy DGM. Interindividual differences in cortical thickness and their genomic underpinnings in autism spectrum disorder. Am J Psychiatry. 2022;179(3):242–54. https://doi.org/10.1176/appi.ajp.2021.20050630.
85. Lin GN, Corominas R, Lemmens I, Yang X, Tavernier J, Hill DE, Vidal M, Sebat J, Iakoucheva LM. Spatiotemporal 16p11.2 protein network implicates cortical late mid-fetal brain development and KCTD13-Cul3-RhoA pathway in psychiatric diseases. Neuron. 2015;85(4):742–54. https://doi.org/10.1016/j.neuron.2015.01.010.
86. Lombardo MV, Eyler L, Pramparo T, Gazestani VH, Hagler DJ, Chen C-H, Dale AM, Seidlitz J, Bethlehem RAI, Bertelsen N, Barnes CC, Lopez L, Campbell K, Lewis NE, Pierce K, Courchesne E. Atypical genomic cortical patterning in autism with poor early language outcome. Sci Adv. 2021;7(36):eabh1663. https://doi.org/10.1126/sciadv.abh1663.
87. Pretzsch CM, Schäfer T, Lombardo MV, Warrier V, Mann C, Bletsch A, Chatham CH, Floris DL, Tillmann J, Yousaf A, Jones E, Charman T, Ambrosino S, Bourgeron T, Dumas G, Loth E, Oakley B, Buitelaar JK, Cliquet F, Ecker C. Neurobiological correlates of change in adaptive behavior in autism. Am J Psychiatry. 2022;179(5):336–49. https://doi.org/10.1176/appi.ajp.21070711.
88. Willsey AJ, Sanders SJ, Li M, Dong S, Tebbenkamp AT, Muhle RA, Reilly SK, Lin L, Fertuzinhos S, Miller JA, Murtha MT, Bichsel C, Niu W, Cotney J, Ercan-Sencicek AG, Gockley J, Gupta AR, Han W, He X, State MW. Coexpression networks implicate human midfetal deep cortical projection neurons in the pathogenesis of autism. Cell. 2013;155(5):997–1007. https://doi.org/10.1016/j.cell.2013.10.020.
89. Kaiser MD, Hudac CM, Shultz S, Lee SM, Cheung C, Berken AM, Deen B, Pitskel NB, Sugrue DR, Voos AC, Saulnier CA, Ventola P, Wolf JM, Klin A, Vander Wyk BC, Pelphrey KA. Neural signatures of autism. Proc Natl Acad Sci U S A. 2010;107(49):21223–8. https://doi.org/10.1073/pnas.1010412107.
90. Klin A, Lin DJ, Gorrindo P, Ramsay G, Jones W. Two-year-olds with autism orient to non-social contingencies rather than biological motion. Nature. 2009;459(7244):257–61. https://doi.org/10.1038/nature07868.
91. Kang HJ, Kawasawa YI, Cheng F, Zhu Y, Xu X, Li M, Sousa AMM, Pletikos M, Meyer KA, Sedmak G, Guennel T, Shin Y, Johnson MB, Krsnik Ž, Mayer S, Fertuzinhos S, Umlauf S, Lisgo SN, Vortmeyer A, Šestan N. Spatio-temporal transcriptome of the human brain. Nature. 2011;478(7370):483–9. https://doi.org/10.1038/nature10523.
92. Fischbach GD, Lord C. The Simons Simplex Collection: a resource for identification of autism genetic risk factors. Neuron. 2010;68(2):192–5. https://doi.org/10.1016/J.NEURON.2010.10.006.
93. Sanders SJ, He X, Willsey AJ, Ercan-Sencicek AG, Samocha KE, Cicek AE, Murtha MT, Bal VH, Bishop SL, Dong S, Goldberg AP, Jinlu C, Keaney JF, Klei L, Mandell JD, Moreno-De-Luca D, Poultney CS, Robinson EB, Smith L, State MW. Insights into autism spectrum disorder genomic architecture and biology from 71 risk loci. Neuron. 2015;87(6):1215–33. https://doi.org/10.1016/j.neuron.2015.09.016.
94. Askham AV. Brain activity patterns may distinguish girls with autism. Spectrum | Autism Research News. 2021. https://www.spectrumnews.org/news/brain-activity-patterns-may-distinguish-girls-with-autism/.
95. Baron-Cohen S. The extreme male brain theory of autism. Trends Cogn Sci. 2002;6(6):248–54. https://doi.org/10.1016/s1364-6613(02)01904-6.
96. Baron-Cohen S, Lombardo MV, Auyeung B, Ashwin E, Chakrabarti B, Knickmeyer R. Why are autism spectrum conditions more prevalent in males? PLoS Biol. 2011;9(6):e1001081. https://doi.org/10.1371/journal.pbio.1001081.
97. Yarkoni T, Poldrack RA, Nichols TE, Van Essen DC, Wager TD. Large-scale automated synthesis of human functional neuroimaging data. Nat Methods. 2011;8(8):665–70. https://doi.org/10.1038/nmeth.1635.

98. Gorgolewski KJ, Varoquaux G, Rivera G, Schwarz Y, Ghosh SS, Maumet C, Sochat VV, Nichols TE, Poldrack RA, Poline J-B, Yarkoni T, Margulies DS. NeuroVault.org: a web-based repository for collecting and sharing unthresholded statistical maps of the human brain. Front Neuroinform. 2015;9:8. https://doi.org/10.3389/fninf.2015.00008.
99. Hawrylycz MJ, Lein ES, Guillozet-Bongaarts AL, Shen EH, Ng L, Miller JA, van de Lagemaat LN, Smith KA, Ebbert A, Riley ZL, Abajian C, Beckmann CF, Bernard A, Bertagnolli D, Boe AF, Cartagena PM, Chakravarty MM, Chapin M, Chong J, Jones AR. An anatomically comprehensive atlas of the adult human brain transcriptome. Nature. 2012;489(7416):391–9. https://doi.org/10.1038/nature11405.
100. Sunkin SM, Ng L, Lau C, Dolbeare T, Gilbert TL, Thompson CL, Hawrylycz M, Dang C. Allen Brain Atlas: an integrated spatio-temporal portal for exploring the central nervous system. Nucleic Acids Res. 2013;41(Database issue):D996–D1008. https://doi.org/10.1093/nar/gks1042.
101. Gupta S, Ellis SE, Ashar FN, Moes A, Bader JS, Zhan J, West AB, Arking DE. Transcriptome analysis reveals dysregulation of innate immune response genes and neuronal activity-dependent genes in autism. Nat Commun. 2014;5(1):1. https://doi.org/10.1038/ncomms6748.
102. Voineagu I, Wang X, Johnston P, Lowe JK, Tian Y, Horvath S, Mill J, Cantor RM, Blencowe BJ, Geschwind DH. Transcriptomic analysis of autistic brain reveals convergent molecular pathology. Nature. 2011;474(7351):380–4. https://doi.org/10.1038/nature10110.
103. Pauli WM, O'Reilly RC, Yarkoni T, Wager TD. Regional specialization within the human striatum for diverse psychological functions. Proc Natl Acad Sci U S A. 2016;113(7):1907–12. https://doi.org/10.1073/pnas.1507610113.
104. Báez-Mendoza R, Schultz W. The role of the striatum in social behavior. Front Neurosci. 2013;7:233. https://doi.org/10.3389/fnins.2013.00233.
105. Haber SN. Corticostriatal circuitry. Dialog Clin Neurosci. 2016;18(1):7–21.
106. Balsters JH, Mantini D, Wenderoth N. Connectivity-based parcellation reveals distinct cortico-striatal connectivity fingerprints in autism spectrum disorder. NeuroImage. 2018;170:412–23. https://doi.org/10.1016/j.neuroimage.2017.02.019.
107. Di Martino A, Kelly C, Grzadzinski R, Zuo XN, Mennes M, Mairena MA, Lord C, Castellanos FX, Milham MP. Aberrant striatal functional connectivity in children with autism. Biol Psychiatry. 2011;69(9):847–56. https://doi.org/10.1016/j.biopsych.2010.10.029.
108. Hughes HK, Moreno RJ, Ashwood P. Innate immune dysfunction and neuroinflammation in autism spectrum disorder (ASD). Brain Behav Immun. 2022;108:245–54. https://doi.org/10.1016/j.bbi.2022.12.001.
109. Lukens JR, Eyo UB. Microglia and neurodevelopmental disorders. Annu Rev Neurosci. 2022;45:425–45. https://doi.org/10.1146/annurev-neuro-110,920-023056.
110. McCarthy MM, Wright CL. Convergence of sex differences and the neuroimmune system in autism spectrum disorder. Biol Psychiatry. 2017;81(5):402–10. https://doi.org/10.1016/j.biopsych.2016.10.004.
111. Madeo AC, Biesecker BB, Brasington C, Erby LH, Peters KF. The relationship between the genetic counseling profession and the disability community: a commentary. Am J Med Genet Part A. 2011;155(8):1777–85. https://doi.org/10.1002/ajmg.a.34054.
112. Miller PS, Levine RL. Avoiding genetic genocide: understanding good intentions and eugenics in the complex dialogue between the medical and disability communities. Genet Med. 2013;15(2):95–102. https://doi.org/10.1038/gim.2012.102.
113. Clements T. The problem with the neurodiversity movement. Quillette; 2017. https://quillette.com/2017/10/15/problem-neurodiversity-movement/.
114. Russell G. Critiques of the neurodiversity movement. In: Kapp SK, editor. Autistic community and the neurodiversity movement: stories from the frontline. Palgrave Macmillan; 2020. https://doi.org/10.1007/978-981-13-8437-0_21.
115. den Houting J. Neurodiversity: an insider's perspective. Autism Int J Res Pract. 2019;23(2):271–3. https://doi.org/10.1177/1362361318820762.
116. Kapp SK. Autistic community and the neurodiversity movement: stories from the frontline. Palgrave Macmillan; 2020. https://doi.org/10.1007/978-981-13-8437-0_21.

117. Oliver M. Social work with disabled people. Macmillan; 1983.
118. Benevides TW, Shore SM, Palmer K, Duncan P, Plank A, Andresen M-L, Caplan R, Cook B, Gassner D, Hector BL, Morgan L, Nebeker L, Purkis Y, Rankowski B, Wittig K, Coughlin SS. Listening to the autistic voice: mental health priorities to guide research and practice in autism from a stakeholder-driven project. Autism Int J Res Pract. 2020;24(4):822–33. https://doi.org/10.1177/1362361320908410.
119. Gotham K, Marvin AR, Taylor JL, Warren Z, Anderson CM, Law PA, Law JK, Lipkin PH. Characterizing the daily life, needs, and priorities of adults with autism spectrum disorder from Interactive Autism Network data. Autism. 2015;19(7):794–804. https://doi.org/10.1177/1362361315583818.
120. Pukki H, Bettin J, Outlaw AG, Hennessy J, Brook K, Dekker M, Doherty M, Shaw SCK, Bervoets J, Rudolph S, Corneloup T, Derwent K, Lee O, Rojas YG, Lawson W, Gutierrez MV, Petek K, Tsiakkirou M, Suoninen A, Yoon W-H. Autistic perspectives on the future of clinical autism research. Autism Adulthood. 2022;4(2):93–101. https://doi.org/10.1089/aut.2022.0017.
121. Pripas-Kapit S. Historicizing Jim Sinclair's "Don't mourn for us": a cultural and intellectual history of neurodiversity's first manifesto. In: Kapp SK, editor. Autistic community and the neurodiversity movement: stories from the frontline. Palgrave Macmillan; 2020.
122. Sinclair J. Don't mourn for us. Our voice, 1 (3). Syracuse: Autism Network; 1993. http://www.autreat.com/dont_mourn.html.
123. Benjamin E, Ziss BE, George BR. Representation is never perfect, but are parents even representatives? Am J Bioethics. 2020;20(4):51–3. https://doi.org/10.1080/15265161.2020.1730505.
124. Buturovic Z. Parents of autistic children are deserving of support. Am J Bioethics. 2020;20(4):54–5. https://doi.org/10.1080/15265161.2020.1733706.
125. Chapman R, Veit W. Representing the autism spectrum. Am J Bioethics. 2020;20(4):46–8. https://doi.org/10.1080/15265161.2020.1730495.
126. McCoy MS, Liu EY, Lutz ASF, Sisti D. Ethical advocacy across the autism spectrum: beyond partial representation. Am J Bioethics. 2020;20(4):13–24. https://doi.org/10.1080/15265161.2020.1730482.
127. Michael C. Is being othered a co-occurring condition of autism? Autism Adulthood. 2021;3(2):118–9. https://doi.org/10.1089/aut.2021.0019.
128. Gillespie-Lynch K, Kapp SK, Brooks PJ, Pickens J, Schwartzman B. Whose expertise is it? Evidence for autistic adults as critical autism experts. Front Psychol. 2017;8:438. https://doi.org/10.3389/fpsyg.2017.00438.
129. Milton DEM, Bracher M. Autistics speak but are they heard? Med Sociol Online. 2013;72(2):61–0.
130. Lory B. For the love of science? Autism Adulthood. 2019;1(1):12–4. https://doi.org/10.1089/aut.2018.0005.
131. Gravino A. I now know what caused my autism, which changes everything—and nothing. CNN—Opinion. 2021. https://www.cnn.com/2021/04/21/opinions/my-autism-cause-changes-everything-and-nothing-gravino/index.html.
132. Williams ZJ. *I Am an Autistic Scientist.* A personal perspective: *I participate in research, and so should you.* Psychology Today. 2022. https://www.psychologytoday.com/us/blog/autistic-lives/202207/i-am-autistic-scientist.
133. Sanderson K. High-profile autism genetics project paused amid backlash. Nature. 2021;598(7879):17–8. https://doi.org/10.1038/d41586-021-02602-7.
134. Boycott Spectrum 10K. Plain text of the full Boycott S10K statement. 2021. https://aucademy.co.uk/2021/09/04/plain-text-of-the-full-boycott-s10k-statement/.
135. Frazier TW, Dawson G, Murray D, Shih A, Sachs JS, Geiger A. Brief report: a survey of autism research priorities across a diverse community of stakeholders. J Autism Dev Disord. 2018;48(11):3965–71. https://doi.org/10.1007/s10803-018-3642-6.
136. Roche L, Adams D, Clark M. Research priorities of the autism community: a systematic review of key stakeholder perspectives. Autism. 2021;25(2):336–48. https://doi.org/10.1177/1362361320967790.

137. Pellicano E, den Houting J. Annual Research Review: shifting from 'normal science' to neurodiversity in autism science. J Child Psychol Psychiatry. 2022;63(4):381–96. https://doi.org/10.1111/jcpp.13534.
138. Baron-Cohen S, Wheelwright S. The empathy quotient: an investigation of adults with Asperger syndrome or high functioning autism, and normal sex differences. J Autism Dev Disord. 2004;34(2):163–75. https://doi.org/10.1023/B:JADD.0000022607.19833.00.
139. Chevallier C, Kohls G, Troiani V, Brodkin ES, Schultz RT. The social motivation theory of autism. Trends Cogn Sci. 2012;16(4):231–8. https://doi.org/10.1016/j.tics.2012.02.007.
140. Delmonte S, Balsters JH, McGrath J, Fitzgerald J, Brennan S, Fagan AJ, Gallagher L. Social and monetary reward processing in autism spectrum disorders. Mol Autism. 2012;3(1):1–13. https://doi.org/10.1186/2040-2392-3-7.
141. Gu X, Eilam-Stock T, Zhou T, Anagnostou E, Kolevzon A, Soorya L, Hof PR, Friston KJ, Fan J. Autonomic and brain responses associated with empathy deficits in autism spectrum disorder. Hum Brain Mapp. 2015;36(9):3323–38. https://doi.org/10.1002/hbm.22840.
142. Fletcher-Watson S, Bird G. Autism and empathy: what are the real links? Autism. 2020;24(1):3–6. https://doi.org/10.1177/1362361319883506.
143. Jaswal VK, Akhtar N. Being versus appearing socially uninterested: challenging assumptions about social motivation in autism. Behav Brain Sci. 2019;42:e82. https://doi.org/10.1017/S0140525X18001826.
144. Kapp SK, Goldknopf E, Brooks PJ, Kofner B, Hossain M. Expanding the critique of the social motivation theory of autism with participatory and developmental research. Behav Brain Sci. 2019;42:e94. https://doi.org/10.1017/S0140525X18002479.
145. Milton DEM. On the ontological status of autism: the 'double empathy problem'. Disabil Soc. 2012;27(6):883–7. https://doi.org/10.1080/09687599.2012.710008.
146. Milton DEM, Gurbuz E, Lopez B. The 'double empathy problem': ten years on. Autism. 2022;26(8):1901–3. https://doi.org/10.1177/13623613221129123.
147. Botha M, Frost DM. Extending the minority stress model to understand mental health problems experienced by the autistic population. Soc Ment Health. 2020;10(1):20–34. https://doi.org/10.1177/2156869318804297.
148. Mitchell P, Sheppard E, Cassidy SA. Autism and the double empathy problem: implications for development and mental health. Br J Dev Psychol. 2021;39(1):1–18. https://doi.org/10.1111/bjdp.12350.
149. Dwyer P. The neurodiversity approach(es): what are they and what do they mean for researchers? Hum Dev. 2022;66(2):73–92. https://doi.org/10.1159/000523723.
150. Gowen E, Poole D, Baimbridge P, Taylor R, Bleazard T, Greenstein A. Guidelines for conducting research studies with the autism community. Autism Policy Pract. 2019;2(1):29.
151. Bottema-Beutel K, Kapp SK, Lester JN, Sasson NJ, Hand BN. Avoiding ableist language: suggestions for autism researchers. Autism Adulthood. 2020;3(1):18–29. https://doi.org/10.1089/aut.2020.0014.
152. Nicolaidis C, Raymaker D, Kapp SK, Baggs A, Ashkenazy E, McDonald K, Weiner M, Maslak J, Hunter M, Joyce A. The AASPIRE practice-based guidelines for the inclusion of autistic adults in research as co-researchers and study participants. Autism. 2019;23(8):2007–19. https://doi.org/10.1177/1362361319830523.
153. Nicolaidis C, Raymaker DM, McDonald KE, Lund EM, Leotti S, Kapp SK, Katz M, Beers LM, Kripke C, Maslak J, Hunter M, Zhen KY. Creating accessible survey instruments for use with autistic adults and people with intellectual disability: lessons learned and recommendations. Autism Adulthood. 2020;2(1):61–76. https://doi.org/10.1089/aut.2019.0074.
154. Ratto AB, Bascom J, DaVanport S, Strang JF, Anthony LG, Verbalis A, Pugliese C, Nadwodny N, Brown LXZ, Cruz M, Hector BL, Kapp SK, Giwa Onaiwu M, Raymaker DM, Robison JE, Stewart C, Stone R, Whetsell E, Pelphrey K, Kenworthy L. Centering the inner experience of autism: development of the self-assessment of autistic traits. Autism Adulthood. 2022;5(1):93–105. https://doi.org/10.1089/aut.2021.0099.

Part III

Psychiatric and Other Medical Comorbidities

6 Internalizing Disorders and Female Autism

Chiara Davico, Ilaria Secci, and Benedetto Vitiello

6.1 Introduction: Internalizing Disorders and Females' Autism

Beyond the core diagnostic symptoms, individuals with ASD have been found to exhibit a range of comorbid psychiatric symptoms that can further and severely interfere with global functioning and overall well-being [1, 2].

It is now well known that people with autism spectrum disorder (ASD) are at higher risk of mental health problems compared to the general population, with 70% of people with ASD being diagnosed with a comorbid psychiatric disorder [1, 3–5].

Internalizing disorders include problems with overcontrolled behavior such as anxiety, depression, and withdrawal. Many studies found that the prevalence of internalizing problems in individuals of all ages with ASD is higher than in non-ASD population [6–14].

Within the typically developing population, research indicates a preponderance of internalizing problem in females, with a strong sex/gender difference emerging during adolescence, probably due to puberty [15–17]. In particular, during early adolescence, sex/gender difference is minimal or nonexistent, but by late adolescence, a strong sex/gender difference in depression emerges once the majority of adolescents have undergone puberty [18, 19]. Similar to depression, anxiety disorders significantly increase in females compared to males during adolescence;

C. Davico (✉) · I. Secci · B. Vitiello
Section of Child and Adolescent Neuropsychiatry, Department of Public Health and Pediatric Sciences, University of Turin, Turin, Italy
e-mail: Chiara.davico@unito.it; ilaria.secci@unito.it; benedetto.Vitiello@unito.it

L. Mazzone et al. (eds.), *Autism Spectrum Disorder: Understanding the Female Phenotype*, https://doi.org/10.1007/978-3-031-62072-0_6

only obsessive-compulsive disorder is an exception, being more prevalent among males [20–22]. Among adults, the prevalence of internalizing disorders tends to grow between 18 and 30 years of age, remain stable between 30 and 50 years, and then decrease after age 50 [23]. Among adults in the general population, internalizing disorders are more prevalent among females, with a reported lifetime cumulative prevalence ranging from 10 to 44% among women and 5 to 26% among men [24].

Females with ASD may be especially vulnerable to internalizing disorders because of the "double hit" conferred by sex/gender and by autistic predisposition to develop these comorbidities [25, 26]. In autistic females, internalizing problems are sometimes heightened by difficulties in asking for help and communicating emotions and thoughts [27].

If we consider internalizing problems in females with autism, it is important to underline that from a methodological point of view, most studies on female autism use sex/gender as a variable to control and not as an independent aspect of ASD that needs to be investigated [9], as well defined by Thomson and Colleagues, "our current understanding of ASD is based on male-centered research" [28].

Given the importance of cognitive level on internalizing comorbidity, some studies have begun to analyze sex/gender differences in homogeneous study samples, as autism cohort with or without intellectual disability [29, 30]. Among difficulties in studying psychiatric comorbidity in female autism, it is important to consider the lower prevalence of ASD among females [31]. All those elements, in addition to a physiological change of internalizing symptoms during development, contribute to the current limitations of the available literature, which often does allow consistent conclusions to be derived. Studies comparing male and female subjects with ASD report divergent results in describing the rate of internalizing symptoms, with some studies reporting similar rates in females as in males, while others reporting a higher prevalence in females, and some others in males [32–34], less [35] or the same level of internalized problems in girls as in boys [36].

Internalizing symptoms in autistic females could also become a reason for misdiagnosis [37, 38]. Some authors point out that autistic females are more difficult to diagnose, because of milder symptom presentation, referral biases, and still more persisting social skills compared to boys [39, 40]. In females, internalizing symptoms, as depression or anxiety, could cover autistic symptoms, making it more difficult to correctly diagnose the main disorder and consequently increasing the possibility to develop secondary comorbidity (Fig. 6.1).

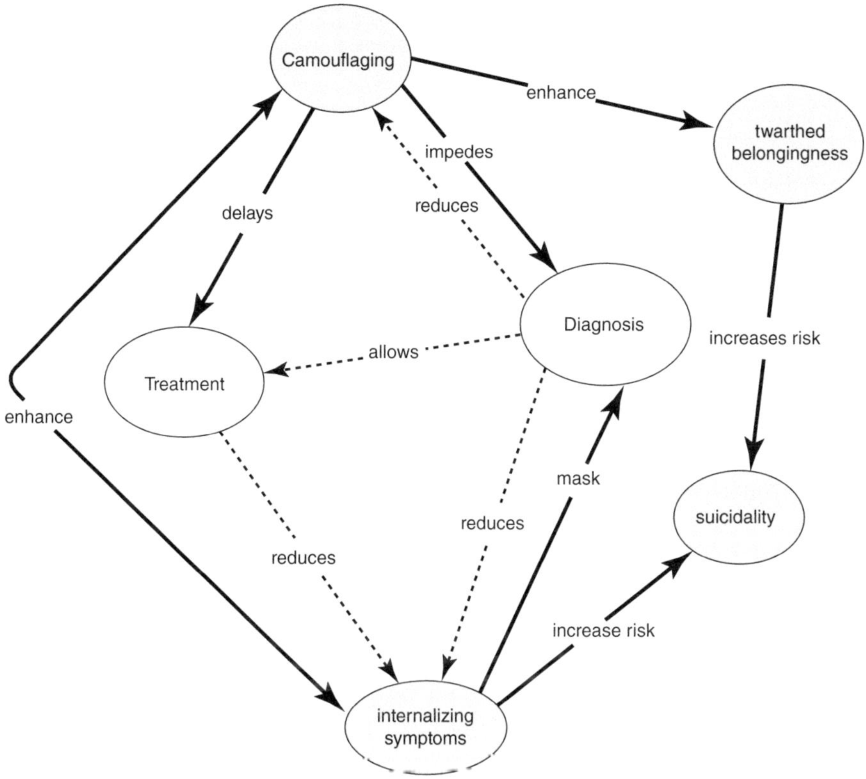

Fig. 6.1 The complex relationship between camouflaging and internalizing symptoms, a theoretical model. *Dashed line*: positive relationship between two elements; *continuous line*: negative relationship between two elements. Circle dimensions and arrows' length do not represent different impacts or links among elements represented in the figure. Camouflaging impedes the possibility of having an autism diagnosis and so delays access to treatment, increasing the feeling of thwarted belongingness, increasing the risk of developing internalizing symptoms, and ultimately increasing the risk of suicidality. A correct diagnosis allows access to the right treatment and contributes to reducing both internalizing symptoms and the need to camouflage. Internalizing symptoms increase the risk of camouflaging and of suicidality, avoiding obtaining a correct diagnosis

6.2 Internalizing Symptoms: The Role of Camouflage Effect

The use of strategies to minimize the visibility of autistic traits in social situations is known as "camouflaging." It has been shown to be associated with poorer mental health in both adults and adolescents with autism [41, 42], and there is now much evidence that camouflaging may be more prominent among autistic females than in autistic males [43, 44]. For example, considering the same level of severity at the Autism Diagnostic Interview-Revised (ADI-R) during adulthood, women tend to show their autistic symptoms less (on the Autism Diagnostic Observation Schedule-ADOS) but perceive them more than men [9], and young girls with autism tend to mimic their peers during play, staying near them during recess, and show fewer problematic behaviors while boys tend to play by themselves [27].

Camouflage effect is one of the factors possibly implied in the underdiagnosis of autistic female [33, 43, 45]: the camouflaging of autistic symptoms often seen in girls makes them appear more "typical," raising less concern in parents and teachers, who consequently less frequently refer them to clinical evaluation.

It has been suggested that camouflaging, despite a potential positive adaptive function, is correlated with higher levels of internalizing symptoms, such as depression, anxiety, and reduced feelings of acceptance, in both autistic and neurotypical adults [41, 44, 46–48], and seems to be associated with poorer mental health in both adults and adolescents with autism [41, 42]. It also seems to be involved in suicidality: in a sample of autistic adults, among other risk factors such as non-suicidal self-injury and unmet needs for support, camouflaging significantly predicted suicidality [49], as detailed below.

Impact of camouflage on well-being seems to differ among males and females with autism. Camouflaging may help autistic people to fit into social contests [46], but males seem to benefit more from camouflaging than females [50]. A significant association between camouflage and stress was found for female autistic adolescents, while this was not confirmed for males [42]. Camouflaging might be particularly impactful for autistic females [51], being mentally exhausting for individuals: autistic females report this experience as "feeling drained." Continually monitoring social situations and measuring how to respond in a way that will be deemed socially appropriate are very energy-consuming [32, 50]. Autistic females interviewed on their feelings regarding camouflage strategies report negative feelings, whereas males were more likely to report that camouflaging was easy, reporting positive or neutral feeling associated [42].

Autistic females may be more aware of the potential social implications of their diagnosis, and this could cause more distress in dealing with other people, with a growing need to camouflage.

Camouflage effect seems to be a key element in understanding the complex relationship between autistic symptoms, female sex/gender, and internalizing symptoms. ASD diagnosis in females is often misinterpreted with other internalizing disorders also, probably, because of camouflage, but at the same time camouflage itself is implied in diagnostic delay (and subsequently delay in activation of therapeutic intervention) and raises the possibility of internalizing symptoms in female autistics with a complex relationship that needs to be further studied.

6.3 Internalizing Symptoms in Females Through Life

6.3.1 Toddlers and Preschool Children

Later in life, young children with ASD exhibit more comorbidity with respect to typically developing (TD) preschoolers [52].

Little is known on the development of internalizing symptoms in preschoolers with ASD and their trajectories up to adolescence. Most studies are cross sectional and therefore not informative of intraindividual changes over time. In most of the cases, the available data on female preschoolers with ASD come from studies that included both sexes, with no specific focus on sex differences or the female sex.

Regarding internalizing comorbidities by sex/gender in toddlers and preschoolers with ASD, studies have reported inconsistent findings: a study in children aged 20–51 months found no sex/gender differences in emotional or behavioral problems [53]. Kirkovski and colleagues suggested that among ASD toddlers, psychiatric comorbidity was clinically significant, but did not present sex/gender differences, which would develop only later [54].

Conversely, another study found that girls with ASD experienced more sleep problems and were more anxious/depressed than boys [55]. But this study was criticized for having accounted for the expected sex/gender differences in the general population [54]. Vaillancourt and colleagues reported that, in a cohort of 392 ASD children (mean age 3 years) consecutively assessed on four occasions, girls presented with clinically elevated levels of internalizing problems [52].

Otherwise, Postorino et al. in a 2-year longitudinal study which examined psychiatric problems with the Child Behavior Checklist (CBCL) among ASD preschoolers (aged 2–5.4 years), found lower scores on anxiety problems subscale at baseline and lower scores at sleep problems subscale in females [56]. Recently, an Italian case-control study (107 females matched with 107 males without impairment in performance IQ) reported that preschool autistic males presented higher internalizing symptom scores than females. In this study, autistic females also reported lower scores on emotionally reactive, anxious-depressed, than males [57].

Further studies are needed to better clarify the role of gender in presenting internalizing comorbidities among very young children with autism, to tailor specific intervention in a very early prevention perspective.

6.3.2 Children and Adolescents

Also concerning children and adolescents, while non-autistic adolescent females report higher levels of anxiety and mood disorders than non-autistic males, there have been contradictory findings regarding sex/gender differences in internalizing comorbidities among autistic adolescents [58], with some studies reporting similar trends by sex/gender, while others indicating no significant differences or even opposite trends [14, 26, 59, 60].

Solomon et al. [25] compared internalizing symptoms [measured with the Behavior Assessment System for Children (BASC-2) and the Children Depression Inventory (CDI)] with autism severity in a small sample of 8–18-year-old boys and girls with ASD and typically developing peers (20 ASD males and 20 ASD females compared with 17 TD males and 19 TD females). While boys and girls with ASD did not differ between themselves on internalizing symptoms in the overall sample, in the subgroup of adolescents (ages 12–18 years), the females had higher levels of anxiety than males and neurotypical girls and higher level of depression than neurotypical girls (while depression symptoms were comparable between males and females with ASD). May et al. [61], in a sample of 7–12-year boys and girls with ASD without intellectual disability (ID), also reported higher parent-rated social anxiety in girls than boys.

William Mandy et al. [29], in a functionally homogeneous sample of youth with ASD, also found higher parent-rated emotional symptoms, measured with the Strengths and Difficulties Questionnaire (SDQ), in girls than boys, with no effect of age on the relationship between sex/gender and SDQ measured symptoms. A recent study on clinical population found that while both male and female psychiatric inpatients with ASD presented with clinically elevated emotion dysregulation compared to general population norms, female inpatients had more severe dysregulation, including higher reactivity and dysphoria, than males [62].

Conversely, Guerrera et al. [63], in a large sample of children and adolescents with ASD not functionally homogeneous (aged 2.6–17.8 years), found higher rates of parent-rated internalizing symptoms (investigated through CBCL) in males than females.

Other studies indicated no sex/gender differences in internalizing symptoms (depression, anxious/depressed, withdrawn) in youth with ASD [30, 34, 56, 64–67]. Park et al. [68] found that children with ASD, as a group, experienced more internalizing and externalizing behaviors than TD children. However, no sex/gender differences were found for internalizing behaviors, as measured by the CBCL, in either ASD or TD groups.

A study by Oswald et al. [26] found that ASD females reported greater levels of parent-reported and adolescent self-reported depressive symptoms than either ASD males or typically developing females in early adolescence. However, by late adolescence, ASD males and females were found to have similar levels of depressive symptoms; in fact, ASD males tended to present a significant increase in depressive symptoms as they became older. Regarding anxiety, in early adolescence, the pattern suggested that females with ASD and typically developing males had significantly higher levels of self-reported separation anxiety and panic than males with ASD or typically developing females, but by late adolescence, both males and females with ASD had higher levels of separation anxiety and panic than neurotypical males and females.

Similar results were found in a recent review and meta-analysis by Hull et al. [50], which investigated sex/gender differences in internalizing and externalizing symptoms in ASD and typically developing samples. Age-related patterns were found for internalizing and externalizing problems: at younger ages, similarly to the neurotypical population, ASD females generally showed greater rates of internalizing problems, while ASD males reported higher levels of externalizing problems. However, at older ages, their levels of internalizing and externalizing problems became more similar, with males with ASD demonstrating increased levels of internalizing problems as they developed.

6.3.3 Adults

Literature regarding adult females is extremely limited, with a significant bias toward childhood and adolescence [69]. A meta-analysis by Hollocks et al. [70] found high rates of comorbid internalizing disorders in adults with ASD, with an estimated prevalence of 27% and 22% of anxiety and depression, respectively, not considering gender.

Some studies examined the developmental trajectory of psychopathology in ASD from late childhood to adulthood. Woodman et al. [71] examined trajectories of co-occurring psychopathology among individuals with ASD (of whom 25% were females) on the internalizing and externalizing scales from the CBCL and found declines in symptoms from late adolescence into adulthood. Characteristics of the adults with ASD, such as female sex, played a smaller role in predicting trajectories of psychopathology. Another study by McCauley et al. [72] used a longitudinal sample of individuals with ASD (of whom 21% were females) diagnosed in childhood to describe the trend of depression and anxiety from childhood to adulthood. For anxiety symptoms, around 30% of current participants had a stable trajectory of elevated anxiety symptoms. For depressive symptoms, over a third of individuals had a high depressive symptom trajectory, characterized by fluctuations peaking at a clinically significant level in early adulthood. Another longitudinal study by Gotham et al. [73], examining the trend of internalizing symptoms from school age to young adulthood in a sample with ASD and non-spectrum developmental disorder, found that in the ASD sample, males showed higher rates of internalizing symptoms at school age, which remain stable throughout adulthood, while females showed a faster increase in adolescence, with no significant sex differences by young adulthood.

A study by Baldwin and Costley [69] investigated, through self-report, the everyday life of a large sample (n = 82) of adult females with ASD without ID and secondly compared the figures with those found in a comparable sample of males with ASD. The study showed high rates of self-reported mental health problems in the sample: 82% of the participants declared to experience stress, while 85% affirmed to suffer from depression or anxiety. The prevalence of mental health problems in females (85%) was significantly higher compared to that found in the male sample (67%). In addition, stress and anxiety seemed to negatively affect all areas of life investigated (such as study, work, and social interaction). Besides, 73% of female participants expressed the need of mental health support, and only 70% of the group seemed to have these needs met. Ee et al. [74] highlighted that autistic adults experienced greater levels of loneliness than non-autistic adults, and female gender was interestingly found to be a protective factor against loneliness, which in turn has been associated with negative psychological conditions, including anxiety and depression. This is confirmed by McGillivray and Evert [75] who also showed high levels of depression, anxiety, and stress in both males and females with ASD, with adult females at particular risk, showing higher levels of stress and depression than same-aged men and younger males and females. A study by Murray et al. [76] highlighted that female gender was a risk factor for anxiety in young to middle adulthood, while no sex/gender difference was reported for depression symptoms, with both males and females showing high rates of depression in young adulthood that later declined. Conversely, Uljarević et al. [77] found that female sex/gender predicted both anxiety and depressive symptoms. Zheng et al. [78] found that young adult females with ASD were more likely than men to have received a depression diagnosis.

6.4 Suicidality Among Autistic Females

Studies suggested that people with ASD are at significantly higher risk of suicidal thoughts and behaviors, and suicide is a leading cause of premature death in this population [79–82]. Autistic traits are also associated with higher rates of suicidality [83–87]. Autism diagnosis and autistic traits have recently indeed been identified as independent risk markers for suicide attempts when controlling for other clinical and demographic risk factors [83]. Further, as mentioned above, other well-known risk factors are also more common in autism, such as depression, social withdrawal, and unemployment. Besides, depression may often be underdiagnosed in autistic people, as it has been suggested in a study by Croen et al. [88], resulting in lack of needed treatment. A recent systematic review on suicide in ASD reported prevalence of suicide attempts from 7 to 47% and suicidal ideation up to 72% across child, adolescent, and adult samples [89]. Hedley et al. [90] reported a prevalence of 36% of recent suicidal ideation in a sample of 185 people with ASD (aged 14–80 years), of whom 50% were females. According to the interpersonal theory of suicidality [91], the simultaneous presence of thwarted belongingness and perceived burdensomeness produce the desire for suicide, which in the presence of acquired capability of suicide can reduce the fear of death and lead to suicide. Pelton and Cassidy applied this theory to ASD people and found that, according to this theoretical background, people with autism seem to be at increased risk of suicide because of autistic symptoms, which in turn were associated with thwarted belongingness [84]. Burdensomeness and thwarted belongingness significantly mediated the relationship between autistic traits and suicidal behavior, and both depression and autistic traits significantly predicted thwarted belongingness and perceived burdensomeness [84]. Thwarted belongingness is related to loneliness: very often, autistic people feel extraneous and distant, as they do not belong to the world. In addition, anxiety can result in social withdrawal, with increasing feelings of being excluded or isolated.

Regarding females, suicide rates among autistic women are reported to be much higher than in other clinical and nonclinical populations [87, 92]. A recent study in a clinical sample of adolescents with ASD found that the risk for suicidality among females was two times higher relative to males [93]. Interestingly, while in the general population women are less likely than men to die by suicide [94], some studies showed that autistic women are as likely, if not more, to die by suicide as autistic men: a 20-year population study by Kirby et al. [81] examined suicidality among individuals diagnosed with ASD in Utah and found that suicide risk in females with

ASD was three times higher than in females without ASD, and even five times higher during the 2013–2017 period. Similarly, Hirvikoski et al. [80] found that females with ASD were over 13 times more likely than females in the general population to die by suicide.

A possible risk factor implied in higher rates of suicidality in autistic females could be camouflaging. As mentioned before, females seem to be more aware than males about their social deficits, and this could lead to a greater sense of loneliness, thwarted belongingness, and a growing need to camouflage. Feelings of isolation may be particularly relevant in undiagnosed autistic females [95, 96].

Camouflaging is also associated with negative feelings and a greater risk of mental health problems, such as stress, depression, and anxiety [41, 42, 46, 97]. A recent study [51], which examined a sample of undiagnosed women with high autistic traits, found that camouflaging was associated with higher distress, suicidality, and poor daily functioning. Interestingly, camouflaging efforts were not linked to the severity of autistic traits. A study by Cassidy et al. [83] found that camouflaging was a unique independent risk factor for suicidal thoughts and behaviors in a sample of autistic adults. However, the study did not highlight any difference in camouflaging between males and females. Another recent study by Cassidy et al. [49] showed that the relationship between autistic traits and suicidality was significantly mediated by camouflaging and feeling of thwarted belongingness.

Besides, difficulty in coping with neurotypical social situations can lead autistic women to experience reduced support in their social networks and thus being less likely to seek help, which in turn increases the likelihood of mental health concern [98]. In the general population, some recent studies suggested that the rates of deaths by suicide may be lower in females due to the fact that they are more willing to ask for help than males, even if females tend to make more attempts. Therefore, the opposite trend in death by suicide observed in ASD samples could possibly be explained by the difficulties in autistic females to seek help, confirming help-seeking behavior to be a crucial element in determining suicide risk.

Hedley et al. [90] examined the potential role of loneliness, social support, and autistic traits in depression and suicidal ideation in a sample of autistic people. They found that autistic females showed higher depression scores than males; however, suicidality did not differ between males and females.

Among other factors implied in these gender differences in suicidality among ASD people, sexual experiences must be taken into account. Females with autism are exposed to a variety of challenges as sexual abuse, social difficulties, and conflicts between ASD traits and feminine identity [32]. Traumatic experiences and identity conflicts are well-known risk factors for suicide in the general population. Regarding sexual experiences, autistic females reported being engaged in sexual behaviors that were later regretted, unwanted, or receiving unwanted sexual advances, but at the same time they reported less sexual interest; this could become a risk factor for being involved in victimization or in sexual abuse [99]. Additionally, gender diversity among autistic individuals has been increasingly explored, with the finding that autistic individuals are more diverse in their gender identities than the wider population [100]. Moreover, autistic individuals experience more gender diverse traits than the wider population, and this is more pronounced among autistic females. This is especially important as gender diversity is a risk factor for suicidal ideation, suicide attempt, and poorer mental health outcome [101]. All these findings underline the necessity of recognizing early internalizing symptoms in females with ASD, who present with increased vulnerability for suicidality and death by suicide relative to males.

6.5 Conclusion

The possibility to summarize clear conclusion about sex differences in internalizing symptomatology among people through ages with ASD is influenced by several variables and limitations among studies that have likely contributed to the disparate results, as the functional heterogeneous vs. homogeneous samples and differences in sample size, age, and measures used across studies. Notwithstanding the current limitations, specific attention to internalizing comorbidities in females with autism is indicated given their clinical relevance and the potential for treatment to reduce functional impairment and improve quality of life.

Key Points

- Females with ASD may be especially vulnerable to internalizing disorders due to a "double hit" conferred by sex/gender and autistic predisposition.
- Internalizing symptoms in females with ASD represent a reason for misdiagnosis: depression and anxiety may cover autistic symptoms.
- The double role of "camouflaging" effect within ASD females: potential positive adaptive function or negative role in the onset internalizing comorbidities?
- Delay in ASD diagnosis due to camouflage may increase the possibility of internalizing symptoms (depression, anxiety).
- Females with ASD report negative feelings regarding camouflaging strategies (energy-consuming and cause of distress), which are associated with negative feelings and greater risk of depression, suicidal behaviors, and thoughts.
- Not considering sex/gender, higher rates of comorbid internalizing disorders have been described in adults with ASD.
- Individuals with ASD are at greater risk of suicidal thoughts and behaviors with suicide representing one of the leading causes of premature death.
- Well-known risk factors for suicide are common in ASD: depression, social withdrawal, and unemployment.
- Suicide rates among women with ASD are reported to be much higher than in other clinical and nonclinical population. Females with autism seem to be more aware than males about their social deficits, leading to a greater sense of loneliness and need to camouflage.

References

1. Gadow KD, Devincent CJ, Pomeroy J, Azizian A. Comparison of DSM-IV symptoms in elementary school-age children with PDD versus clinic and community samples. Autism. 2005;9(4):392–415. https://doi.org/10.1177/1362361305056079.
2. Volker MA, Lopata C, Smerbeck AM, Knoll VA, Thomeer ML, Toomey JA, Rodgers JD. BASC-2 PRS profiles for students with high-functioning autism spectrum disorders. J Autism Dev Disord. 2010;40(2):188–99. https://doi.org/10.1007/s10803-009-0849-6.
3. Leyfer OT, Folstein SE, Bacalman S, Davis NO, Dinh E, Morgan J, Tager-Flusberg H, Lainhart JE. Comorbid psychiatric disorders in children with autism: interview development and rates of disorders. J Autism Dev Disord. 2006;36(7):849–61. https://doi.org/10.1007/s10803-006-0123-0.
4. Simonoff E, Pickles A, Charman T, Chandler S, Loucas T, Baird G. Psychiatric disorders in children with autism spectrum disorders: prevalence, comorbidity, and associated factors in a population-derived sample. J Am Acad Child Adolesc Psychiatry. 2008;47(8):921–9. https://doi.org/10.1097/CHI.0b013e318179964f.
5. van Steensel FJA, Bögels SM, de Bruin EI. Psychiatric comorbidity in children with autism spectrum disorders: a comparison with children with ADHD. J Child Fam Stud. 2013;22(3):368–76. https://doi.org/10.1007/s10826-012-9587-z.
6. Hossain MM, Khan N, Sultana A, Ma P, McKyer ELJ, Ahmed HU, Purohit N. Prevalence of comorbid psychiatric disorders among people with autism spectrum disorder: an umbrella review of systematic reviews and meta-analyses. Psychiatry Res. 2020;287:112922. https://doi.org/10.1016/j.psychres.2020.112922.
7. Smith IC, White SW. Socio-emotional determinants of depressive symptoms in adolescents and adults with autism spectrum disorder: a systematic review. Autism. 2020;24(4):995–1010. https://doi.org/10.1177/1362361320908101.
8. Mazzone L, Ruta L, Reale L. Psychiatric comorbidities in Asperger syndrome and high functioning autism: diagnostic challenges. Ann Gen Psychiatry. 2012;11(1):16. https://doi.org/10.1186/1744-859X-11-16.
9. Young H, Oreve M-J, Speranza M. Clinical characteristics and problems diagnosing autism spectrum disorder in girls. Arch Pédiatrie. 2018;25(6):399–403. https://doi.org/10.1016/j.arcped.2018.06.008.
10. Howlin P, Moss P. Adults with autism spectrum disorders. Can J Psychiatry. 2012;57(5):275–83. https://doi.org/10.1177/070674371205700502.
11. Keith JM, Jamieson JP, Bennetto L. The importance of adolescent self-report in autism spectrum disorder: integration of questionnaire and autonomic measures. J Abnorm Child Psychol. 2019;47(4):741–54. https://doi.org/10.1007/s10802-018-0455-1.
12. van Steensel FJA, Bögels SM, Perrin S. Anxiety disorders in children and adolescents with autistic spectrum disorders: a meta-analysis. Clin Child Fam Psychol Rev. 2011;14(3):302–17. https://doi.org/10.1007/s10567-011-0097-0.
13. Mertens J, Zane ER, Neumeyer K, Grossman RB. How anxious do you think I am? Relationship between state and trait anxiety in children with and without ASD during social tasks. J Autism Dev Disord. 2017;47(12):3692–703. https://doi.org/10.1007/s10803-016-2979-y.
14. Rynkiewicz A, Łucka I. Autism spectrum disorder (ASD) in girls. Co-occurring psychopathology. Sex differences in clinical manifestation. Psychiatr Pol. 2018;52(4):629–39. https://doi.org/10.12740/PP/OnlineFirst/58837.
15. Angold A, Rutter M. Effects of age and pubertal status on depression in a large clinical sample. Dev Psychopathol. 1992;4(1):5–28. https://doi.org/10.1017/S0954579400005538.
16. Van Oort FVA, Greaves-Lord K, Verhulst FC, Ormel J, Huizink AC. The developmental course of anxiety symptoms during adolescence: the TRAILS study. J Child Psychol Psychiatry. 2009;50(10):1209–17. https://doi.org/10.1111/j.1469-7610.2009.02092.x.

17. Zahn-Waxler C, Shirtcliff EA, Marceau K. Disorders of childhood and adolescence: gender and psychopathology. Annu Rev Clin Psychol. 2008;4(1):275–303. https://doi.org/10.1146/annurev.clinpsy.3.022806.091358.
18. Hankin BL, Abramson LY, Moffitt TE, Silva PA, McGee R, Angell KE. Development of depression from preadolescence to young adulthood: emerging gender differences in a 10-year longitudinal study. J Abnorm Psychol. 1998;107(1):128.
19. Alloy LB, Hamilton JL, Hamlat EJ, Abramson LY. Pubertal development, emotion regulatory styles, and the emergence of sex differences in internalizing disorders and symptoms in adolescence. Clin Psychol Sci. 2016;4(5):867–81. https://doi.org/10.1177/2167702616643008.
20. Angst J, Dobler-Mikola A. The Zurich study: VI. A continuum from depression to anxiety disorders? Eur Arch Psychiatry Neurol Sci. 1985;235(3):179–86. https://doi.org/10.1007/BF00380990.
21. Bruce SE, Yonkers KA, Otto MW. Influence of psychiatric comorbidity on recovery and recurrence in generalized anxiety disorder, social phobia, and panic disorder: a 12-year prospective study. Am J Psychiatry. 2005;162:1179–87.
22. Regier DA, Narrow WE, Rae DS. The epidemiology of anxiety disorders: the epidemiologic catchment area (ECA) experience. J Psychiatr Res. 1990;24:3–14. https://doi.org/10.1016/0022-3956(90)90031-K.
23. van Loo HM, Beijers L, Wieling M, de Jong TR, Schoevers RA, Kendler KS. Prevalence of internalizing disorders, symptoms, and traits across age using advanced nonlinear models. Psychol Med. 2021;53:78–87. https://doi.org/10.1017/S0033291721001148.
24. Boyd A, Van de Velde S, Vilagut G, de Graaf R, O'Neill S, Florescu S, Alonso J, Kovess-Masfety V. Gender differences in mental disorders and suicidality in Europe: results from a large cross-sectional population-based study. J Affect Disord. 2015;173:245–54. https://doi.org/10.1016/j.jad.2014.11.002.
25. Solomon M, Miller M, Taylor SL, Hinshaw SP, Carter CS. Autism symptoms and internalizing psychopathology in girls and boys with autism spectrum disorders. J Autism Dev Disord. 2012;42(1):48–59. https://doi.org/10.1007/s10803-011-1215-z.
26. Oswald TM, Winter-Messiers MA, Gibson B, Schmidt AM, Herr CM, Solomon M. Sex differences in internalizing problems during adolescence in autism spectrum disorder. J Autism Dev Disord. 2016;46(2):624–36. https://doi.org/10.1007/s10803-015-2608-1.
27. Dean M, Harwood R, Kasari C. The art of camouflage: gender differences in the social behaviors of girls and boys with autism spectrum disorder. Autism. 2017;21(6):678–89. https://doi.org/10.1177/1362361316671845.
28. Thompson T, Caruso M, Ellerbeck K. Sex matters in autism and other developmental disabilities. J Learn Disabil. 2003;7(4):345–62. https://doi.org/10.1177/1469004703074003.
29. Mandy W, Chilvers R, Chowdhury U, Salter G, Seigal A, Skuse D. Sex differences in autism spectrum disorder: evidence from a large sample of children and adolescents. J Autism Dev Disord. 2012;42(7):1304–13. https://doi.org/10.1007/s10803-011-1356-0.
30. Nasca BC, Lopata C, Donnelly JP, Rodgers JD, Thomeer ML. Sex differences in externalizing and internalizing symptoms of children with ASD. J Autism Dev Disord. 2020;50(9):3245–52. https://doi.org/10.1007/s10803-019-04132-8.
31. Loomes R, Hull L, Mandy WPL. What is the male-to-female ratio in autism spectrum disorder? A systematic review and meta-analysis. J Am Acad Child Adolesc Psychiatry. 2017;56(6):466–74. https://doi.org/10.1016/j.jaac.2017.03.013.
32. Bargiela S, Steward R, Mandy W. The experiences of late-diagnosed women with autism spectrum conditions: an investigation of the female autism phenotype. J Autism Dev Disord. 2016;46(10):3281–94. https://doi.org/10.1007/s10803-016-2872-8.
33. Rynkiewicz A, Schuller B, Marchi E, Piana S, Camurri A, Lassalle A, Baron-Cohen S. An investigation of the 'female camouflage effect' in autism using a computerized ADOS-2 and a test of sex/gender differences. Mol Autism. 2016;7(1):10. https://doi.org/10.1186/s13229-016-0073-0.
34. Pisula E, Pudło M, Słowińska M, Kawa R, Strząska M, Banasiak A, Wolańczyk T. Behavioral and emotional problems in high-functioning girls and boys with autism spectrum disorders:

parents' reports and adolescents' self-reports. Autism. 2017;21(6):738–48. https://doi.org/10.1177/1362361316675119.
35. McLennan JD, Lord C, Schopler E. Sex differences in higher functioning people with autism. J Autism Dev Disord. 1993;23(2):217–27. https://doi.org/10.1007/BF01046216.
36. Lai M-C, Lombardo MV, Pasco G, Ruigrok ANV, Wheelwright SJ, Sadek SA, Chakrabarti B, MRC AIMS Consortium, Baron-Cohen S. A behavioral comparison of male and female adults with high functioning autism spectrum conditions. PLoS One. 2011;6(6):e20835. https://doi.org/10.1371/journal.pone.0020835.
37. Kopp S, Gillberg C. Girls with social deficits and learning problems: autism, atypical Asperger syndrome or a variant of these conditions. Eur Child Adolesc Psychiatry. 1992;1(2):89–99. https://doi.org/10.1007/BF02091791.
38. Mandy W, Tchanturia K. Do women with eating disorders who have social and flexibility difficulties really have autism? A case series. Mol Autism. 2015;6(1):6. https://doi.org/10.1186/2040-2392-6-6.
39. Posserud M-B, Lundervold AJ, Gillberg C. Autistic features in a total population of 7–9-year-old children assessed by the ASSQ (Autism Spectrum Screening Questionnaire). J Child Psychol Psychiatry. 2006;47(2):167–75. https://doi.org/10.1111/j.1469-7610.2005.01462.x.
40. Constantino JN, Todd RD. Autistic traits in the general population: a twin study. Arch Gen Psychiatry. 2003;60(5):524. https://doi.org/10.1001/archpsyc.60.5.524.
41. Hull L, Mandy W, Lai M-C, Baron-Cohen S, Allison C, Smith P, Petrides KV. Development and validation of the camouflaging autistic traits questionnaire (CAT-Q). J Autism Dev Disord. 2019;49(3):819–33. https://doi.org/10.1007/s10803-018-3792-6.
42. Bernardin CJ, Mason E, Lewis T, Kanne S. "You must become a Chameleon to survive": adolescent experiences of camouflaging. J Autism Dev Disord. 2021;51(12):4422–35. https://doi.org/10.1007/s10803-021-04912-1.
43. Hull L, Lai M-C, Baron-Cohen S, Allison C, Smith P, Petrides K, Mandy W. Gender differences in self-reported camouflaging in autistic and non-autistic adults. Autism. 2020a;24(2):352–63. https://doi.org/10.1177/1362361319864804.
44. Lai M-C, Szatmari P. Sex and gender impacts on the behavioural presentation and recognition of autism. Curr Opin Psychiatry. 2020;33(2):117–23. https://doi.org/10.1097/YCO.0000000000000575.
45. Hull L, Petrides KV, Mandy W. The female autism phenotype and camouflaging: a narrative review. Rev J Autism Dev Disord. 2020b;7(4):306–17. https://doi.org/10.1007/s40489-020-00197-9.
46. Cage E, Troxell-Whitman Z. Understanding the reasons, contexts and costs of camouflaging for autistic adults. J Autism Dev Disord. 2019;49(5):1899–911. https://doi.org/10.1007/s10803-018-03878-x.
47. Livingston LA, Shah P, Happé F. Compensatory strategies below the behavioural surface in autism: a qualitative study. Lancet Psychiatry. 2019;6(9):766–77. https://doi.org/10.1016/S2215-0366(19)30224-X.
48. Lai M-C, Lombardo MV, Ruigrok AN, Chakrabarti B, Auyeung B, Szatmari P, Happé F, Baron-Cohen S, MRC AIMS Consortium. Quantifying and exploring camouflaging in men and women with autism. Autism. 2017;21(6):690–702. https://doi.org/10.1177/1362361316671012.
49. Cassidy SA, Gould K, Townsend E, Pelton M, Robertson AE, Rodgers J. Is camouflaging autistic traits associated with suicidal thoughts and behaviours? Expanding the interpersonal psychological theory of suicide in an undergraduate student sample. J Autism Dev Disord. 2020;50(10):3638–48. https://doi.org/10.1007/s10803-019-04323-3.
50. Hull L, Mandy W, Petrides K. Behavioural and cognitive sex/gender differences in autism spectrum condition and typically developing males and females. Autism. 2017;21(6):706–27. https://doi.org/10.1177/1362361316669087.
51. Beck JS, Lundwall RA, Gabrielsen T, Cox JC, South M. Looking good but feeling bad: "Camouflaging" behaviors and mental health in women with autistic traits. Autism. 2020;24(4):809–21. https://doi.org/10.1177/1362361320912147.

52. Vaillancourt T, Haltigan JD, Smith I, Zwaigenbaum L, Szatmari P, Fombonne E, Waddell C, Duku E, Mirenda P, Georgiades S, Bennett T, Volden J, Elsabbagh M, Roberts W, Bryson S. Joint trajectories of internalizing and externalizing problems in preschool children with autism spectrum disorder. Dev Psychopathol. 2017;29(1):203–14. https://doi.org/10.1017/S0954579416000043.
53. Herring S, Gray K, Taffe J, Tonge B, Sweeney D, Einfeld S. Behaviour and emotional problems in toddlers with pervasive developmental disorders and developmental delay: associations with parental mental health and family functioning. J Intellect Disabil Res. 2006;50(12):874–82. https://doi.org/10.1111/j.1365-2788.2006.00904.x.
54. Kirkovski M, Enticott PG, Fitzgerald PB. A review of the role of female gender in autism spectrum disorders. J Autism Dev Disord. 2013;43(11):2584–603. https://doi.org/10.1007/s10803-013-1811-1.
55. Hartley SL, Sikora DM. Sex differences in autism spectrum disorder: an examination of developmental functioning, autistic symptoms, and coexisting behavior problems in toddlers. J Autism Dev Disord. 2009;39(12):1715–22. https://doi.org/10.1007/s10803-009-0810-8.
56. Postorino V, Fatta LM, De Peppo L, Giovagnoli G, Armando M, Vicari S, Mazzone L. Longitudinal comparison between male and female preschool children with autism spectrum disorder. J Autism Dev Disord. 2015;45(7):2046–55. https://doi.org/10.1007/s10803-015-2366-0.
57. Prosperi M, Turi M, Guerrera S, Napoli E, Tancredi R, Igliozzi R, Apicella F, Valeri G, Lattarulo C, Gemma A, Santocchi E, Calderoni S, Muratori F, Vicari S. Sex differences in autism spectrum disorder: an investigation on core symptoms and psychiatric comorbidity in preschoolers. Front Integr Neurosci. 2021;14:594082. https://doi.org/10.3389/fnint.2020.594082.
58. Merikangas KR, He JP, Brody D, Fisher PW, Bourdon K, Koretz DS. Prevalence and treatment of mental disorders among US children in the 2001–2004 NHANES. Pediatrics. 2010;125(1):75–81. https://doi.org/10.1542/peds.2008-2598.
59. Margari L, Palumbi R, Peschechera A, Craig F, de Giambattista C, Ventura P, Margari F. Sex-gender comparisons in comorbidities of children and adolescents with high-functioning autism spectrum disorder. Front Psychiatry. 2019;10:159. https://doi.org/10.3389/fpsyt.2019.00159.
60. Mattila M-L, Hurtig T, Haapsamo H, Jussila K, Kuusikko-Gauffin S, Kielinen M, Linna S-L, Ebeling H, Bloigu R, Joskitt L, Pauls DL, Moilanen I. Comorbid psychiatric disorders associated with Asperger syndrome/high-functioning autism: a community- and clinic-based study. J Autism Dev Disord. 2010;40(9):1080–93. https://doi.org/10.1007/s10803-010-0958-2.
61. May T, Cornish K, Rinehart N. Does gender matter? A 1 year follow-up of autistic, attention and anxiety symptoms in high-functioning children with autism spectrum disorder. J Autism Dev Disord. 2014;44(5):1077–86. https://doi.org/10.1007/s10803-013-1964-y.
62. Wieckowski AT, Luallin S, Pan Z, Righi G, Gabriels RL, Mazefsky C. Gender differences in emotion dysregulation in an autism inpatient psychiatric sample. Autism Res. 2020;13(8):1343–8. https://doi.org/10.1002/aur.2295.
63. Guerrera S, Menghini D, Napoli E, Di Vara S, Valeri G, Vicari S. Assessment of psychopathological comorbidities in children and adolescents with autism spectrum disorder using the child behavior checklist. Front Psychiatry. 2019;10:535. https://doi.org/10.3389/fpsyt.2019.00535.
64. Brereton AV, Tonge BJ, Einfeld SL. Psychopathology in children and adolescents with autism compared to young people with intellectual disability. J Autism Dev Disord. 2006;36(7):863–70. https://doi.org/10.1007/s10803-006-0125-y.
65. Holtmann M, Bölte S, Poustka F. Autism spectrum disorders: sex differences in autistic behaviour domains and coexisting psychopathology. Dev Med Child Neurol. 2007;49(5):361–6. https://doi.org/10.1111/j.1469-8749.2007.00361.x.
66. Kuusikko S, Pollock-Wurman R, Jussila K, Carter AS, Mattila M-L, Ebeling H, Pauls DL, Moilanen I. Social anxiety in high-functioning children and adolescents with autism and Asperger syndrome. J Autism Dev Disord. 2008;38(9):1697–709. https://doi.org/10.1007/s10803-008-0555-9.

67. Worley JA, Matson JL. Psychiatric symptoms in children diagnosed with an autism spectrum disorder: an examination of gender differences. Res Autism Spectr Disord. 2011;5(3):1086–91. https://doi.org/10.1016/j.rasd.2010.12.002.
68. Park S, Cho S-C, Cho IH, Kim B-N, Kim J-W, Shin M-S, Chung U-S, Park T-W, Son J-W, Yoo HJ. Sex differences in children with autism spectrum disorders compared with their unaffected siblings and typically developing children. Res Autism Spectr Disord. 2012;6(2):861–70. https://doi.org/10.1016/j.rasd.2011.11.006.
69. Baldwin S, Costley D. The experiences and needs of female adults with high-functioning autism spectrum disorder. Autism. 2016;20(4):483–95. https://doi.org/10.1177/1362361315590805.
70. Hollocks MJ, Lerh JW, Magiati I, Meiser-Stedman R, Brugha TS. Anxiety and depression in adults with autism spectrum disorder: a systematic review and meta-analysis. Psychol Med. 2019;49(4):559–72. https://doi.org/10.1017/S0033291718002283.
71. Woodman AC, Mailick MR, Greenberg JS. Trajectories of internalizing and externalizing symptoms among adults with autism spectrum disorders. Dev Psychopathol. 2016;28(2):565–81. https://doi.org/10.1017/S095457941500108X.
72. McCauley JB, Elias R, Lord C. Trajectories of co-occurring psychopathology symptoms in autism from late childhood to adulthood. Dev Psychopathol. 2020;32(4):1287–302. https://doi.org/10.1017/S0954579420000826.
73. Gotham K, Brunwasser SM, Lord C. Depressive and anxiety symptom trajectories from school age through young adulthood in samples with autism spectrum disorder and developmental delay. J Am Acad Child Adolesc Psychiatry. 2015;54(5):369–376.e3. https://doi.org/10.1016/j.jaac.2015.02.005.
74. Ee D, Hwang YI, Reppermund S, Srasuebkul P, Trollor JN, Foley K-R, Arnold SRC. Loneliness in adults on the autism spectrum. Autism Adulthood. 2019;1(3):182–93. https://doi.org/10.1089/aut.2018.0038.
75. McGillivray JA, Evert HT. Exploring the effect of gender and age on stress and emotional distress in adults with autism spectrum disorder. Focus Autism Dev Disabil. 2018;33(1): 55–64. https://doi.org/10.1177/1088357614549317.
76. Murray C, Kovshoff H, Brown A, Abbott P, Hadwin JA. Exploring the anxiety and depression profile in individuals diagnosed with an autism spectrum disorder in adulthood. Res Autism Spectr Disord. 2019;58:1–8. https://doi.org/10.1016/j.rasd.2018.11.002.
77. Uljarević M, Hedley D, Rose-Foley K, Magiati I, Cai RY, Dissanayake C, Richdale A, Trollor J. Anxiety and depression from adolescence to old age in autism spectrum disorder. J Autism Dev Disord. 2020;50(9):3155–65. https://doi.org/10.1007/s10803-019-04084 z.
78. Zheng S, Adams R, Taylor JL, Pezzimenti F, Bishop SL. Depression in independent young adults on the autism spectrum: demographic characteristics, service use, and barriers. Autism. 2021;25:1960–72. https://doi.org/10.1177/13623613211008276.
79. Raja M. Suicide risk in adults with Asperger's syndrome. Lancet Psychiatry. 2014;1(2):99–101. https://doi.org/10.1016/S2215-0366(14)70257-3.
80. Hirvikoski T, Mittendorfer-Rutz E, Boman M, Larsson H, Lichtenstein P, Bölte S. Premature mortality in autism spectrum disorder. Br J Psychiatry. 2016;208(3):232–8. https://doi.org/10.1192/bjp.bp.114.160192.
81. Kirby AV, Bakian AV, Zhang Y, Bilder DA, Keeshin BR, Coon H. A 20-year study of suicide death in a statewide autism population. Autism Res. 2019;12(4):658–66. https://doi.org/10.1002/aur.2076.
82. Richards G, Kenny R, Griffiths S, Allison C, Mosse D, Holt R, O'Connor RC, Cassidy S, Baron-Cohen S. Autistic traits in adults who have attempted suicide. Mol Autism. 2019;10(1):26. https://doi.org/10.1186/s13229-019-0274-4.
83. Cassidy S, Bradley L, Shaw R, Baron-Cohen S. Risk markers for suicidality in autistic adults. Mol Autism. 2018;9(1):42. https://doi.org/10.1186/s13229-018-0226-4.
84. Pelton MK, Cassidy SA. Are autistic traits associated with suicidality? A test of the interpersonal-psychological theory of suicide in a non-clinical young adult sample: are autistic traits associated with suicidality? Autism Res. 2017;10(11):1891–904. https://doi.org/10.1002/aur.1828.

85. Paquette-Smith M, Weiss J, Lunsky Y. History of suicide attempts in adults with Asperger syndrome. Crisis. 2014;35(4):273–7. https://doi.org/10.1027/0227-5910/a000263.
86. Takara K, Kondo T. Comorbid atypical autistic traits as a potential risk factor for suicide attempts among adult depressed patients: a case–control study. Ann Gen Psychiatry. 2014;13(1):33. https://doi.org/10.1186/s12991-014-0033-z.
87. Cassidy S, Bradley P, Robinson J, Allison C, McHugh M, Baron-Cohen S. Suicidal ideation and suicide plans or attempts in adults with Asperger's syndrome attending a specialist diagnostic clinic: a clinical cohort study. Lancet Psychiatry. 2014;1(2):142–7. https://doi.org/10.1016/S2215-0366(14)70248-2.
88. Croen LA, Zerbo O, Qian Y, Massolo ML, Rich S, Sidney S, Kripke C. The health status of adults on the autism spectrum. Autism. 2015;19(7):814–23. https://doi.org/10.1177/1362361315577517.
89. Zahid S, Upthegrove R. Suicidality in autistic spectrum disorders: a systematic review. Crisis. 2017;38(4):237–46. https://doi.org/10.1027/0227-5910/a000458.
90. Hedley D, Uljarević M, Foley K-R, Richdale A, Trollor J. Risk and protective factors underlying depression and suicidal ideation in autism spectrum disorder. Depress Anxiety. 2018;35(7):648–57. https://doi.org/10.1002/da.22759.
91. Van Orden KA, Witte TK, Cukrowicz KC, Braithwaite SR, Selby EA, Joiner TE. The interpersonal theory of suicide. Psychol Rev. 2010;117(2):575–600. https://doi.org/10.1037/a0018697.
92. Hirvikoski T, Boman M, Chen Q, D'Onofrio BM, Mittendorfer-Rutz E, Lichtenstein P, Bölte S, Larsson H. Individual risk and familial liability for suicide attempt and suicide in autism: a population-based study. Psychol Med. 2020;50(9):1463–74. https://doi.org/10.1017/S0033291719001405.
93. Holden R, Mueller J, McGowan J, Sanyal J, Kikoler M, Simonoff E, Velupillai S, Downs J. Investigating bullying as a predictor of suicidality in a clinical sample of adolescents with autism spectrum disorder. Autism Res. 2020;13(6):988–97. https://doi.org/10.1002/aur.2292.
94. Hedegaard H. Suicide mortality in the United States, 1999–2019. National Center for Health Statistics; 2021. https://doi.org/10.15620/cdc:101761.
95. Hickey A, Crabtree J, Stott J. 'Suddenly the first fifty years of my life made sense': experiences of older people with autism. Autism. 2018;22(3):357–67. https://doi.org/10.1177/1362361316680914.
96. Leedham A, Thompson AR, Smith R, Freeth M. 'I was exhausted trying to figure it out': the experiences of females receiving an autism diagnosis in middle to late adulthood. Autism. 2020;24(1):135–46. https://doi.org/10.1177/1362361319853442.
97. Milner V, McIntosh H, Colvert E, Happé F. A qualitative exploration of the female experience of autism spectrum disorder (ASD). J Autism Dev Disord. 2019;49(6):2389–402. https://doi.org/10.1007/s10803-019-03906-4.
98. Howlin P, Magiati I. Autism spectrum disorder: outcomes in adulthood. Curr Opin Psychiatry. 2017;30(2):69–76. https://doi.org/10.1097/YCO.0000000000000308.
99. Pecora LA, Hancock GI, Mesibov GB, Stokes MA. Characterising the sexuality and sexual experiences of autistic females. J Autism Dev Disord. 2019;49(12):4834–46. https://doi.org/10.1007/s10803-019-04204-9.
100. George R, Stokes MA. Gender identity and sexual orientation in autism spectrum disorder. Autism. 2018;22(8):970–82. https://doi.org/10.1177/1362361317714587.
101. Chew D, Tollit MA, Poulakis Z, Zwickl S, Cheung AS, Pang KC. Youths with a non-binary gender identity: a review of their sociodemographic and clinical profile. Lancet Child Adolesc Health. 2020;4(4):322–30. https://doi.org/10.1016/S2352-4642(19)30403-1.

Female Autism and Externalizing Disorders

7

Chiara Davico, Caterina Lux, and Benedetto Vitiello

7.1 Introduction

Beyond the core diagnostic symptoms, individuals with autism spectrum disorder (ASD) are more likely to experience a heavier burden of psychiatric comorbidity than typically developing peers [1]. It is reported that nearly 70% of people with ASD present at least one comorbid psychiatric disorder, whereas nearly 40% individuals may have two or more psychiatric disorders [2]. The wide range of psychiatric symptoms can further interfere with the difficulties in adaptive responses and daily functioning, worsening problems like restlessness, passivity, social isolation, aggressiveness, and irritability [3].

Externalizing disorders include attention deficit/hyperactivity disorder (ADHD), oppositional defiant disorder (ODD), and conduct disorder [4]. In addition, aggression, delinquency, and substance use are considered under the umbrella term of externalizing behaviors.

The current literature about the prevalence by sex/gender of externalizing and internalizing symptoms in ASD is rather limited, and heterogeneous, with often conflicting findings among studies. Some authors reported higher levels of parent-rated aggression, hyperactivity, and inattention in boys than in girls with ASD [5], while others found higher levels of irritability and externalizing behaviors in girls [6], and still others reported no sex/gender differences in externalizing disorders among individuals with ASD [7–10]. It has been suggested that these inconsistent findings may be due to methodological factors: sample size and inclusion of wide range of cognitive/functional levels of participants, which could mask sex differences [11, 12].

C. Davico (✉) · C. Lux · B. Vitiello
Section of Child and Adolescent Neuropsychiatry, Department of Public Health and Pediatric Sciences, University of Turin, Turin, Italy
e-mail: Chiara.davico@unito.it; caterinamaria.lux@unito.it; Benedetto.Vitiello@unito.it

L. Mazzone et al. (eds.), *Autism Spectrum Disorder: Understanding the Female Phenotype*, https://doi.org/10.1007/978-3-031-62072-0_7

7.2 Externalizing Disorders in the General Population

Epidemiological surveys in the general population have consistently documented a higher rate of any lifetime externalizing disorders among males than females [13]. Several biologic and psychosocial hypotheses have been proposed to explain this difference, including that of gender role hypothesis, according to which this difference in prevalence is due to the difference in the typical stressors, coping resources, and opportunity structures for expressing psychologic distress made available differentially to males and females in different countries.

Sex/gender differences in externalizing (e.g., substance use) and internalizing (e.g., depression) seem to decrease in countries where roles of men and women are more equal [14]. There are no significant sex/gender differences in the median age of onset of externalizing problems, with an immediate increase in cumulative proportion with increasing age, occurring roughly at the median age of onset, for both men and women [13].

Most of the externalizing problems, as aggressiveness, oppositional behavior, and ADHD, tend to follow a parabolic curve over time and to decline as individuals age, except for substance use and delinquency that increase with age [15, 16].

7.3 Externalizing Disorders and Intellectual Disability

When considering sex/gender differences in externalizing symptoms in ASD, it is crucial to consider the role of intellectual disability (ID).

The most widely reported data on the prevalence by sex of ASD indicate a male-to-female ratio of about 4–5:1 in the general ASD population, but lower in individuals with intellectual disability and higher in individuals with low support needs [17, 18]. The association with cognitive competences, as a higher proportion of females have concurrent intellectual disability, has long been considered having etiological implications, such as a higher liability threshold for females to develop autism [19, 20]. Recent large-scale epidemiological studies and meta-analyses suggest that the male-to-female ratio in ASD prevalence may in fact be lower, more in the range of 2–5:1 [21–23], and that the sex ratio is not influenced by intellectual disability [24, 25]. These reports of a lower sex ratio than previously known, independently from intellectual disability, may be due to the greater success of recent studies in identifying females with ASD, particularly individuals with low support needs [26]. Nevertheless, even studies that accounted for these issues still found a 2–5:1 male predominance, with the clinically identified females with ASD having, on average, lower intelligence than males. Given the inverse correlation between IQ and both autistic symptomatology [27] and externalizing symptoms [28], intelligence is to be considered as a potential confounding variable in the studies of sex/gender differences, highlighting the need to control for its effects [12].

Longitudinal studies suggest that there are dynamic associations between cognitive ability and behavioral difficulties in the general child population [29–32]. Causal links are bidirectional. High levels of externalizing problems interfere with a child's normative development and consequently with the acquisition of age-appropriate cognitive skills [33]. Moreover, lack of self-control, sustained attention deficits, and difficulties in following directions make learning difficult and reduce opportunities to strengthen a broad range of cognitive abilities [34]. At the same time, there is also evidence in support of the opposite causal direction of the association between cognition and externalizing behaviors. For example, frontally mediated deficits in executive functions [35, 36] and general neurocognitive deficits can be both risk factors [37] and outcomes of psychopathology [38].

The interconnection between cognitive ability and behavioral problems is further reinforced by sharing some among the most important risk factors for both, such as low socio-economic status [39], low parental education [40], maternal psychopathology [41], and low birth weight [42].

Concerning the time course, increasing levels of externalizing symptoms throughout childhood and until middle adolescence seem to be associated with both an increase in internalizing symptoms and a decline in cognitive ability. However, it remains to be determined if the decline in cognitive skills and/or increase in internalizing symptoms are causally linked to the increases in externalizing symptoms, or if it is the increase in externalizing symptoms that leads to a decline in cognitive skills and increase in internalizing symptoms, or if other variables account for the externalizing symptoms changing in parallel with both internalizing symptoms and cognitive difficulties [28].

Available evidence indicates that these associations described in general child samples are present also in ASD, where externalizing problems tend to be associated with lower intelligence and greater ASD symptom severity [43]. Particularly, most of the literature about children with ASD suggests that higher ASD symptom severity, poorer intellectual functioning, and being male would predict high stable trajectory for externalizing problems, while a pattern of increasing internalizing problems would be predicted by lower ASD symptom severity, better intellectual functioning, and female sex (Fig. 7.1). Low socio-economic status appears to be a common risk factor for both externalizing and internalizing symptoms. With respect to sex/gender differences, studies more specifically aimed at identifying this discrepancy suggest that girls with ASD are as affected as boys with ASD in terms of

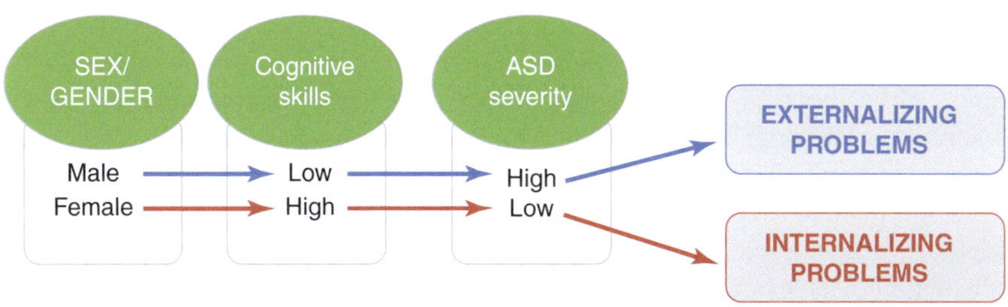

Fig. 7.1 Main predictors of externalizing and internalizing problems according to sex/gender, level of cognitive skills, and level of autism symptom's severity

externalizing problems but are likely more affected than typically developing girls [16], while decreases in disruptive behaviors over time seem to be actually associated with an average IQ and being female [43].

7.4 Aggressive Behaviors in People with ASD

As well summarized by Tsiouris [44], "aggressive behaviors can be normal for the person's chronological or mental age and sex, proactive (offensive) or reactive (defensive), planned (premeditated) or impulsive (affective or disinhibited), cyclical or constant, setting-dependent or setting-independent, and transient or chronic, and their patterns can change depending on the variables initiating, maintaining, or blocking them. Aggressive behaviors can serve the function of establishing dominance, defending a territory, getting attention, retaining isolation, communicating needs, satisfying wishes and needs, or avoiding tasks/demands/places."

Aggressive problems are frequent among children with ASD and constitute a primary reason for concern among caregivers and teachers and a main reason for residential placement [45]. The presence of severe aggressive behavior in youth with ASD was found to increase the likelihood of psychiatric hospitalization by nearly fivefold compared to non-ASD peers. Aggression, irritability, tantrums, and noncompliance are strongly associated with parental stress [46, 47] among children and adolescents, from a very young age [48]. These problems are very frequent in ASD, with prevalence estimates ranging from 16.6% [49] to 78.5% [50], based on age, with rates decreasing with age, and on the assessment measures that were used. Studies using more detailed and specific psychometric tools, such as the Child Behavior Checklist [51, 52], rather than single selected items of the Autism Diagnostic Interview (ADI-R) or Autism Diagnostic Observation Schedule (ADOS), are more reliable and tend to report lower prevalence estimates, with 8–23% of children with ASD presenting with aggressive behavior [53, 54].

Aggressive behaviors in ASD seem to be influenced by several factors, as the severity of a child's ASD symptoms [55] and the presence of intellectual disability, as detailed below, or level of expressive language as they cannot relate, communicate, plan, or solve problems in another way. At the same time, aggressive behaviors in children with ASD strongly impact adaptive functioning, quality of life, parental stress, and general long-term outcome.

Externalizing problems in ASD have been studied mainly in children and adolescents, while the available literature on adults with ASD is relatively scarce. As described in children, also in adults with ASD, aggressive behaviors represent a serious concern and constitute a main reason for requiring a restrictive environment for some patients [44, 56–59]. It seems to be especially frequent among young adults with severe intellectual disability and/or an associated genetic condition or personality disorder. Aggression can be distinguished in verbal or physical aggression and can be directed toward others or the self, with the latter being especially frequent in ASD. Aggressive behavior toward other people or objects was found to be more common among young adults with severe to profound ID. Verbal aggression was associated with younger age in samples with mild to moderate ID, while physical aggression toward self was associated with ASD in general, and especially in females with severe to profound ID and/or ASD [56, 60–67].

In both children and adults with ASD, aggressive behaviors can be due to unresolved medical problems such as pain, constipation, or epilepsy that cause discomfort and arousal problems. Discomfort due to unresolved medical problems or pain may reduce the threshold for tolerance of environmental stimuli that could act as triggers of aggression [59, 68, 69], as it happens with sensory/perceptual overload, which can be a trigger for aggressive behaviors in ASD people. Among a large sample of adults with ASD, triggers of aggression such as frustration, discomfort, change in the physical/social environment, and defensive reactions have been studied, and they are associated with an increasing number of psychiatric disorders such as anxiety disorder, depression, mood disorder, or psychosis [67].

When managing aggression in both children and adults with ASD, especially those with a high burden of ASD symptoms and severe intellectual disability, possible medical conditions must be considered together with the possibility of newly onset psychiatric comorbidity.

7.5 Aggressive Behaviors in Females with ASD

Specific literature regarding aggressive behaviors among females with autism is still extremely scarce. Sex/gender has consistently not been associated with aggressive behavior in children with ASD [47, 54, 70–74]. Self-directed aggression is more common in females with severe ID [66, 75] [69, 76, 77].

Recently, Neuhaus and colleagues investigated child/family factors and communicative skills in relation to aggression among 145 individuals with ASD (65 female; ages 8–17 years), with specific regards to sex/gender differences. They found that whereas aggressive behavior was higher when males were younger and had lower communication skills, the same factors did not appear to be associated with aggression in ASD females: this raised some questions about the possibility of different mechanisms (e.g., temperamental traits, impulsivity) or functions (e.g., escape, protest) underlying aggression among males and females in verbal youth with ASD [78] [79].

Another field unexplored in females with autism is the relationship between aggression, or more in general externalizing behaviors, and menstrual cycle, about which really little is currently known. Premenstrual syndrome has a wide variety of signs and symptoms, including mood swings, breast tenderness, food cravings, fatigue, irritability, and depression, and, especially in low-functioning patients, dysmenorrhea could become a trigger for externalizing behaviors. Exploring aggression and its mechanism or functions in females with ASD remains an important challenge in need of further research and possible development of specific interventions.

7.6 Attention Deficit/Hyperactivity Disorder in Girls with ASD

In the fifth edition of the *Diagnostic and Statistical Manual of Mental Disorders* (DSM-5), ADHD is included in the category of neurodevelopmental disorders, whereas in the DSM-IV-TR, ADHD was classified as a disruptive behavior disorder [80]. Furthermore, the DSM-5, unlike DSM-IV-TR, allows a diagnosis of ADHD to be made in people with ASD [81]. The goal behind these changes is to create a category that represents the developmental trajectories of these disorders and a diagnostic system that accurately accommodates the plasticity of neurodevelopment over the lifespan [82].

The co-occurrence of ADHD among people with ASD is reported to range from 25% to 65% [2], and ADHD is one of the most common comorbidities both in children [83–85] and in adults with ASD [86].

In both ASD and ADHD, most research has predominantly focused on males than on females. This disparity is justified by the male prevalence in clinically identified population with ASD, as mentioned above, and the same phenomenon occurs in the ADHD population, where sex ratio is 3:1 male to female [81, 87] [88].

Some studies identified female sex as a protective factor for ADHD, and for oppositional defiant disorder and tic disorder too [84, 89, 90]. These findings are in contrast with other studies that found equal vulnerability for ADHD in males and females with ASD [7, 91], suggesting a shared neurobiological impairment, supported by twin studies [92, 93], which overrides the usual relative neurodevelopmental resilience of females but shares the same decline in prevalence during postpubertal brain maturation [7]. Beyond genetics, recent meta-analyses, based on neuroimaging findings [94, 95], also supported the concept of ASD and ADHD as disorders of large-scale connectivity, with little overlap in specific regions [96, 97].

Concerning the clinical presentation, overlapping characteristics between ASD and ADHD have been identified in social impairment [98], especially in social function, social perception abilities [99], and social interactions. Also, about the executive functions, there are findings of deficits in both ASD and ADHD, compared to typical-development population [100]. Although each disorder seems to a have a specific profile of executive dysfunction, with ASD showing more severe impairment in cognitive flexibility and ADHD in planning and working memory, subjects with both ASD and ADHD are more severely impaired in all domains [101].

The presence of overlapping symptomatology between ASD and ADHD involves the risk of misdiagnosis or delays in diagnosis [98, 102, 103]. Moreover, research with the specific aim to evaluate if the diagnostic scales that are considered best practices for ASD or ADHD are valid also for diagnosing comorbidities between disorders is still scarce. Specifically, a delay in ASD diagnosis is frequent in children and adolescents with a previous diagnosis of ADHD; this delay seems to be greater for females than for males (2.6 years vs. 1.8 years) [103], consistently with data reported in global ASD population [104].

7.7 Substance Use Disorder and Delinquency in People with ASD

Even though substance use disorder (SUD) is one of the psychiatric comorbidities less frequently diagnosed in people with ASD, a prevalence ranging from 1.3% to 36% was reported in a recent meta-analysis [105]. Specifically, tobacco, alcohol, and cannabis are the substances most commonly selected [106, 107].

Recent research suggests that most of the well-established risk factors for substance abuse in the general population are shared with ASD population [108]. Furthermore, the social impairment and the maladaptive coping strategies frequently present in people with ASD represent specific risk factors for substance use disorder in autism [109]. Anxiolytic effect of alcohol and cannabis indeed could act as social facilitators and help to suppress social anxiety and to better cope with social events [110, 111]. Furthermore, some studies suggest an association between higher autistic traits and increased risk of substance abuse [107, 112]. Also, mood disorders, consistently with the general population, may increase the risk of substance abuse in people with ASD [113].

The combination of these characteristics, together with the higher perception of social deficit in females with ASD, makes sex/gender differences in substance use disorders an interesting field that requires further research in ASD.

Concerning delinquency in ASD, a recent review reported a prevalence ranging from 5% to 26%, while ASD was found in 2–18% of the forensic population studied. Some symptoms of autism, such as the overactive sense of right and wrong and the unwillingness to break the law, tend to act as protective factors from committing criminal behavior. On the other hand, other symptoms of ASD, such as a tendency to misunderstand the behavior of others, represent risks factors for offending behaviors [114]. The diagnosis of ASD has been described as one of the psychiatric disorders more prevalent among individuals who have committed some sex offences, whereas ASD is less prevalent among offenders convicted of other categories of offence, such as property crimes [115]. It seems that some autistic characteristics, such as idiosyncratic interpretations and obsessions, could be related to the motive for the offence. As for TD individuals, in ASD people who exhibit violent offending behaviors, adverse childhood experiences as neglect and child abuse might be significant risk factors [116]. To our knowledge, no specific literature is available on females with ASD as crime perpetrators, while there is some evidence for being the victims of violence. Also in this field, further research is required.

Key Points

- Nearly 70% of people with ASD present at least one comorbid psychiatric disorder.
- Greater symptom severity, lower IQ, and male sex/gender are associated with externalizing problems.
- Prevalence of aggressive behaviors in ASD ranges from 16.6% to 78.5%.
- Self-directed aggression is more common in females with severe ID.
- Medical conditions (with particular regard to menstrual symptoms in females) causing discomfort and arousal problems have to be considered when managing aggression in individuals with ASD.
- ADHD represents the common comorbidity in both children and adults with ASD (co-occurrence rate ranging from 25% to 65%).
- A greater delay in ASD diagnosis is frequent in female children with a previous diagnosis of ADHD.
- The overactive sense of right and the unwillingness to break the law act as protective factors from committing criminal behavior.
- Some autistic characteristics such as tendency to misunderstand others' behavior, idiosyncratic interpretations, and obsessions could represent risk factors for offending behaviors.

References

1. Romero M, et al. Psychiatric comorbidities in autism spectrum disorder: A comparative study between DSM-IV-TR and DSM-5 diagnosis. Int J Clin Heal Psychol. 2016;16:266–75.
2. Hossain MM, et al. Prevalence of comorbid psychiatric disorders among people with autism spectrum disorder: an umbrella review of systematic reviews and meta-analyses. Psychiatry Res. 2020;287:112922.
3. Fitzpatrick SE, Srivorakiat L, Wink LK, Pedapati EV, Erickson CA. Aggression in autism spectrum disorder: presentation and treatment options. Neuropsychiatr Dis Treat. 2016;12:1525–38.
4. Vaillancourt, T. & Boylan, K. Behavioural and emotional disorders of childhood and adolescence. in *Abnormal Psychology: Perspectives, DSM-5 Update Edition (5th ed.)* Pearson Education:Toronto, ON, (2015).
5. Giarelli E, et al. Sex differences in the evaluation and diagnosis of autism spectrum disorders among children. Disabil Health J. 2010;3:107–16.
6. Frazier TW, Georgiades S, Bishop SL, Hardan AY. Behavioral and cognitive characteristics of females and males with autism in the Simons simplex collection. J Am Acad Child Adolesc Psychiatry. 2014;53:329–40.
7. Brereton AV, Tonge BJ, Einfeld SL. Psychopathology in children and adolescents with autism compared to young people with intellectual disability. J Autism Dev Disord. 2006;36:863–70.
8. Simonoff E, et al. Psychiatric disorders in children with autism spectrum disorders: prevalence, comorbidity, and associated factors in a population-derived sample. J Am Acad Child Adolesc Psychiatry. 2008;47:921–9.
9. Postorino V, et al. Longitudinal comparison between male and female preschool children with autism spectrum disorder. J Autism Dev Disord. 2015;45:2046–55.

10. Prosperi M, et al. Sex differences in autism Spectrum disorder: an investigation on Core symptoms and psychiatric comorbidity in preschoolers. Front Integr Neurosci. 2021;14:594082.
11. Lai MC, et al. A behavioral comparison of male and female adults with high functioning autism spectrum conditions. PLoS One. 2011;6:e20835.
12. Mandy W, et al. Sex differences in autism spectrum disorder: evidence from a large sample of children and adolescents. J Autism Dev Disord. 2012;42:1304–13.
13. Boyd A, et al. Gender differences in mental disorders and suicidality in Europe: results from a large cross-sectional population-based study. J Affect Disord. 2015;173:245–54.
14. Seedat S, et al. Cross-national associations between gender and mental disorders in the World Health Organization world mental health surveys. Arch Gen Psychiatry. 2009;66:785–95.
15. Shattuck PT, et al. Change in autism symptoms and maladaptive behaviors in adolescents and adults with an autism spectrum disorder. J Autism Dev Disord. 2007;37:1735–47.
16. Vaillancourt T, et al. Joint trajectories of internalizing and externalizing problems in preschool children with autism spectrum disorder. Dev Psychopathol. 2017;29:203–14.
17. Fombonne E. Epidemiology of pervasive developmental disorders. Pediatr Res. 2009;65:591–8.
18. Maenner MJ, Warren Z, Williams AR, et al. Prevalence and characteristics of autism Spectrum disorder among children aged 8 years — autism and developmental disabilities monitoring network, 11 sites, United States, 2020. MMWR Surveill Summ. 2023;72(SS-2):1–14. https://doi.org/10.15585/mmwr.ss7202a1.
19. Tsai L, Stewart MA, August G. Implication of sex differences in the familial transmission of infantile autism. J Autism Dev Disord. 1981;11:165–73.
20. Wing L. Sex ratios in early childhood autism and related conditions. Psychiatry Res. 1981;5:129–37.
21. Baird G, et al. Prevalence of disorders of the autism spectrum in a population cohort of children in South Thames: the special needs and autism project (SNAP). Lancet (London, England). 2006;368:210–5.
22. Baio J, et al. Prevalence of autism spectrum disorder among children aged 8 years - autism and developmental disabilities monitoring network, 11 sites, United States, 2014. MMWR Surveill Summ. 2018;67:1–23.
23. Loomes R, Hull L, Mandy WPL. What is the male-to-female ratio in autism Spectrum disorder? A systematic review and meta-analysis. J Am Acad Child Adolesc Psychiatry. 2017;56:466–74.
24. Mattila M-L, et al. Autism spectrum disorders according to DSM-IV-TR and comparison with DSM-5 draft criteria: an epidemiological study. J Am Acad Child Adolesc Psychiatry. 2011;50:583–592.e11.
25. Idring S, et al. Autism spectrum disorders in the Stockholm youth cohort: design, prevalence and validity. PLoS One. 2012;7:e41280.
26. Lai MC, Lombardo MV, Auyeung B, Chakrabarti B, Baron-Cohen S. Sex/gender differences and autism: setting the scene for future research. J Am Acad Child Adolesc Psychiatry. 2015;54:11–24.
27. Skuse DH, et al. Social communication competence and functional adaptation in a general population of children: preliminary evidence for sex-by-verbal IQ differential risk. J Am Acad Child Adolesc Psychiatry. 2009;48:128–37.
28. Papachristou E, Flouri E. The codevelopment of internalizing symptoms, externalizing symptoms, and cognitive ability across childhood and adolescence. Dev Psychopathol. 2020;32:1375–89.
29. Emerson E. Prevalence of psychiatric disorders in children and adolescents with and without intellectual disability. J Intellect Disabil Res. 2003;47:51–8.
30. Emerson E, Hatton C. Mental health of children and adolescents with intellectual disabilities in Britain. Br J Psychiatry. 2007;191:493–9.
31. Van Der Ende J, Verhulst FC, Tiemeier H. The bidirectional pathways between internalizing and externalizing problems and academic performance from 6 to 18 years. Dev Psychopathol. 2016;28:855–67.

32. Flouri E, et al. Developmental cascades of internalising symptoms, externalising problems and cognitive ability from early childhood to middle adolescence. Eur Psychiatry. 2019;57:61–9.
33. Campbell SB. Behavior problems in preschool children: clinical and developmental issues. New York: Guilford Press; 2002.
34. Rimm-Kaufman SE, Pianta RC, Cox MJ. Teachers' judgments of problems in the transition to kindergarten. Early Child Res Q. 2000;15:147–66.
35. Sergeant JA, Geurts H, Oosterlaan J. How specific is a deficit of executive functioning for attention-deficit/hyperactivity disorder? Behav Brain Res. 2002;130:3–28.
36. Van der Meere J, Marzocchi GM, De Meo T. Response inhibition and attention deficit hyperactivity disorder with and without oppositional defiant disorder screened from a community sample. Dev Neuropsychol. 2005;28:459–72.
37. Koenen KC, et al. Childhood IQ and adult mental disorders: a test of the cognitive reserve hypothesis. Am J Psychiatry. 2009;166:50–7.
38. Wood SJ, et al. Cognitive decline following psychosis onset: data from the PACE clinic. Br J Psychiatry Suppl. 2007;51:s52–7.
39. Flouri E, Midouhas E. Environmental adversity and children's early trajectories of problem behavior: the role of harsh parental discipline. J Fam Psychol. 2017;31:234–43.
40. Noble KG, et al. Family income, parental education and brain structure in children and adolescents. Nat Neurosci. 2015;18:773–8.
41. Bjørnebekk A, et al. Development of children born to mothers with mental health problems: subcortical volumes and cognitive performance at 4½ years. Eur Child Adolesc Psychiatry. 2015;24:115–8.
42. Farajdokht F, et al. Very low birth weight is associated with brain structure abnormalities and cognitive function impairments: A systematic review. Brain Cogn. 2017;118:80–9.
43. Gray K, et al. Trajectory of behavior and emotional problems in autism. Am J Intellect Dev Disabil. 2012;117:121–33.
44. Tsiouris JA. Pharmacotherapy for aggressive behaviours in persons with intellectual disabilities: treatment or mistreatment? J Intellect Disabil Res. 2010;54:1–16.
45. Mandell DS. Psychiatric hospitalization among children with autism spectrum disorders. J Autism Dev Disord. 2008;38:1059–65.
46. Lecavalier L, Leone S, Wiltz J. The impact of behaviour problems on caregiver stress in young people with autism spectrum disorders. J Intellect Disabil Res. 2006;50:172–83.
47. Mazurek MO, Kanne SM, Wodka EL. Physical aggression in children and adolescents with autism spectrum disorders. Res Autism Spectr Disord. 2013;7:455–65.
48. Giovagnoli G, et al. Behavioral and emotional profile and parental stress in preschool children with autism spectrum disorder. Res Dev Disabil. 2015;45–46:411–21.
49. Mayes SD, et al. Explosive, oppositional, and aggressive behavior in children with autism compared to other clinical disorders and typical children. Res Autism Spectr Disord. 2012;6:1–10.
50. Medeiros K, Kozlowski AM, Beighley JS, Rojahn J, Matson JL. The effects of developmental quotient and diagnostic criteria on challenging behaviors in toddlers with developmental disabilities. Res Dev Disabil. 2012;33:1110–6.
51. Achenbach TM, Rescorla LA. Manual for the ASEBA Preschool Forms & Profiles Child Behaviour Checklist (CBCL) ages 1 1/2 - 5. In: Manual for the ASEBA Preschool Forms and Profiles; 2000. p. 74–100.
52. Achenbach TM, Rescorla L. Manual for the ASEBA school-age forms & profiles : an integrated system of multi-informant assessment. Burlington: ASEBA; 2001.
53. Georgiades S, et al. Phenotypic overlap between core diagnostic features and emotional/ behavioral problems in preschool children with autism spectrum disorder. J Autism Dev Disord. 2011;41:1321–9.
54. Hartley SL, Sikora DM, McCoy R. Prevalence and risk factors of maladaptive behaviour in young children with autistic disorder. J Intellect Disabil Res. 2008;52:819–29.
55. Jang J, Dixon DR, Tarbox J, Granpeesheh D. Symptom severity and challenging behavior in children with ASD. Res Autism Spectr Disord. 2011;5:1028–32.

56. Crocker AG, et al. Prevalence and types of aggressive behaviour among adults with intellectual disabilities. J Intellect Disabil Res. 2006;50:652–61.
57. Crocker AG, Mercier C, Allaire J-F, Roy M-E. Profiles and correlates of aggressive behaviour among adults with intellectual disabilities. J Intellect Disabil Res. 2007;51:786–801.
58. Cohen IL, Yoo JH, Goodwin MS, Moskowitz L. Assessing challenging behaviors in autism Spectrum disorders: prevalence, rating scales, and autonomic indicators. In: Matson JL, Sturmey P, editors. International handbook of autism and pervasive developmental disorders. New York: Springer; 2011. p. 247–70. https://doi.org/10.1007/978-1-4419-8065-6_15.
59. Tsiouris JA, Kim SY, Brown WT, Cohen IL. Association of aggressive behaviours with psychiatric disorders, age, sex and degree of intellectual disability: a large-scale survey. J Intellect Disabil Res. 2011;55:636–49.
60. Moss S, et al. Psychiatric symptoms in adults with learning disability and challenging behaviour. Br J Psychiatry. 2000;177:452–6.
61. McClintock K, Hall S, Oliver C. Risk markers associated with challenging behaviours in people with intellectual disabilities: A meta-analytic study. J Intellect Disabil Res. 2003;47:405–16.
62. Rojahn J, Matson JL, Naglieri JA, Mayville E. Relationships between psychiatric conditions and behavior problems among adults with mental retardation. Am J Ment Retard. 2004;109:21–33.
63. Holden B, Gitlesen JP. A total population study of challenging behaviour in the county of Hedmark, Norway: prevalence, and risk markers. Res Dev Disabil. 2006;27:456–65.
64. Cooper S-A, van der Speck R. Epidemiology of mental ill health in adults with intellectual disabilities. Curr Opin Psychiatry. 2009;22:431–6.
65. Cooper S-A, et al. Adults with intellectual disabilities: prevalence, incidence and remission of self-injurious behaviour, and related factors. J Intellect Disabil Res. 2009;53:200–16.
66. Cohen IL, et al. A large scale study of the psychometric characteristics of the IBR modified overt aggression scale: findings and evidence for increased self-destructive behaviors in adult females with autism spectrum disorder. J Autism Dev Disord. 2010;40:599–609.
67. Cohen IL, Tsiouris JA. Triggers of aggressive behaviors in intellectually disabled adults and their association with autism, medical conditions, psychiatric disorders, age and sex: A large-scale study. J Autism Dev Disord. 2020;50:3748–62.
68. Barnhill LJ. The diagnosis and treatment of individuals with mental illness and developmental disabilities: an overview. Psychiatry Q. 2008;79:157–70.
69. Tsiouris JA, Cohen IL, Patti PJ, Korosh WM. Treatment of previously undiagnosed psychiatric disorders in persons with developmental disabilities decreased or eliminated self-injurious behavior. J Clin Psychiatry. 2003;64:1081–90.
70. Sikora DM, Hall TA, Hartley SL, Gerrard-Morris AE, Cagle S. Does parent report of behavior differ across ADOS-G classifications: analysis of scores from the CBCL and GARS. J Autism Dev Disord. 2008;38:440–8.
71. Murphy O, Healy O, Leader G. Risk factors for challenging behaviors among 157 children with autism spectrum disorder in Ireland. Res Autism Spectr Disord. 2009;3:474–82.
72. Kanne SM, Mazurek MO. Aggression in children and adolescents with ASD: prevalence and risk factors. J Autism Dev Disord. 2011;41:926–37.
73. Farmer CA, Aman MG. Aggressive behavior in a sample of children with autism spectrum disorders. Res Autism Spectr Disord. 2011;5:317–23.
74. Kozlowski AM, Matson JL, Rieske RD. Gender effects on challenging behaviors in children with autism spectrum disorders. Res Autism Spectr Disord. 2012;6:958–64.
75. Cooper S-A, et al. Adults with intellectual disabilities: prevalence, incidence and remission of aggressive behaviour and related factors. J Intellect Disabil Res. 2009;53:217–32.
76. Marston GM, Perry DW, Roy A. Manifestations of depression in people with intellectual disability. J Intellect Disabil Res. 1997;41(Pt 6):476–80.
77. Hemmings CP, Gravestock S, Pickard M, Bouras N. Psychiatric symptoms and problem behaviours in people with intellectual disabilities. J Intellect Disabil Res. 2006;50:269–76.

78. Neuhaus E, et al. Language and aggressive behaviors in male and female youth with autism Spectrum disorder. J Autism Dev Disord. 2021;52:454–62. https://doi.org/10.1007/s10803-020-04773-0.
79. Neuhaus E, Webb SJ, Bernier RA. Linking social motivation with social skill: the role of emotion dysregulation in autism spectrum disorder. Dev Psychopathol. 2019;31:931–43.
80. Doernberg E, Hollander E. Neurodevelopmental disorders (ASD and ADHD): DSM-5, ICD-10, and ICD-11. CNS Spectr. 2016;21:295–9.
81. American Psychiatric Association. *Diagnostic and statistical manual of mental disorders.* 5th ed *(DSM 5)*; 2013.
82. Wilson CE, et al. Comparison of ICD-10R, DSM-IV-TR and DSM-5 in an adult autism spectrum disorder diagnostic clinic. J Autism Dev Disord. 2013;43:2515–25.
83. Yerys BE, Wallace GL, Jankowsi KF, Bollich A, Kenworthy L. Impaired consonant trigrams test (CTT) performance relates to everyday working memory difficulties in children with autism spectrum disorders. Child Neuropsychol. 2011;17:391–9.
84. Salazar F, et al. Co-occurring psychiatric disorders in preschool and elementary school-aged children with autism Spectrum disorder. J Autism Dev Disord. 2015;45:2283–94.
85. Joshi G, et al. Symptom profile of ADHD in youth with high-functioning autism Spectrum disorder: A comparative study in psychiatrically referred populations. J Atten Disord. 2017;21:846–55.
86. Lugo-Marín J, et al. Prevalence of psychiatric disorders in adults with autism spectrum disorder: A systematic review and meta-analysis. Res Autism Spectr Disord. 2019;59:22–33.
87. Sayal K, Prasad V, Daley D, Ford T, Coghill D. ADHD in children and young people: prevalence, care pathways, and service provision. Lancet Psychiatry. 2018;5:175–86.
88. Levy F, Hay DA, Bennet KS, McStephen M. Gender differences in ADHD subtype comorbidity. J Am Acad Child Adolesc Psychiatry. 2005;44:368–76.
89. May T, Cornish K, Rinehart NJ. Gender profiles of behavioral attention in children with autism Spectrum disorder. J Atten Disord. 2016;20:627–35.
90. Hull L, Mandy W, Petrides KV. Behavioural and cognitive sex/gender differences in autism spectrum condition and typically developing males and females. Autism. 2017;21:706–27.
91. Gadow KD, Devincent CJ, Pomeroy J, Azizian A. Comparison of DSM-IV symptoms in elementary school-age children with PDD versus clinic and community samples. Autism. 2005;9:392–415.
92. Jokiranta-Olkoniemi E, et al. Risk of psychiatric and neurodevelopmental disorders among siblings of probands with autism spectrum disorders. JAMA Psychiatry. 2016;73:622–9.
93. Ghirardi L, et al. The familial co-aggregation of ASD and ADHD: A register-based cohort study. Mol Psychiatry. 2018;23:257–62.
94. Di Martino A, et al. Shared and distinct intrinsic functional network centrality in autism and attention-deficit/hyperactivity disorder. Biol Psychiatry. 2013;74:623–32.
95. Bethlehem RAI, Romero-Garcia R, Mak E, Bullmore ET, Baron-Cohen S. Structural covariance networks in children with autism or ADHD. Cereb Cortex. 2017;27:4267–76.
96. Dougherty CC, Evans DW, Myers SM, Moore GJ, Michael AM. A comparison of structural brain imaging findings in autism Spectrum disorder and attention-deficit hyperactivity disorder. Neuropsychol Rev. 2016;26:25–43.
97. Rommelse N, Buitelaar JK, Hartman CA. Structural brain imaging correlates of ASD and ADHD across the lifespan: a hypothesis-generating review on developmental ASD–ADHD subtypes. J Neural Transm. 2017;124:259–71.
98. Antshel KM, Russo N. Autism Spectrum disorders and ADHD: overlapping phenomenology, diagnostic issues, and treatment considerations. Curr Psychiatry Rep. 2019;21:34.
99. Baribeau DA, et al. Examining and comparing social perception abilities across childhood-onset neurodevelopmental disorders. J Am Acad Child Adolesc Psychiatry. 2015;54:479–486.e1.
100. Craig F, et al. A review of executive function deficits in autism spectrum disorder and attention-deficit/hyperactivity disorder. Neuropsychiatr Dis Treat. 2016;12:1191–202.

101. Colombi C, Ghaziuddin M. Neuropsychological characteristics of children with mixed autism and ADHD. Autism Res Treat. 2017;2017:1–5.
102. Stevens T, Peng L, Barnard-Brak L. The comorbidity of ADHD in children diagnosed with autism spectrum disorder. Res Autism Spectr Disord. 2016;31:11–8.
103. Kentrou V, de Veld DMJ, Mataw KJK, Begeer S. Delayed autism spectrum disorder recognition in children and adolescents previously diagnosed with attention-deficit/hyperactivity disorder. Autism. 2019;23:1065–72.
104. Lai M-C, Baron-Cohen S. Identifying the lost generation of adults with autism spectrum conditions. Lancet Psychiatry. 2015;2:1013–27.
105. Ressel M, et al. Systematic review of risk and protective factors associated with substance use and abuse in individuals with autism spectrum disorders. Autism. 2020;24:899–918.
106. Sizoo B, van den Brink W, van Eenige MG, van der Gaag RJ. Personality characteristics of adults with autism Spectrum disorders or attention deficit hyperactivity disorder with and without substance use disorders. J Nerv Ment Dis. 2009;197:450–4.
107. De Alwis D, et al. ADHD symptoms, autistic traits, and substance use and misuse in adult Australian twins. J Stud Alcohol Drugs. 2014;75:211–21.
108. Butwicka A, et al. Increased risk for substance use-related problems in autism Spectrum disorders: A population-based cohort study. J Autism Dev Disord. 2017;47:80–9.
109. Kronenberg LM, Goossens PJJ, Van Busschbach J, Van Achterberg T, Van den Brink W. Coping styles in substance use disorder (SUD) patients with and without co-occurring attention deficit/hyperactivity disorder (ADHD) or autism spectrum disorder (ASD). BMC Psychiatry. 2015;15:1–8.
110. Kronenberg LM, Slager-Visscher K, Goossens PJJ, van den Brink W, van Achterberg T. Everyday life consequences of substance use in adult patients with a substance use disorder (SUD) and co-occurring attention deficit/hyperactivity disorder (ADHD) or autism spectrum disorder (ASD): A patient's perspective. BMC Psychiatry. 2014;14:1–9.
111. Clarke T, Tickle A, Gillott A. Substance use disorder in Asperger syndrome: an investigation into the development and maintenance of substance use disorder by individuals with a diagnosis of Asperger syndrome. Int J Drug Policy. 2016;27:154–63.
112. Mulligan RC, Reiersen AM, Todorov AA. Attention-deficit/hyperactivity disorder, autistic traits, and substance use among Missouri adolescents. Scand J child Adolesc psychiatry Psychol. 2014;2:86–92.
113. Lalanne L, Weiner L, Trojak B, Berna F, Bertschy G. Substance-use disorder in high-functioning autism: clinical and neurocognitive insights from two case reports. BMC Psychiatry. 2015;15:1–5.
114. Rutten AX, Vermeiren RRJM, Van Nieuwenhuizen C. Autism in adult and juvenile delinquents: A literature review. Child Adolesc Psychiatry Ment Health. 2017;11:1–12.
115. 't Hart-Kerkhoffs, L. A. *et al.* Autism spectrum disorder symptoms in juvenile suspects of sex offenses. J Clin Psychiatry 70, 266–272 (2009).
116. Allely CS, et al. Violence is rare in autism: when it does occur, is it sometimes extreme? J Psychol. 2017;151:49–68.

Sex Differences in Epilepsy and Other Medical Comorbidities

8

Laurie A. Brenner, Erika J. Axeen, and Katheryn F. Frazier

8.1 Introduction

Medical comorbidities are more common in autism spectrum disorder (ASD) than in the general population [1, 2]. Comorbid conditions with an especially high prevalence in ASD include epilepsy, sleep disturbance, digestive disorders (e.g., constipation), and feeding issues. For autistic females, there is also growing evidence that hormonal and reproductive challenges may occur more often than in non-autistic females [3]. This chapter focuses on epilepsy because it is one of the most common medical comorbidities in ASD [1], and autistic females are at higher risk for epilepsy than males [3, 4]. We also provide general information about the co-occurrence and management of sleep disturbances, digestive disorders, feeding issues, and reproductive challenges that can accompany ASD. Timely diagnosis and treatment of co-occurring medical conditions are essential to overall health and well-being. Accurate diagnosis can be complicated by autism-related symptoms, such as communication difficulties and atypical behaviors [5], as well as co-occurring cognitive conditions such as intellectual disability [6]. A good understanding of commonly occurring medical conditions and related signs and symptoms enables early intervention when problems arise to minimize the negative impact on the quality of life. In the sections below, we summarize current research and share a novel, multidisciplinary treatment approach to managing care for these individuals.

L. A. Brenner (✉) · E. J. Axeen
Department of Neurology, University of Virginia, Charlottesville, VA, USA
e-mail: Lb3sj@virginia.edu

K. F. Frazier
Department of Pediatrics, University of Virginia, Charlottesville, VA, USA

L. Mazzone et al. (eds.), *Autism Spectrum Disorder: Understanding the Female Phenotype*, https://doi.org/10.1007/978-3-031-62072-0_8

8.2 ASD and Epilepsy

The median prevalence of epilepsy in ASD is 12% [7] compared to a 1% epilepsy prevalence in the general population [8, 9]. The pathophysiological link between ASD and epilepsy is not known. In ASD, as in the general population, epilepsy is an etiologically and clinically heterogeneous condition with variable ages of onset [7, 10, 11]. Compared to ASD only, autistic individuals with epilepsy tend to have lower intelligence, lower adaptive functioning [12–14], increased healthcare utilization [15], and increased risk of death [16]. For individuals first diagnosed with ASD, the onset of seizures is associated with a decline in daily living skills [13], indicating greater dependence on caregivers to accomplish basic self-care activities in the home. Greater reliance on caregivers is associated with higher levels of caregiver stress [17], and mothers of children with both ASD and epilepsy report a lower perceived quality of life when compared to mothers of children with ASD alone [18].

The comorbidity of ASD and epilepsy can be a "double burden" for families. There are frequent visits to a neurologist for medication management and often additional medical tests such as electroencephalogram (EEG) and neuroimaging that can be stressful for a person on the autism spectrum. Some of these medical visits include physical contact that can be unpleasant or painful (e.g., electrode placement, physical exam, blood draw), and the environment is often characterized by bright lights, unusual noises, and unfamiliar faces. Medications used to treat seizures may have side effects that exacerbate mood or behavior problems or are associated with cognitive slowing. Many families also cope with sleep disruption if seizures are nocturnal, visits to the emergency department, anxiety/fear about the risk of physical injury or sudden unexplained death in epilepsy (SUDEP), general uncertainty about when the subsequent seizure will occur, and occupational/childcare issues if a child misses school on account of seizures.

When ASD and epilepsy co-occur, complex symptom-symptom and symptom-treatment interactions can differ from either condition in isolation. Understanding both conditions—in isolation and combination—is essential for providing high-quality, comprehensive, and patient-centered care. In the sections below, we summarize current research on clinical presentation and potential etiologies and discuss how a multidisciplinary approach to diagnosis and management can improve outcomes.

8.2.1 Clinical Characteristics and Sex Differences

In autistic individuals, the age of seizure onset has a bimodal distribution, with the first peak in early childhood and a second possibly higher peak in adolescence [19–21]. A population-based study reported 10% or lower prevalence rates in children under 12, increasing to 26.2% by adolescence [14]. Other studies have not shown an increased risk in adolescence [22, 23], possibly due to differences in study design. Epilepsy within ASD is heterogeneous; no specific seizure type or epilepsy syndrome is associated with autism [22, 23]. Both focal and generalized seizures are common [22].

Clinical characteristics that may differentiate ASD with epilepsy from ASD only include higher rates of intellectual disability [12] and higher levels of hyperactivity and repetitive and/or sensory behaviors [24, 25]. Adaptive functioning is lower overall [13, 14], even in patients who do not have an intellectual disability diagnosis. There is also a higher percentage of patients who are nonverbal or minimally verbal than in the ASD-only population [26].

Autistic females may be disproportionately affected by epilepsy. Although there are reports to the contrary [12, 21], the preponderance of evidence suggests that the male:female ratio is lower in ASD with epilepsy compared to ASD only [22, 23]. For example, a meta-analysis [4] found a male:female ratio in autism with epilepsy of 2:1 compared to 3.5:1 in autism only. Furthermore, autistic females with epilepsy may be more likely to present with neuroimaging abnormalities and to have a higher risk of medication-resistant epilepsy than males [27]. One potential confounding factor is the higher rate of intellectual disability in autistic females [28, 29]. Intellectual disability is independently associated with epilepsy [30] and could conceivably explain the different sex/gender ratio in ASD with epilepsy. Interestingly, in the study by Blackmon et al. [27], there were no sex/gender differences in intellectual ability even though females had a more severe epilepsy phenotype. Although there is still much to be discovered about the presentation of epilepsy in autistic females, existing research highlights the importance of modeling sex/gender differences when examining risk factors for epilepsy as well as treatment response.

8.2.2 Etiology

Despite a high rate of co-occurrence [7], the casual mechanisms of ASD with epilepsy are not fully understood. Severe epilepsy types such as developmental and epileptic encephalopathy (DEE) may contribute to ASD symptom manifestation or exacerbation. In other cases, ASD is evident in early childhood, but seizures do not develop until adolescence or adulthood. The overlap and temporal variability in symptom manifestation raise the possibility of common neurobiological pathways predisposing to seizures and ASD symptoms. Proposed etiologies include genetic and nongenetic factors [31–35].

Genetic syndromes and single-gene disorders associated with high rates of ASD and epilepsy include fragile X, Angelman, Phelan-McDermid, and tuberous sclerosis complex (TSC), among others. TSC is a multisystem neurocutaneous syndrome caused by pathogenic variants in the *TSC1* and *TSC2* genes, which are part of the mammalian target of rapamycin—"mTOR"—signaling pathway that regulates cell growth. Clinical features of TSC include hamartomas (overgrowths) in various organs, such as the skin and central nervous system and associated neurological and neuropsychiatric disorders [36, 37]. ASD and epilepsy occur alone and as comorbid features in TSC. Earlier seizure onset and higher seizure frequency are each associated with having an ASD diagnosis [38, 39]. From a treatment standpoint, early intervention and better management of seizures in TSC reduce the risk of ASD [40]. Therefore, TSC provides an interesting model in which there is an underlying genetic etiology and the potential for symptom exacerbation as a function of specific neurobiological characteristics.

Advances in genetic technology have increased our understanding of risk beyond the more well-known genetic syndromes. For example, genes involved in synaptic function and structure (e.g., *NRX1, SHANK3*) and neurotransmission (e.g., *SYNGAP1, GABRG1*) could predispose to one or both conditions, with emergent phenotype contingent upon gene-gene and/or gene-environment interactions [41]. Many of these genes have been implicated in ASD, epilepsy, or both. In addition to *TSC1/TSC2*, other mTOR signaling pathway genes regulate neuron development, synaptic properties, and white matter connectivity. The spectrum of aberrant developmental outcomes associated with mTOR dysregulation includes focal cortical dysplasia and hemimegalencephaly [32], which are associated with epilepsy and may also increase the risk for ASD/autistic traits. Genetics is a rapidly advancing field; as basic science uncovers new links between genetic variants and symptom expression, findings can be translated into the clinical realm to clarify their clinical significance for individual patients. The discovery of new genetic candidates in ASD and epilepsy will open the door to clinical trials that assess whether specific treatments are more effective for certain genetic profiles.

Evidence reviewed here and elsewhere [32] supports the hypothesis of a genetic pathogenesis in at least a subset of individuals with autism and epilepsy; however, other etiologies could lead to similar clinical outcomes via their effects on brain development and function. Among the possible candidates for shared pathogenesis are maternal immune activation [42], postnatal immune dysfunction and/or inflammation [33, 43], premature birth and associated complications [34, 35, 44], and cortical malformation [31]. Cortical malformations, such as dysplasia, heterotopia, or megalencephaly, are often associated with genetic etiologies but in the case of a somatic mutation may not be detectable by routine genetic test panels [45]. In conclusion, there are undoubtedly multiple underlying etiologies, both genetic and nongenetic, that can result in ASD and epilepsy. Future research may gain traction by identifying the relationship between underlying etiology and phenotypic expression, such as epilepsy type, language development, and/or severity of repetitive and restricted behaviors. Ultimately, zeroing in on subtypes of the autism-epilepsy spectrum will be informative for clinical trials that lead to precision medicine approaches to optimize treatment response.

8.2.3 Clinical Management

The intersection of ASD and epilepsy creates a unique clinical presentation with potentially complex diagnostic and treatment needs. Providers well versed in both conditions are more likely to recognize concerning symptoms and refer for additional evaluation. Access to multidisciplinary care increases the odds of accurate diagnosis and appropriate treatment.

In patients first diagnosed with ASD, autistic symptoms may obscure seizures and delay an epilepsy diagnosis. For example, nonepileptic stereotypies, common in the ASD phenotype, are a potential confounding factor that can complicate diagnosis. Other complicating factors include the absence of self-report (e.g., description of seizure aura) in nonverbal patients with severe intellectual disability. Familiarity with typical seizure semiology and how that differs from other repetitive or stereotyped behaviors is essential. Additional data used to evaluate epilepsy include an electroencephalogram (EEG) and sometimes neuroimaging. In the setting of ASD, clinical interpretation of EEG findings is complicated by high base rates of electrographic abnormalities without a clinical correlate. In individuals with no seizure history, interictal epileptiform discharges occur at ~5% in non-autistic individuals [46], whereas the rate may be as high as 20–60% in autistic individuals [47–49]. A thorough clinical history and video recording of behavioral events, in addition to EEG, can increase diagnostic precision.

Epilepsy alone is associated with cognitive dysfunction [50], and delays or deficits in the domains of language and executive function can overlap with the clinical phenotype of ASD. In patients first diagnosed with epilepsy, social, language, and behavioral difficulties may be assumed secondary to the epilepsy syndrome, reducing the likelihood that other diagnoses such as ASD are considered in the differential. Children with epilepsy may also present with more dynamic features of ASD when compared to the more classic ASD phenotype suggested by the Diagnostic and Statistical Manual of Mental Disorders-fifth Edition [51]. In children with DEE, symptoms of ASD may only appear after the onset of the encephalopathy, and the associated developmental regression can occur at a later age than the regression seen in ASD without epilepsy. While most will have a stable profile of ASD characteristics from early in childhood, others may see a worsening or improvement in their ASD traits over time, and members of the treatment team should reassess at various time points to see whether the current diagnoses are still appropriate.

Evaluation of ASD in a patient with epilepsy should be conducted by providers familiar with both conditions, as many widely available standardized diagnostic tools were developed for idiopathic ASD using predominately male populations without co-occurring complex medical conditions. Developmentally appropriate assessment is optimized in a multidisciplinary team setting where a thorough assessment of language, cognition, and adaptive functioning can be completed in addition to an extended developmental history focused on social communication and atypical and/or maladaptive behaviors. Unfortunately, many resource-poor areas do not have access to such a team, and many children do not receive accurate diagnoses.

Accurate diagnosis of ASD and/or intellectual disability is essential to connect individuals and families with appropriate treatments and school supports. For example, an ASD diagnosis will qualify a child for applied behavior analysis (ABA) or other behavioral support that may not be available with the epilepsy diagnosis alone. In the case of intellectual disability, it can facilitate access to community resources and help the school identify an appropriate educational approach that is centered on functional academics and life skills to maximize independence and self-actualization. Accurate diagnosis is also helpful for family members and for the child's treatment team as it allows the family and others to understand what types of support may be needed beyond anti-seizure medications to improve communication, behavior, and general functioning.

From a medical standpoint, individuals with both autism and epilepsy provide an extra level of complexity when treating their seizures and/or their behaviors with medications. As will be discussed below, sleep disorders often occur in ASD, and poor sleep can exacerbate seizure frequency in those with epilepsy. If the individual has nocturnal seizures, that can also interfere with sleep, making seizure control and daytime behaviors more difficult.

Medications used for behavior often do not work as well in those with both ASD and epilepsy as compared to those with ASD only or to those who are typically developing [52]. Furthermore, in more medically complex patients, providers must closely monitor for drug-drug interactions. Many of the antipsychotic medications used to treat aggressive behavior and irritability in ASD may increase or decrease levels of seizure medication in the blood, affecting seizure management. Additionally, some medications such as bupropion, a selective norepinephrine reuptake inhibitor used for depression, can lower the seizure threshold [53]. Stimulant medications, used for the treatment of comorbid attention problems, which are common in both ASD and epilepsy, have been shown not to affect seizure frequency in patients with epilepsy [54]; however, families may need reassurance and education on research findings when they are reluctant to add a stimulant medication.

8.3 Other Medical Comorbidities

Many autistic individuals are affected by more than one medical comorbidity, with accumulating evidence that females have more medical comorbidities compared to autistic males or typically developing females. Medication interactions and side effects can complicate treatment decisions. For example, some seizure medications can exacerbate behavioral problems, and deciding to adjust dosing, switch medications, or add another medication requires good communication among providers.

8.3.1 Sleep

Sleep-related problems are the most commonly reported comorbidity in ASD, with up to 80% of patients affected over the lifespan. Multiple aspects of sleep can be affected, including sleep onset, maintenance, efficiency, and total sleep time. Difficulty with sleep onset is one of the most common presenting symptoms. Autistic individuals can also have significant behavioral challenges around the transition to sleep. The lack of quality sleep significantly affects daytime behavior, ability to communicate, and daily living activities and can impact other physical and mental health issues such as seizure occurrence and mood symptoms. The effects are often passed along to the caregiver, who also gets little sleep as a result, affecting the entire family's quality of life [55].

8.3.2 Gastrointestinal Disorders

Gastrointestinal disorders are extremely common in ASD and can affect individuals across the lifespan. Abdominal pain, constipation, and diarrhea are reported at higher levels in those with ASD than those without [56]. Children with ASD and gastrointestinal symptoms are more likely to have high levels of irritability and affective symptoms compared to those with ASD without gastrointestinal symptoms [57]. Chronic functional constipation is the most frequently reported symptom, particularly among those with more impairing levels of ASD and intellectual disability. The etiology of constipation is multifactorial, but sensory processing differences, difficulties with toilet training secondary to communication or cognitive delays, and poor nutritional intake can all play a role.

8.3.3 Feeding Behaviors

Problematic feeding behaviors are more commonly seen in autistic patients compared to those who are typically developing. Autistic children are more likely to have food selectivity, with a low number of acceptable foods they will eat, often due to texture difficulties or the need for sameness in appearance or presentation. In addition, they can have more aberrant behaviors surrounding mealtime, such as food refusal, throwing food, or refusing to sit for mealtime. Maladaptive feeding behavior can lead to significant stress for caregivers and puts those with ASD at risk of nutritional deficiencies and growth failure [58, 59].

8.3.4 Reproductive and Endocrine Concerns

A recent review of health concerns in autistic females highlights the increased risk of reproductive and endocrine disorders compared to typically developing females. Autistic females have reported higher levels of autism-specific sensory and emotional symptoms in relation to their menstrual cycles, along with higher rates of dysmenorrhea and cycle irregularity [60]. In addition, higher rates of thyroid disease, polycystic ovarian syndrome, ovarian cancer, and difficulties during pregnancy (including preeclampsia and preterm birth) have all been reported in studies using electronic medical records or health registry data [3].

8.4 Treatment Models

Effective management of medical comorbidities requires timely access to specialists and open communication channels to coordinate treatments and address medication interactions and side effects. Patients with complex needs can benefit from a "medical home" that is patient centered, comprehensive, coordinated, accessible, culturally sensitive, and committed to quality and safety [61].

To be patient and family centered, it is helpful if at least one member of the medical team has specialized knowledge about ASD [62], particularly for lower functioning patients with cognitive limitations or who are minimally verbal, so that decision-making respects the needs, wants, and preferences of the patient within the family context. A team member with ASD experience may also decrease the risk of diagnostic overshadowing, e.g., recognizing when the ASD diagnosis does NOT encompass an ASD patient's repetitive behaviors and referring to a neurologist to evaluate possible seizures. To be comprehensive and coordinated, the team of relevant specialists must be organized to facilitate communication and data integration so that decisions are not made in isolation. Accessibility is one of the biggest challenges for medically complex patients served by multiple specialists, with visits typically scheduled on different days in different locations. Multidisciplinary or interdisciplinary clinics, where multiple specialists see families in a single clinic visit, can improve accessibility for families and communication among providers. Clinics situated in a broader health system can be particularly effective because other specialists are readily available, and results can be easily reviewed or shared via the medical record system. Quality and safety are maximized when multiple specialists work together in an adequately resourced health system to address the complex needs and preferences of the patient.

With these criteria in mind, the authors of this chapter developed a new clinic—Clinic for Autism Plus Epilepsy (CAPE)—to serve patients with ASD, epilepsy, and other comorbidities. Core providers include a developmental pediatrician, an epileptologist (neurologist with specialized epilepsy training), a neuropsychologist, and a care coordinator. The clinic is situated at an academic medical center in a level 4 epilepsy center. One of the strengths of our clinic model is that we continue to follow patients through adolescence and into early adulthood. We use standardized measures, such as the Autism Impact Measure [63–65] and Aberrant Behavior Checklist [66, 67], to track symptoms and inform medical decision-making.

Our developmental pediatrician and neuropsychologist have experience diagnosing, assessing, and managing children on the autism spectrum. The epileptologist has neurogenetics training and extensive experience as part of our epilepsy surgery team in identifying patients with medically refractory epilepsy who may be good candidates for surgical intervention. The care coordinator provides essential support for scheduling, answering patient questions, referrals to other specialists, and interfacing with insurance companies for authorization purposes. Patients are scheduled to see the developmental pediatrician and epileptologist at every visit. The neuropsychologist sees patients for an initial visit and is then available for follow-up as needed. Common reasons for follow-up with neuropsychology include assessment of nonverbal intelligence in a minimally verbal patient, pre-surgical baseline, or more extensive profiling of strengths and weaknesses to supplement the school's psychoeducational evaluation. Other specialists who are not officially part of the clinic but who are readily accessible include a social worker, educational specialist, autism family navigator, pediatric gastroenterologist, psychologist, sleep specialist, endocrinologist, and genetic counselor.

Treatment guidelines for seizures do not differ for someone with ASD compared to someone without; however, in clinical practice, it is often necessary to consider treatment-related exacerbation of mood, behavior, and/or sleep issues as well as medication interactions, which must be factored into medical decision-making. One in three youth with epilepsy is medically refractory [68], meaning seizures persist despite multiple medication trials. Less complex epilepsy patients can be managed by a general neurologist, but when seizures become medically refractory, the quality-of-care standard is for patients to be referred to a comprehensive epilepsy center for evaluation. Pre-surgical evaluation to determine whether the individual is a good candidate for surgery or other procedure (e.g., laser ablation) includes neuroimaging, long-term EEG monitoring, and neuropsychological testing. Special considerations relevant to epilepsy patients with ASD may include sedation for a positron emission tomography (PET) scan, difficulty complying with prolonged EEG monitoring, and/or a different approach to the intracranial monitoring phase depending on the individual's functional and intellectual level. We provide two case examples below to illustrate how our clinic can assist with comprehensive care.

Example 1 Patient 1 is a 16-year-old female with autism diagnosed at 2 years of age and seizure onset at 9 years of age. She is minimally verbal and requires assistance with most activities of daily living, including bathing and dressing. Seizures were managed by a neurologist in private practice until puberty, when seizure severity and frequency increased significantly. At her initial CAPE visit, seizures were medically refractory, and she was having monthly episodes of status epilepticus with associated breathing difficulties necessitating a trip to the emergency department. A Phase 1 pre-surgical evaluation revealed multifocal seizures, and she was not deemed appropriate for surgical resection. Her CAPE epileptologist made several significant changes to her medication regimen, including switching her to new medications and adjusting doses to bring seizures under better control. Medication decision-making was complicated by worsening of autistic symptoms (particularly repetitive behaviors), sleep disturbance, aggression, and elopement. The epileptologist and developmental pediatrician worked closely together to track symptoms, treat symptom exacerbation, and manage other comorbidities such as sleep disturbance. Patient 1 continues to have seizures, but they are much less severe (now focal impaired awareness rather than status epilepticus) and do not require visits to the emergency department. Managing behavior and sleep continues to be a challenge, but with her epilepsy stable, the family is in a better position to partner with school specialists and therapists to target maladaptive behaviors.

Patient 1 exemplifies the complex issues that can arise for patients with ASD and medical comorbidities. The epileptologist was able to leverage her expertise to develop a more effective treatment plan, resulting in improved family quality of life and reduced risk for morbidity. The multidisciplinary team helped evaluate the most likely contributors to behavior change (seizure frequency vs. seizure medication vs. stressors at school/home vs. sleep deprivation vs. other medical issues) and plan treatment accordingly. Regular follow-ups, and the data from rating scales administered at each visit, helped monitor response to treatment and facilitate frequent communication among providers so that adjustments to the treatment plan could be made to optimize benefit and minimize undesirable side effects.

Example 2 Patient 2 is a 13-year-old male with seizure onset at 18 months of age and autism diagnosis at 8 years of age. He was seen for neuropsychological evaluation and diagnosed with mild intellectual disability and attention deficit/hyperactivity disorder (ADHD). He has mild anxiety. Medical history is notable for status epilepticus, right mesial temporal sclerosis, and right temporal cortical dysplasia. Seizure type is focal impaired awareness with and without secondary generalization. He has an individualized education plan for school. The family lives over an hour away from their medical home, so streamlining visits in a single clinic was more convenient for them and less disruptive to work and school schedules.

Patient 2 continued to have seizures despite multiple medication trials. His epileptologist referred him for a Phase 1 epilepsy pre-surgical evaluation, and he subsequently underwent stereotactic laser ablation of the mesial temporal lobe. He has been seizure free since the laser ablation, and the epileptologist is gradually weaning him off his epilepsy medication. The developmental pediatrician plays a key role in managing his ADHD, monitoring anxiety, coordinating access to the educational specialist as needed to advocate for appropriate special education services, and ensuring that the family is connected to autism resources in the area. The care coordinator plays an essential role in orchestrating schedules to minimize travel time and missed school/work. He is scheduled for follow-up with neuropsychology to assess progress and update recommendations as he prepares for the transition to high school.

Patient 2 illustrates the value added by multiple specialists participating in an individual's care to manage comorbidities across the lifespan and to identify potential candidates for epilepsy surgery. The CAPE clinic facilitated communication among the epileptologist, developmental pediatrician, and neuropsychologist to ensure that the patient and his family understood their options and the care team was working together to respect their wishes. By sharing information openly, we were better able to anticipate future needs and to create a timetable for follow-up and medication change relative to major life events (e.g., laser ablation procedure, transition to high school).

8.5 Key Points

In summary, we highlight the following key points about autism spectrum disorder (ASD) and the co-occurrence of epilepsy and other medical comorbidities:

- Epilepsy is the most common comorbid medical condition, and it disproportionately affects autistic females.
- Although there is substantial heterogeneity in clinical characteristics, individuals with both ASD and epilepsy tend to have a higher level of support needs (lower

intelligence, greater dependence on caregivers) than individuals who have ASD but not epilepsy, and this can have a substantial impact on the family's quality of life.

- The diagnosis and management of ASD and epilepsy are optimized when providers have familiarity with both conditions alone *and in combination* because ASD may present differently in the context of epilepsy and vice versa.
- No seizure type or underlying etiology is associated with ASD plus epilepsy. Possible mechanisms for shared pathogenesis include genetic, metabolic, immunological, and complications related to premature birth.
- Other common medical comorbidities in ASD, such as sleep disturbance and gastrointestinal and/or feeding issues, can complicate care and require consideration of drug-drug interactions and side effects that can exacerbate other symptoms.
- Multidisciplinary care teams help identify and address symptoms promptly and monitor behavior over time to optimize the treatment regimen. Frequent communication among providers improves the quality of patient care, particularly for more medically complex patients. Care teams in a more extensive healthcare system are well positioned to coordinate with other specialists and facilitate access to resources.

References

1. Brondino N, Fusar-Poli L, Miccli E, Di Stefano M, Damiani S, Rocchetti M, et al. Prevalence of medical comorbidities in adults with autism Spectrum disorder. J Gen Intern Med. 2019;34(10):1992–4.
2. Al-Beltagi M. Autism medical comorbidities. World J Clin Pediatr. 2021;10(3):15–28.
3. Kassee C, Babinski S, Tint A, Lunsky Y, Brown HK, Ameis SH, et al. Physical health of autistic girls and women: a scoping review. Mol Autism. 2020;11(1):84.
4. Amiet C, Gourfinkel-An I, Bouzamondo A, Tordjman S, Baulac M, Lechat P, et al. Epilepsy in autism is associated with intellectual disability and gender: evidence from a meta-analysis. Biol Psychiatry. 2008;64(7):577–82.
5. Association AP. Diagnostic and statistical manual of mental disorders, vol. xliv. 5th ed. Arlington, VA; 2013. p. 947.
6. Matson JL, Shoemaker M. Intellectual disability and its relationship to autism spectrum disorders. Res Dev Disabil. 2009;30(6):1107–14.
7. Lukmanji S, Manji SA, Kadhim S, Sauro KM, Wirrell EC, Kwon CS, et al. The co-occurrence of epilepsy and autism: a systematic review. Epilepsy Behav. 2019;98(Pt A):238–48.
8. Forsgren L, Beghi E, Oun A, Sillanpaa M. The epidemiology of epilepsy in Europe - a systematic review. Eur J Neurol. 2005;12(4):245–53.
9. Zack MM, Kobau R. National and state estimates of the numbers of adults and children with active epilepsy - United States, 2015. MMWR Morb Mortal Wkly Rep. 2017;66(31):821–5.
10. Spence SJ, Schneider MT. The role of epilepsy and epileptiform EEGs in autism spectrum disorders. Pediatr Res. 2009;65(6):599–606.
11. Alaimo H, Geller E, Mahalingam R, Rodriguez A, Goldberg R, Bojko A, et al. Ictal EEG in patients with autistic spectrum disorder and epilepsy. Epilepsy Res. 2020;168:106482.

12. Woolfenden S, Sarkozy V, Ridley G, Coory M, Williams K. A systematic review of two outcomes in autism spectrum disorder - epilepsy and mortality. Dev Med Child Neurol. 2012;54(4):306–12.
13. Capal JK, Macklin EA, Lu F, Barnes G. Factors associated with seizure onset in children with autism Spectrum disorder. Pediatrics. 2020;145:S117–S25.
14. Viscidi EW, Triche EW, Pescosolido MF, McLean RL, Joseph RM, Spence SJ, et al. Clinical characteristics of children with autism spectrum disorder and co-occurring epilepsy. PLoS One. 2013;8(7):e67797.
15. Kohane IS, McMurry A, Weber G, MacFadden D, Rappaport L, Kunkel L, et al. The co-morbidity burden of children and young adults with autism spectrum disorders. PLoS One. 2012;7(4):e33224.
16. Gillberg C, Billstedt E, Sundh V, Gillberg IC. Mortality in autism: a prospective longitudinal community-based study. J Autism Dev Disord. 2010;40(3):352–7.
17. Postorino V, Gillespie S, Lecavalier L, Smith T, Johnson C, Swiezy N, et al. Clinical correlates of parenting stress in children with autism Spectrum disorder and serious behavioral problems. J Child Fam Stud. 2019;28(8):2069–77.
18. Celik H, Acikel SB, Ozdemir FMA, Aksoy E, Oztoprak U, Cucu E, et al. Evaluation of the anxiety level of mothers of children with epilepsy during the COVID-19 pandemic period. Eur Neurol. 2021;84(3):192–9.
19. Volkmar FR, Nelson DS. Seizure disorders in autism. J Am Acad Child Adolesc Psychiatry. 1990;29(1):127–9.
20. Kawasaki Y, Yokota K, Shinomiya M, Shimizu Y, Niwa S. Brief report: electroencephalographic paroxysmal activities in the frontal area emerged in middle childhood and during adolescence in a follow-up study of autism. J Autism Dev Disord. 1997;27(5):605–20.
21. Hara H. Autism and epilepsy: a retrospective follow-up study. Brain and Development. 2007;29(8):486–90.
22. Jokiranta E, Sourander A, Suominen A, Timonen-Soivio L, Brown AS, Sillanpaa M. Epilepsy among children and adolescents with autism spectrum disorders: a population-based study. J Autism Dev Disord. 2014;44(10):2547–57.
23. Danielsson S, Gillberg IC, Billstedt E, Gillberg C, Olsson I. Epilepsy in young adults with autism: a prospective population-based follow-up study of 120 individuals diagnosed in childhood. Epilepsia. 2005;46(6):918–23.
24. Cuccaro ML, Tuchman RF, Hamilton KL, Wright HH, Abramson RK, Haines JL, et al. Exploring the relationship between autism spectrum disorder and epilepsy using latent class cluster analysis. J Autism Dev Disord. 2012;42(8):1630–41.
25. Viscidi EW, Johnson AL, Spence SJ, Buka SL, Morrow EM, Triche EW. The association between epilepsy and autism symptoms and maladaptive behaviors in children with autism spectrum disorder. Autism. 2014;18(8):996–1006.
26. Bolton PF, Carcani-Rathwell I, Hutton J, Goode S, Howlin P, Rutter M. Epilepsy in autism: features and correlates. Br J Psychiatry. 2011;198(4):289–94.
27. Blackmon K, Bluvstein J, MacAllister WS, Avallone J, Misajon J, Hedlund J, et al. Treatment resistant epilepsy in autism Spectrum disorder: increased risk for females. Autism Res. 2016;9(2):311–20.
28. Loomes R, Hull L, Mandy WPL. What is the male-to-female ratio in autism Spectrum disorder? A systematic review and meta-analysis. J Am Acad Child Adolesc Psychiatry. 2017;56(6):466–74.
29. Posserud MB, Skretting Solberg B, Engeland A, Haavik J, Klungsoyr K. Male to female ratios in autism spectrum disorders by age, intellectual disability and attention-deficit/hyperactivity disorder. Acta Psychiatr Scand. 2021;144:635–46.
30. Morgan CL, Baxter H, Kerr MP. Prevalence of epilepsy and associated health service utilization and mortality among patients with intellectual disability. Am J Ment Retard. 2003;108(5):293–300.
31. Blackmon K. Structural MRI biomarkers of shared pathogenesis in autism spectrum disorder and epilepsy. Epilepsy Behav. 2015;47:172–82.

32. Specchio N, Di Micco V, Trivisano M, Ferretti A, Curatolo P. The epilepsy-autism spectrum disorder phenotype in the era of molecular genetics and precision therapy. Epilepsia. 2021;63:6–21.
33. Lewis ML, Kesler M, Candy SA, Rho JM, Pittman QJ. Comorbid epilepsy in autism spectrum disorder: implications of postnatal inflammation for brain excitability. Epilepsia. 2018;59(7):1316–26.
34. Allen L, Leon-Attia O, Shaham M, Shefer S, Gabis LV. Autism risk linked to prematurity is more accentuated in girls. PLoS One. 2020;15(8):e0236994.
35. Li W, Peng A, Deng S, Lai W, Qiu X, Zhang L, et al. Do premature and postterm birth increase the risk of epilepsy? An updated meta-analysis Epilepsy Behav. 2019;97:83–91.
36. Henske EP, Jozwiak S, Kingswood JC, Sampson JR, Thiele EA. Tuberous sclerosis complex. Nat Rev Dis Primers. 2016;2:16035.
37. Northrup H, Krueger DA. International tuberous sclerosis complex consensus G. Tuberous sclerosis complex diagnostic criteria update: recommendations of the 2012 Iinternational tuberous sclerosis complex consensus conference. Pediatr Neurol. 2013;49(4):243–54.
38. Numis AL, Major P, Montenegro MA, Muzykewicz DA, Pulsifer MB, Thiele EA. Identification of risk factors for autism spectrum disorders in tuberous sclerosis complex. Neurology. 2011;76(11):981–7.
39. Specchio N, Pietrafusa N, Trivisano M, Moavero R, De Palma L, Ferretti A, et al. Autism and epilepsy in patients with tuberous sclerosis complex. Front Neurol. 2020;11:639.
40. Bombardieri R, Pinci M, Moavero R, Cerminara C, Curatolo P. Early control of seizures improves long-term outcome in children with tuberous sclerosis complex. Eur J Paediatr Neurol. 2010;14(2):146–9.
41. Lo-Castro A, Curatolo P. Epilepsy associated with autism and attention deficit hyperactivity disorder: is there a genetic link? Brain and Development. 2014;36(3):185–93.
42. Pineda E, Shin D, You SJ, Auvin S, Sankar R, Mazarati A. Maternal immune activation promotes hippocampal kindling epileptogenesis in mice. Ann Neurol. 2013;74(1):11–9.
43. Vargas DL, Nascimbene C, Krishnan C, Zimmerman AW, Pardo CA. Neuroglial activation and neuroinflammation in the brain of patients with autism. Ann Neurol. 2005;57(1):67–81.
44. Hirschberger RG, Kuban KCK, O'Shea TM, Joseph RM, Heeren T, Douglass LM, et al. Co-occurrence and severity of neurodevelopmental burden (cognitive impairment, cerebral palsy, autism Spectrum disorder, and epilepsy) at age ten years in children born extremely preterm. Pediatr Neurol. 2018;79:45–52.
45. Nishioka M, Bundo M, Iwamoto K, Kato T. Somatic mutations in the human brain: implications for psychiatric research. Mol Psychiatry. 2019;24(6):839–56.
46. Eeg-Olofsson O, Petersen I, Sellden U. The development of the electroencephalogram in normal children from the age of 1 through 15 years. Paroxysmal activity. Neuropadiatric. 1971;2(4):375–404.
47. Rossi PG, Parmeggiani A, Bach V, Santucci M, Visconti P. EEG features and epilepsy in patients with autism. Brain and Development. 1995;17(3):169–74.
48. Hughes SW, Crunelli V. Thalamic mechanisms of EEG alpha rhythms and their pathological implications. Neuroscientist. 2005;11(4):357–72.
49. Hughes JR, Melyn M. EEG and seizures in autistic children and adolescents: further findings with therapeutic implications. Clin EEG Neurosci. 2005;36(1):15–20.
50. Badawy RA, Johnson KA, Cook MJ, Harvey AS. A mechanistic appraisal of cognitive dysfunction in epilepsy. Neurosci Biobehav Rev. 2012;36(8):1885–96.
51. Holmes H, Sawer F, Clark M. Autism spectrum disorders and epilepsy in children: a commentary on the occurrence of autism in epilepsy; how it can present differently and the challenges associated with diagnosis. Epilepsy Behav. 2021;117:107813.
52. Besag F, Aldenkamp A, Caplan R, Dunn DW, Gobbi G, Sillanpää M. Psychiatric and Behavioural disorders in children with epilepsy (ILAE task force report): epilepsy and autism. Epileptic Disord. 2016;18(s1):S16–23.

53. Johnston JA, Lineberry CG, Ascher JA, Davidson J, Khayrallah MA, Feighner JP, et al. A 102-center prospective study of seizure in association with bupropion. J Clin Psychiatry. 1991;52(11):450–6.
54. Dunn D, Williams A, Giust J, Kronenberger W. Epilepsy and attention-deficit hyperactivity disorder: links, risks, and challenges. Neuropsychiatr Dis Treat. 2016;12:287.
55. Feng S, Huang H, Wang N, Wei Y, Liu Y, Qin D. Sleep disorders in children with autism Spectrum disorder: insights from animal models, especially non-human primate model. Front Behav Neurosci. 2021;15:673372.
56. McElhanon BO, McCracken C, Karpen S, Sharp WG. Gastrointestinal symptoms in autism Spectrum disorder: a meta-analysis. Pediatrics. 2014;133(5):872–83.
57. Chaidez V, Hansen RL, Hertz-Picciotto I. Gastrointestinal problems in children with autism, developmental delays or typical development. J Autism Dev Disord. 2014;44(5):1117–27.
58. Ledford JR, Gast DL. Feeding problems in children with autism Spectrum disorders. Focus Autism Other Dev Disabil. 2006;21(3):153–66.
59. Curtin C, Hubbard K, Anderson SE, Mick E, Must A, Bandini LG. Food selectivity, mealtime behavior problems, spousal stress, and family food choices in children with and without autism Spectrum disorder. J Autism Dev Disord. 2015;45(10):3308–15.
60. Steward R, Crane L, Mairi Roy E, Remington A, Pellicano E. "Life is much more difficult to manage during periods": autistic experiences of menstruation. J Autism Dev Disord. 2018;48(12):4287–92.
61. AHRQ. Agency for Healthcare Research and Quality. U.S. Department of Health & Human Services. https://pcmh.ahrq.gov/page/defining-pcmh.
62. Farmer JE, Clark MJ, Mayfield WA, Cheak-Zamora N, Marvin AR, Law JK, et al. The relationship between the medical home and unmet needs for children with autism Spectrum disorders. Matern Child Hlth J. 2014;18(3):672–80.
63. Mazurek MO, Carlson C, Baker-Ericzen M, Butter E, Norris M, Kanne S. Construct validity of the autism impact measure (AIM). J Autism Dev Disord. 2020;50(7):2307–19.
64. Mazurek MO, Carlson C, Baker-Ericzen M, Butter E, Norris M, Barr C, et al. The autism impact measure (AIM): examination of sensitivity to change. Autism Res. 2020;13(11):1867–79.
65. Kanne SM, Mazurek MO, Sikora D, Bellando J, Branum-Martin L, Handen B, et al. The autism impact measure (AIM): initial development of a new tool for treatment outcome measurement. J Autism Dev Disord. 2014;44(1):168–79.
66. Kaat AJ, Zelko F, Wilkening G, Berg AT. Evaluation of the aberrant behavior checklist for developmental and epileptic encephalopathies. Epilepsy Behav. 2021;119:107958.
67. Kaat AJ, Lecavalier L, Aman MG. Validity of the aberrant behavior checklist in children with autism spectrum disorder. J Autism Dev Disord. 2014;44(5):1103–16.
68. Kalilani L, Sun X, Pelgrims B, Noack-Rink M, Villanueva V. The epidemiology of drug-resistant epilepsy: a systematic review and meta-analysis. Epilepsia. 2018;59(12):2179–93.

Part IV

Treatment

9 The Role of Sex and Gender Differences in Psychosocial Treatment Strategies for Autism Spectrum Disorder

Julia Zhong, Eliya Ahmad, Carla B. Kalvin, and Denis G. Sukhodolsky

9.1 Gender Differences in Autism and Implications for Treatment

There has been increasing recognition of sex and gender differences in autism spectrum disorder (ASD), including ongoing research on the "female autism phenotype," which describes how the manifestation of autism symptoms in girls and women may differ from the common expression of autism in boys and men, on which the diagnostic criteria and research have focused [1]. The behavioral expressions of autism in girls represent similar symptoms to those in the current diagnostic criteria, including difficulties with social communication and interaction, restricted interests and repetitive behaviors, and sensory sensitivities, but they may be expressed in ways that differ from the traditional diagnostic criteria [2]. For instance, girls on the spectrum often demonstrate stronger social motivation, fewer signs of repetitive behaviors, and narrow interests, and they tend to focus more on social information and learning while making more efforts towards social coping than boys on the spectrum [1]. They are often more able to demonstrate reciprocal conversation and can be more motivated to initiate friendships [3]. Special interests may go unnoticed in girls since topics may focus on interests similar to those of neurotypical peers [4].

Furthermore, females with ASD may also express other behaviors or characteristics, such as camouflaging or "masking," i.e., hiding their ASD-related impairments, not currently considered in the ASD diagnostic criteria [2]. These behavioral differences, in addition to gender biases in the diagnostic criteria, position females with ASD at an elevated risk of being undiagnosed or misdiagnosed compared to

J. Zhong · E. Ahmad · C. B. Kalvin · D. G. Sukhodolsky (✉)
Yale University School of Medicine, Child Study Center, New Haven, CT, USA
e-mail: denis.sukhodolsky@yale.edu

L. Mazzone et al. (eds.), *Autism Spectrum Disorder: Understanding the Female Phenotype*, https://doi.org/10.1007/978-3-031-62072-0_9

males with ASD. In fact, in adult ASD diagnostic services, the gender ratio is lower (2 males to 1 female) than in child services up to 11 years of age (5 males to 1 female), demonstrating that ASD diagnosis in females is often missed in early development [5]. This chapter addresses how sex differences in autistic behavioral phenotypes can be incorporated into clinical conceptualization and treatment planning.

Girls on the spectrum can also be affected by societal gender expectations and social norms, which contribute to the development of autistic girls. Autistic girls may feel pressured to conform to gender-related expectations of a neurotypical world where society expects girls and women to be empathetic, communicative, and emotionally expressive and where society disapproves of neurotypical women who do not conform to those standards. Thus, girls on the spectrum can feel the pressure to "camouflage" or "mask" their symptoms to fit in with these social expectations [1, 6]. In fact, "masking" is common among ASD females due to the demand to fit in with the neurotypical world and to disguise social interaction difficulties such as feelings of unease and anxiety in social situations [4]. Camouflaging or masking can be exhausting and contribute to poorer mental health due to the excessive effort required to maintain the expected behavior [4]. Indeed, camouflaging is linked to increased self-reported stress and anxiety compared to those who do not mask their autistic traits [7, 8]. Gender-based norms and expectations also impact peer socializing practices in ways that can uniquely impact autistic girls. Due to sex/gender differences in exposure to and reinforcement for social behavior beginning in early childhood, girls and boys learn to socialize with peers differently. Among girls, peer socialization focuses more on interpersonal relationships, emotions, and sharing stories about oneself, all of which require nuanced social communication skills. Consequently, language and social communication deficits conferred by ASD may represent more of an impediment to everyday peer interactions for girls than boys and thus may be more detrimental to girls' social development than boys [9].

Societal expectations can also play a role in the elevated levels of co-occurring psychopathologies for females on the autism spectrum. Adolescent girls with ASD exhibit more internalizing symptoms, such as anxiety and depression, than typically developing girls and boys with ASD [10, 11]. Adolescent girls on the spectrum with self-care skills below those of same-aged peers or more limited social interactions or relationships can also develop a negative self-perception, elevating the risk of manifesting internalizing symptoms [12].

Other key gender differences concern the age of diagnosis and access to services. Compared to men with ASD, women on the autism spectrum are often diagnosed later in life, precluding them from accessing essential services early in development. Further, since most interventions and therapies for autism are directed to children and early adolescents, autistic women diagnosed in late adolescence or adulthood have far fewer services available to them when they are most likely to seek help [6]. In a recent study, Gesi et al. found that in a sample of 61 adults with ASD, females experienced a significantly greater delay in both referral to mental health services and an older age of ASD diagnosis (mean age of diagnosis being 29.4 years) compared to males (19.8 years) [13]. Similarly, within a large, population-based cohort of children with ASD, females received a formal diagnosis later than their age-equivalent males [14]. Relatedly, many services for autistic children are accessed through education and school services; without a diagnosis, many girls on the spectrum cannot utilize these resources. Although most studies of autism include small sample sizes of girls, making it challenging to assess gender equity in services, Yianni-Coudurier et al. found that girls with ASD had higher placement levels into regular versus self-contained classes [15]. Similarly, May et al. found that significantly fewer females received integration-aide support at school in a sample of equal numbers of boys and girls on the spectrum [16]. Concerns salient to women, such as reproductive health and parenting, have almost no empirical autism research [17, 18]. Unique challenges for females with ASD include maintaining long-term friendships, navigating puberty, and fearing exploitation in romantic and sexual relationships [4, 19, 20].

Given the differences in the expressions and experiences of girls on the spectrum, it is critical to consider how autism treatments may need to be tailored to be accessible and effective and address the unique needs of girls with ASD. This chapter reviews some of the more common interventions for autism symptoms and associated conditions with particular attention to sex/gender considerations and how existing interventions could be tailored to the unique needs of girls on the spectrum.

9.2 Applied Behavior Analysis and Related Treatments

Applied behavior analysis, or ABA, was one of the earliest interventions for people with autism and is currently the most commonly practiced intervention for ASD. Based on the principles of behaviorism, ABA relies on operant conditioning to change behaviors. Specifically, the antecedents and consequences of behaviors are analyzed and modified as needed to change behavior. There are many components to specific ABA interventions, and certain aspects of ABA have given way to new interventions that use principles of ABA without adhering to strict ABA models. Despite differences in the structure, format, and emphasis of different ABA-based interventions, most ABA-based interventions demonstrate moderate to high levels of efficacy, with improvements most consistently shown in communication, expressive language, and socialization [21]. The following section describes the main ABA and ABA-based interventions, including relevant findings and implications for gender differences in treatment delivery and response.

9.2.1 Discrete Trial Training

Discrete trial training, or DTT, is one of the earliest ABA approaches based on breaking skills down into specific tasks. For example, a child with autism may be taught how to communicate using sign language by teaching the child to use a specific sign in a specific circumstance and then expanding the skill to different settings, as was done successfully by Carr and Dores [22]. Correct responses are positively reinforced to increase their occurrence. Specific reinforcement strategies vary depending on the child's age and developmental stage and can include praise or access to a preferred item, among others [23]. Other DTT techniques include prompting and prompt fading when teaching new skills; prompts may include verbal, visual, and physical prompts.

Discrete trial training was pioneered by Dr. O. Ivar Lovaas and has since been studied in various settings [24]. For example, a 2012 study assessed the effectiveness of DTT in mainstream preschool settings and found that DTT generated greater improvements in adaptive and intellectual functioning compared to a control group receiving treatment as usual [25]. A review of 22 studies assessing DTT was conducted in 2016 and demonstrated that children in high-intensity DTT programs showed greater improvements in multiple areas, including intellectual functioning, adaptive skills, expressive and receptive language, visual-spatial skills, social skills, nonverbal communication, and play skills, as compared to control groups [26].

Despite the popularity of DTT, no studies have tested the impacts of sex/gender on the efficacy of DTT, and the studies that list the gender breakdown of their participants have typically included significantly more boys than girls. However, one pilot study testing a DTT-based intervention in an all-female sample of minimally verbal girls with ASD has demonstrated promising results. Of the ten preschool-aged girls in the study, those randomized to the intervention group, demonstrated improvements in social initiation [27]. Still, despite these promising results, more research is needed to assess whether DTT is equally effective in boys and girls. One obvious conclusion from the literature is that boys are more likely to be enrolled in clinical studies of DTT than girls. Until the sample sizes of girls in the randomized trials are sufficient for statistical hypothesis testing, it would be informative if future studies documented specific tasks and skills that are targeted in female participants as well as any clinical observations about the type of antecedents, rewards, and implementation of DTT techniques with girls.

Early intensive behavioral intervention (EIBI) (also known as early intensive behavioral treatment) is an early intervention model for young children with autism based on the principles of ABA. EIBI interventions, which typically comprise between 15 and 40 h per week, can be implemented across settings, such as home and school, and can utilize various teaching methods, such as discrete trial training and other ABA-based interventions. Studies have shown that children receiving EIBI when implemented early and at a high intensity have more positive outcomes than children receiving other intervention methods [24]. In a 2020 study, higher intensity EIBI was associated with more positive outcomes than EIBI delivered with fewer intervention hours. Yet, even an EIBI program with fewer than recommended intervention hours was more effective than an eclectic treatment comparison group [28]. According to a 2018 review, studies of EIBI consistently demonstrate improvements in adaptive behavior, IQ, and expressive and language skills. However, many of the studies of EIBI either have small sample sizes or utilize suboptimal designs, limiting the power to draw conclusions [29]. Further research using more rigorous study designs must be conducted to draw stronger conclusions regarding the efficacy of EIBI. Additionally, of all the included studies that reported the sex/gender breakdown of their participants, the vast majority were male; further research should investigate whether sex/gender significantly impacts the efficacy of EIBI.

9.2.2 Pivotal Response Treatment

Pivotal response treatment (or PRT, also known as pivotal response training) is a naturalistic behavioral intervention based on the principles of ABA. Like ABA, PRT utilizes the principle of operant conditioning to build desired skills. However, instead of targeting individual behaviors, PRT focuses on "pivotal" areas of development, including motivation, self-initiation, responsiveness to multiple cues, and self-regulation of behavior [30]. Instead of focusing on the adult-directed practice of specific tasks, PRT is delivered through naturally occurring situations in a child's daily life, such as play, and utilizes naturally occurring positive reinforcement. As such, progress made through PRT may be more generalizable to broader contexts compared to other forms of applied behavior analysis [31].

Initial studies of PRT aimed to improve language skills by utilizing naturally occurring conditions [31]. This was later expanded to other domains, including social reciprocity and adaptive behavior. Numerous studies have demonstrated the benefits of PRT across many different domains. A 2016 meta-analysis analyzed 34 studies of PRT for individuals with ASD and reported improvements across multiple domains, including play skills, social skills, and academic skills. All studies found that PRT was effective and generated improvements in the domains studied [32]. Of note, across the 34 studies included in the meta-analysis, 71.2% of participants were male.

While most studies of PRT have not analyzed sex/gender differences in treatment response, a 2007 study tested the efficacy of PRT across different demographics, including sex/gender. One hundred and fifty-eight families participated in a 12-week intervention in which parents were trained to implement PRT. While both boys and girls significantly improved daily living skills, socialization, and adaptive behaviors, only boys significantly improved communications skills [33]. These findings indicate that while PRT is generally effective for both boys and girls, there may be differences in the efficacy for girls, specifically in areas of communication. A recent study by Terroso and colleagues tested sex/gender differences in the effects of PRT on co-occurring symptoms of externalizing and internalizing disorders [34]. Participants included 30 children with ASD (10 girls and 20 boys aged 4–11 years) who received 6 h of PRT per week for 16 weeks. Emotional and behavioral symptoms were assessed before and after treatment using the Child Behavior Checklist (CBCL). Results indicated no sex/gender differences in comorbid symptoms at baseline, and both girls and boys showed improvement in emotional and behavioral problems following PRT. While this study supports the efficacy of PRT as a treatment for emotional and behavioral symptoms in boys and girls with ASD, clearly, more research on sex/gender differences in PRT treatment outcomes, particularly in the area of communication, needs to be conducted.

9.2.3 Early Start Denver Model (Early Intervention, ABA-Based, Naturalistic, Parent-Led)

The Early Start Denver Model (ESDM) was developed as an early intervention program for toddlers and young children diagnosed with ASD [35]. ESDM targets areas of development impacted by ASD, including language skills and interpersonal communication, by integrating principles of ABA with developmental approaches and play therapy. ESDM can be implemented in a wide variety of settings. Typically, trained professionals teach ESDM principles to parents, who implement it in naturalistic settings. Parents can select priority objectives on which to focus therapeutic attention, generating a high degree of individualization for each child's treatment plan. Regarding empirical support, the efficacy of ESDM was tested in a randomized controlled trial against a control group who received interventions in the community; 48 children between the ages of 18 months and 30 months who had ASD diagnoses were assigned to receive either an ESDM intervention or interventions through community providers. Over 2 years, the ESDM group received 20 h of therapy per week from trained clinicians and an average of 16.3 h per week of parent-implemented therapy. Compared to children in the community control group, children who received ESDM showed a significant increase in cognitive abilities and more adaptive developmental trajectories in social skills and daily living skills [35]. The male-female ratio of participants was 3.5:1, but no data analysis of sex/gender differences was reported.

A 2020 meta-analysis of 12 studies of ESDM reported moderate effect sizes for improvements in cognition ($g = 0.412$) and language ($g = 0.408$) but no significant effects for measures of autism symptomatology, adaptive behavior, social communication, or restrictive and repetitive behaviors. Approximately 80% of subjects in studies of ESDM were male, but no analysis of the effects of sex on treatment outcomes was reported. Importantly, the researchers noted that the high proportion of male participants could obscure potential differences in outcomes for girls, since autism symptoms often present differently in girls than boys, even as infants and toddlers [36].

9.2.4 Floortime Therapy (Early Intervention, Naturalistic, Play-Based, Child-Led)

Floortime therapy, or DIRFloortime, is a play-based intervention stemming from the developmental, individual-difference, relationship-based model, or DIR, framework developed by Dr. Stanley Greenspan [37]. Designed for children with developmental delays such as ASD, the DIR model focuses on strengthening developmental foundations leading to developing new skills rather than directly teaching new skills. During Floortime, adults engage children in unstructured play while encouraging growth in capacities such as communication, problem-solving, and engagement. Several studies of Floortime, ranging from two single-subject designs to a 2-year study of 200 children receiving Floortime, have demonstrated positive outcomes in the areas of communication, shared engagement, emotional functioning, problem-solving, and daily living skills [37–39]. However, many of these and other studies of Floortime use less rigorous experimental methods. A meta-analysis conducted in 2017 analyzed the methods and results of ten studies assessing Floortime therapy. While all studies showed favorable results for DIR/Floortime, only half utilized a comparison group or randomized trial design. Of those that did, the intensity of the experimental and comparison interventions was not equivalent, limiting the conclusiveness of the study results [40]. Further research with more experimental rigor must be conducted before Floortime therapy can be considered an evidence-based treatment, although preliminary research seems favorable.

9.2.5 Joint Attention

Joint attention, which consists of nonverbally communicating about an object or event with another person through eye contact and gestures, is a frequent deficit of people with autism [41]. Such deficits are thought to be connected to other deficits common in ASD, namely in language and social abilities [42]. Interventions have been developed to target joint attention and improve joint attention behaviors in people with autism. Typically, joint attention training interventions utilize principles of ABA, including discrete trial training and pivotal response training. Since joint attention behaviors do not usually develop in typically developing children until around 14–18 months of age, most joint attention interventions for children with ASD are aimed at children with mental ages around this range [43]. In a single-subject design study from 2000, behavioral and developmental approaches were used to teach joint attention initiations to a child with ASD, indicating that the teaching of joint attention is possible [44]. In another study utilizing principles of ABA to target multiple aspects of joint attention, the target behaviors (responding to showing, pointing, and gaze shifting of adults; coordinated gaze shifting; and pointing) were successfully taught to 4-year-olds with a mental age over 14 months and were generalized to other contexts outside the study [45]. Parent-training models of joint attention training, in which parents are taught to implement joint attention training interventions, have also been shown to be effective with 1- to 2-year-old children [46]. In addition to demonstrating improvements in joint attention, studies of joint attention training have also been linked to improvements in expressive language and social-communicative characteristics [47]. Many of the studies assessing joint attention training did not mention the sex/gender breakdown of the participants, and those that did included more boys than girls.

A naturalistic developmental behavioral intervention called JASPER, which stands for "Joint Attention, Symbolic Play, Engagement, and Regulation," aims to improve social-communication skills for minimally verbal children with ASD. JASPER facilitates joint attention through play routines and consequently promotes targeted communication skills. Supporting the efficacy of JASPER, in a

2012 study of the intervention delivered to 3- to 5-year-old minimally verbal children with ASD, children who received a 12-week version of JASPER showed greater improvements in play diversity and gesture initiation compared to children receiving treatment as usual [48]. Regarding treatment mechanisms of JASPER, preliminary evidence suggests that improvements in joint engagement may mediate improvements in initiated joint attention and later improvements in language when delivered to 2- through 5-year-old children [49].

9.3 Cognitive Behavioral Therapies

Cognitive behavioral therapy (CBT) can be a useful treatment option for autistic individuals who experience comorbid mental health conditions, such as anxiety, depression, or irritability. CBT teaches new skills for coping with negative emotions, such as monitoring negative thoughts and replacing them with more adaptive ones [50]. CBT approaches often utilize structured treatment manuals that feature specific techniques for building coping skills and problem-solving or behavioral exposure exercises that have been modified for individuals with ASD [51]. Unlike other interventions for children with ASD, which focus on early childhood and have been primarily studied and tested in the period from infancy through preschool, CBT is typically used with elementary- and middle-school-aged children and has been primarily studied in children in this age range.

9.3.1 Cognitive Behavioral Therapy (CBT) for Anxiety in Autism

Comorbid anxiety disorders are common in children and adolescents with autism spectrum disorder, with prevalence rates ranging between 11% and 84% [52, 53]. Higher levels of anxiety symptoms in ASD are associated with more behavioral problems and can negatively impact the quality of life [54]. Cognitive-behavioral therapy (CBT) has been shown to be highly effective in reducing symptoms of anxiety disorders in typically developing children [55], and there is a growing body of evidence of its effectiveness for children with ASD who can engage in verbal communication [50, 56, 57].

Examples of structured CBT programs for anxiety include Coping Cat [58], Coping Koala [59], and Skills for Academic and Social Success [60]. To adapt standard CBT for anxiety programs for children with ASD, several CBT interventions have been developed that include modifications and additions to the standard CBT format. Common modifications include the use of visual stimuli or strategies (e.g., emotion "thermometers," cue cards related to circumscribed interests), motivating metaphors, social stories, modules on social skills, increased number of exposures, extended psychoeducation for parents, and school collaboration [56]. Other useful modifications include focusing on social skills deficits, encouraging the development of daily living skills, and capitalizing on children's specialized interests for greater therapy engagement.

Results of two meta-analyses of CBT treatments for anxiety in children with ASD (including both adapted and non-adapted treatments) have demonstrated promising results. When compared to children in control conditions, children with ASD receiving CBT for anxiety showed greater reductions in anxiety, with moderate effect sizes [50, 57]. In addition, parent involvement in treatment was linked to higher levels of improvement [57].

Regarding the issue of adapting treatment for children with ASD, several studies support the utility of modifying treatment for this population. In their study comparing the effectiveness of a standard CBT treatment for anxiety in children with and without ASD, van Steensel and Bogels found that, although standard CBT for anxiety disorders was effective for children with ASD, it was less effective in reducing anxiety and improving quality of life than it was for children without ASD. These results indicate that standard CBT may be insufficient for children with ASD [54]. Relatedly, in the meta-analyses conducted by Perihan et al. (2020), interventions of longer duration had a greater effect on reducing anxiety symptoms for children with ASD [57]. This result suggests that children with ASD may need greater intervention dosages to obtain comparable effects to their non-ASD peers, potentially due to the longer duration of time needed for those with ASD to understand and apply strategies for coping. Further supporting the use of adapted treatments, in their randomized controlled trial comparing a standard CBT program, an adapted CBT program for ASD, and treatment as usual, Wood and colleagues found that CBT adapted for ASD outperformed the other conditions on internalizing symptom scales, social-communication symptoms, and anxiety-associated social functioning [51]. Lastly, results from a randomized controlled trial of an adapted CBT program implemented in a general child psychiatric hospital in Denmark suggest the potential for adapted CBT for ASD programs to be an effective cross-cultural treatment in community settings.

Studies have not examined the effects of gender on the effectiveness of CBT for anxiety in children with ASD, nor the themes or topics of anxiety across gender in this population. Given the higher prevalence of anxiety in girls in both the general and ASD populations compared to boys, CBT for anxiety is likely to be a particularly pertinent therapy for girls with ASD. For example, given the use of masking and its association with anxiety in girls with ASD, exploration of how thoughts and behaviors related to masking may perpetuate anxiety (e.g., thought "I will sound dumb" and behavior of staying quiet in class perpetuates fear of speaking in class) may be useful to address in therapy. In addition, social challenges reported by girls with ASD, such as difficulty initiating and maintaining relationships, problems resolving conflicts with friends [4], and experiences of peer exclusion and isolation, may be linked to social anxiety and/or contribute to problems in everyday functioning [9]. As such, supplementing standard CBT practices with a focus on building social skills and enhancing social problem-solving may represent a helpful addition to therapy. Further, exposure exercises involving challenging social situations may be particularly useful when carried out in addition to other exposure exercises targeted in CBT. In these situations, continued practice of social skills in challenging social situations, paired with coaching and feedback conducted by a skilled therapist, is likely to lead to the development of important social skills, enhanced social competence, increased self-efficacy, and reduced anxiety and/or avoidance of otherwise stressful social situations. Lastly, given that girls on the autism spectrum are subject to societal sex/gender expectations that can lead to stress and anxiety, to the extent that sex/gender stereotypes and expectations are relevant for a given individual, it may be useful to address those issues and concerns in the context of therapy sessions.

9.3.2 Cognitive Behavioral Therapy for Irritability in Autism

Children with ASD present with high rates of co-occurring irritability, which is characterized by frequent and developmentally inappropriate anger outbursts and can confer greater functioning impairment than the core symptoms of the ASD itself [61]. Childhood irritability can present itself as a range of externalizing behaviors, from temper tantrums and screaming to physical aggression that could harm oneself or others, and its mood component can constitute enduring and intense anger [61]. CBT has been found to be an effective treatment for children and adolescents with disruptive behavior disorders such as conduct disorder and oppositional defiant disorder [62].

However, the use of CBT for disruptive behavior in autistic children and adolescents is still relatively novel. Similar to CBT for anxiety, which has been adapted for the needs of autistic individuals, CBT for disruptive behavior and autism includes modifications tailored to this population. One of the early trials of CBT for anger management in 52 children aged 10–14 with Asperger's syndrome was conducted by Sofronoff et al. [63]. Participants who received CBT showed significantly fewer anger outbursts and an increased ability to generate appropriate coping strategies.

CBT for irritability and aggression targets deficits in emotion regulation and social problem-solving skills associated with aggressive behavior. Common strategies and techniques used in this treatment include identifying antecedents and consequences of aggressive behavior, learning strategies for recognizing and regulating anger expression, and practicing cognitive problem-solving skills and socially appropriate behaviors that can replace angry and aggressive reactions [61].

Ongoing efforts are to adapt and test a transdiagnostic CBT treatment manual for irritability in adolescents with autism [64]. This treatment begins with a detailed assessment of the frequency (i.e., number of episodes per week), duration (i.e., time), and intensity (i.e., risk of injury, property damage, and impact on family) of anger outbursts and aggressive behaviors. Two to three of the most pressing behavioral problems are identified as target symptoms and are used to tailor therapeutic techniques. CBT for irritability comprises three modules: emotion regulation, social problem-solving, and development of social skills for preventing and resolving conflict situations. The first module focuses on identifying anger triggers, developing prevention strategies, and learning emotion regulation skills like cognitive reappraisal and relaxation training. The second module covers problem-solving skills, such as generating multiple solutions and considering consequences for different courses of action in conflicts. Finally, the third module helps children develop skills for preventing or resolving potentially anger-provoking situations with friends, siblings, parents, and teachers [65]. Each session also contains a parent component, in which parents are taught about the skills their children are learning, and a plan is devised to allow for practicing the skills for that week. Throughout the treatment, parents serve as coaches to facilitate skills acquisition and reward nonaggressive behaviors. The manual also contains treatment fidelity checklists to aid in evaluating treatment adherence [65].

Although sex/gender differences exist in the prevalence of disruptive behavior disorders in that males are more often diagnosed than females with conduct disorder and oppositional defiant disorder [66], it is important to note that this discrepancy does not mean that girls and women do not experience anger, irritability, or frustration. CBT for irritability can offer valuable tools for helping neurotypical and autistic girls recognize and express their anger and frustration in socially adaptive ways. It is also important to recognize that sex/gender expectations and stereotypes may perpetuate notions that females should not express their anger or can manage their emotions of frustration on their own without help. Furthermore, it is important to consider how societal sex/gender expectations can impact the expression of externalizing behaviors. Boys and men are more socially acceptable to outwardly express their angry moods, whereas girls and women are expected to internalize them. Thus, autistic girls may experience and express their feelings of irritability and anger in different ways than autistic boys do. There might also be important sex and gender differences in the antecedents of anger or events and situations that may lead to anger in autistic girls. For example, autistic girls have reported higher levels of relational aggression within their friendships, which may indicate difficulty in identifying and managing conflict within friendships and a topic that can be addressed in the treatment [67]. The role of co-occurring conditions, such as ADHD and anxiety, may have similar effects on the experience of anger in all children, but exposure to traumatic events poses a twofold risk of irritability in girls relative to boys [68]. Although research on the treatment of anger in girls has been sorely lacking [69], clinical observations and case reports indicate that CBT could be a helpful treatment for girls with clinically significant levels of irritability [70].

9.4 Social Skills Trainings

Social skills training (SST) programs are a common and widely used evidence-based group-based intervention for autistic school-aged children, adolescents, and adults. Based on social learning theory, SST programs aim to address social impairment and foster social skills through behavioral and social learning techniques. The group-based component allows autistic individuals to practice newly learned skills in a relatively naturalistic context [71]. Many SST programs have been developed, but intervention content, teaching strategy, mode of delivery, and intensity of therapy vary immensely [72]. For instance, some didactic manualized programs teach social skills through behavioral modeling, role play, and individualized feedback, whereas other didactic models may only teach social skills without practice. Other performance-based programs aim to elicit skills through play [72]. Programs also vary in their use of a combination of parent, teacher, or peer involvement, with some peer programs exclusively including peers with ASD and some programs also including typically developing peers. Recent research indicates that the extent to which a certain type of program is beneficial may depend on the child's characteristics. For example, in a study testing the relative efficacy of a didactic social skills group with all ASD peers to an activity-based social skills group with ASD and typically developing peers, the degree to which one group was more beneficial than the other varied depending on the child's quality of relationship with his or her teacher [73]. Content also varies from program to program. Among the five randomized control trial studies included in their meta-analysis, Wolstencroft et al. found that each program's syllabus differed from one another and emphasized different domains of social skills, including social knowledge, communication, cognition, and emotion [72]. Didactic interventions can include instruction on topics ranging from cognitive skills (i.e., cognitive social skills and flexibility) to verbal and nonverbal social skills (i.e., rules and cues, eye contact, facial expression, social perception, or perspective taking) to language skills.

Meta-analyses of SST programs reveal moderate to large effect sizes [72, 74, 75]. In a meta-analysis of randomized control trials of SST programs for autistic children and adolescents, Gates et al. found that group-based SST interventions led to moderate overall improvements in social competence and knowledge but that this knowledge did not carry over into changes in actual social behavior [74]. The authors concluded that basic, didactic teaching of social skills may not provide opportunities to allow for skill application and rehearsal of behaviors. However, in their systematic review and meta-analysis, Wolstencroft et al. found large effect sizes for improved social communication following treatment and moderate effect sizes for improved social skills for children with ASD [72]. In their meta-analysis of studies of adult SST programs, Dubreucq et al. found similar levels of efficacy and further demonstrated the utility of implementing SST programs for adults in enriched and more naturalistic environments to allow for more skill generalization [75]. Furthermore, programs that included parent groups and were more intensive and longer lasting were found to be more effective [72].

While Gates et al. found that sex/gender did not moderate the efficacy of SST programs for autistic children and adolescents, it is important to note that in most of the included studies, the participant samples were majority (50% to >90%) male [74]. Similarly, in the Dubreucq et al.'s meta-analysis, most of the participants were men (55.8–96.8%), and the small number of studies included precluded analysis of moderation by gender [75].

Below, we describe three social skills training programs that may be more applicable and effective for autistic girls and women based on the ways in which the programs address the needs of individuals in this population and their families.

PEERS Training.

The *Program for the Education and Enrichment of Relational Skills (PEERS)* is a social skills intervention that has been well validated by multiple sites and in cross-cultural contexts through clinical trials and randomized controlled trials [76–83] and that has shown long-term maintenance of social skills gains even 1–5 years after intervention [84]. Developed by Laugeson et al., the UCLA PEERS Program is a parent-assisted manualized social skills group intervention originally designed for high-functioning autistic adolescents but has now been demonstrated to also be effective in the young adult population [77, 79, 83]. The program consists of 14 weekly 90-min sessions, in which teenagers or young adults on the spectrum and their parents attend simultaneous separate group sessions where social skills are taught utilizing psychoeducational and cognitive behavioral therapy treatment techniques [85]. For adolescents and young adults, sessions consist of a didactic lesson on a specific social skill, followed by a role-playing demonstration and behavioral rehearsals with performance feedback. Separately, the parent group completes a review handout on the topic. Homework is then assigned for the next week, and parents are responsible for assisting their children with the socialization homework and providing coaching at home. Topics for these lessons include conversational skills, electronic forms of communication, developing friendship networks, appropriate use of humor, peer entry and exit strategies, how to have successful get-togethers, good sportsmanship, handling teasing and bullying, changing reputations, resolving arguments with friends, and handling rumors and gossip [83]. The young adult manual includes four additional topics related to dating etiquette and strategies, such as showing romantic interest, handling rejection, and general dating guidelines [77].

PEERS has been shown to be effective in increasing overall social skills. Laugeson et al. found an overall improvement in social skills with improvement maintained at a 14-week follow-up assessment in a group of 28 middle and high school students (ages 12–17; 23 male and 5 female), half of whom received *PEERS* intervention immediately and the other half after a delay period [83]. Participants showed decreased ASD symptoms relating to social responsiveness, increased knowledge of social skills, and increased frequency of hosted get-togethers. Blinded teacher ratings also demonstrated significant improvements in social functioning after 14 weeks [83]. These results were further replicated in an autistic young adult population (ages 18–24, 75–78% male) [77]. These improvements were also seen with implementing *PEERS* in an educational setting. *The Program for the Education and Enrichment of Relational Skills (PEERS) Curriculum for School-Based Professionals*, a teacher-facilitated daily social skills class (30 min per day for 14 weeks), was found to be more effective than another manualized social skills intervention (*Super Skills*, Coucouvanis, 2005) [86] in improving overall social responsiveness, social cognition, frequency of hosted and invited get-togethers, and social skills knowledge [76].

While *PEERS* has been well validated, the samples of these studies have been predominantly male (77–83%). Cross-cultural studies of PEERS in East Asian countries also contain heavily male samples (21% female in Shum et al. [80] and 32% female in Yamada et al. [81]), which may potentially limit generalizability to adolescent autistic females. In an effort to test the efficacy of PEERS in an all-female sample, Wolstencroft and colleagues [87] delivered the intervention to a sample of seven adolescent girls with Turner syndrome complicated by social communication problems. Following the delivery of PEERS, which was delivered via a hybrid in-person/online delivery format, the participants demonstrated improvements in several areas related to social communication, as well as reductions in ASD-related symptomatology [87].

To examine whether gender moderates the efficacy of the PEERS program, McVey et al. investigated if changes in social behavior among autistic female adolescents and young adults differed from autistic males who participated in the same PEERS program [88]. The researchers found that there were no differences in patterns of improvement between the genders, demonstrating that PEERS for adolescents and PEERS for young adults are a beneficial social skills program for girls on the spectrum [88]. This study is also noteworthy for a large sample of 177 participants, including 27 (15%) who were female.

McVey et al. suggested that future studies should consider an all-female PEERS group to examine interpersonal engagement in this population and which sections or aspects of PEERS may be more beneficial to autistic girls [88]. Indeed, in the all-female study of PEERS by Wolstencroft and colleagues, participant feedback revealed that some of the discussion topics (such as coaching of "good sportsmanship") were perceived as less relevant for girls [87]. Furthermore, given the unique challenges autistic girls often experience regarding socialization with neurotypical girls, topics within the PEERS curriculum could be tailored to emphasize social-emotional needs of this population, including social skills related to understanding nuances in communication and sharing personal or emotional experiences with others. Furthermore, it could be beneficial for the young adult curriculum on dating to include a more in-depth section on sexual health and consent.

9.4.1 Girls Night out

Girls Night Out (GNO), developed by Jamison and Schuttler at the University of Kansas Medical Center, is a social skills and self-care program designed to address the unique needs of adolescent females and young women with ASD and other developmental disabilities. The overall goal of GNO is to improve participants' social-emotional health through empowerment and improvement in self-perception and confidence [12]. The manualized intervention program is peer-mediated, incorporating typically developing peers as mediators, and occurs within natural and community settings to facilitate the generalization of skills. The program consists of a core curriculum that reflects feedback from focus groups and participant data and the opportunity for tailored and individualized interventions.

GNO is based on a theoretical framework that improving self-perception and self-confidence will increase one's likelihood of engaging in social entry skills and social activities. In a cyclical manner, this increased engagement in socialization will allow for improved social skills and increased competence, further reinforcing greater self-perception, confidence, and positive social-emotional health. The program promotes the empowerment of autistic women's self-awareness and ownership of goal setting and monitoring.

The curriculum itself consists of three core areas for improvement: (a) relating to others, (b) self-care, and (c) self-determination in social competence and self-perception. These topics are targeted through empirically based strategies of instruction and practice of social and self-care behaviors (i.e., reciprocal conversation, shared interests, independence) within age-appropriate activities. Sessions take place in multiple community contexts and settings to create a meaningful social experience for the participants and to enhance generalizability. The program is women-led, with female facilitators, participants, and community partners to create a safe environment and to set the tone for positive female interactions. GNO consists of 2-h weekly sessions over the course of 12–16 weeks, and sessions target one or more of the core curriculum concepts in natural community settings and locations. Participant groups consist of 4–6 participants with ASD and other developmental disabilities and at least an equal number of trained typically developing peers. This group composition allows both girls with and without ASD to develop acceptance and appreciation of each other's differences, develop skills in navigating those differences, and build long-term relationships.

Skills addressed in the core area of relating to others consist of conversation "entry" skills and relationship-building skills and concepts. Self-care skills are tailored to the individual; each participant's relevant self-care needs and activities are determined based on their values, needs, and interests. Following this, attention is placed on developing and improving the skills needed to complete the targeted activities (i.e., selecting appropriate clothing and caring for one's body and health). Finally, participants' strengths and desired growth areas are identified to improve self-determination in social competence and self-perception. GNO then provides opportunities to practice these social and self-care skills across multiple settings with planned practice sessions, homework, and individually designed support.

Preliminary findings from Jamison and Schuttler's analysis of self-report measures of a combined sample of five GNO groups from 2013 to 2017 (N = 34) revealed significant improvements in autistic participants' overall social competence and perceived quality of life as well as high satisfaction with the program and its activities from both participants and their parents [12]. Significant improvements were found for measures of empathy, engagement, and cooperation, and near-significant improvements were found for global self-perception following the intervention. Significant decreases in internalizing symptoms were also reported. However, due to the study's small sample size, definitive conclusions about GNO would best be supported by replication with a large sample. Still, the medium and large effect sizes found in the study's small sample suggest meaningful changes in perceived quality of life and evidence for the social validity of the program. GNO's curriculum is based on research on conversation skills identified as important for adolescent females and informal discussions with typically developing adolescent females. The curriculum has since been modified with feedback from program participants through focus groups and data, allowing for a program that promotes a high degree of social validity. Furthermore, GNO has seen low rates of participant attrition (6%) and extremely positive anecdotal reports, written feedback, and high satisfaction, indicating that this program is a service that autistic young women, adolescents, and their families value and need.

GNO is one of the first interventions designed for autistic girls and women. The program utilizes a consumer-driven approach that promotes a high degree of social validity and increases the likelihood of engagement for participants, thus allowing for a meaningful program. It addresses the unique social needs and daily living skills of autistic women by empowering its participants and has the potential for broad dissemination.

9.4.2 Healthy Relationship Skills and Sexual Health for Autistic Youth Programs

Although autistic women report more unmet needs with respect to mental health and vocational services, as well as a higher risk of sexual abuse, issues of reproductive and sexual health remain fairly under-investigated in this population [89]. In their review of 27 studies to assess the current state of care for autistic women in romantic relationships and reproductive health, Dubreucq and Dubreucq identified loneliness, negative self-perception, self-stigma, sensory sensitivity, and impaired social communication related to dating as barriers to romantic relationships for individuals with ASD. They further identified decrypting dating situations and adopting assertive behaviors in intimate relationships as challenges unique to women with ASD.

Only two SST interventions addressing romantic relationships in ASD have explored the role of gender in program outcomes: PEERS for Young Adults (described above) [88] and the Tackling Teenage Training program [90]. Studies on both interventions found that gender did not moderate behavioral, content knowledge, or cognitive outcomes. Additionally, in their systematic review of three randomized controlled trials of programs on dating and relationships for individuals with autism, Holmes et al. reported that all programs increased content knowledge, but only one improved social and behavioral functioning [91]. However, participants in the interventions included in both reviews were majority (75%) male. As such, the curriculums and topics may not have addressed the unique challenges of autistic women, and the predominance of men may have induced sex/gender-related biases in the development of these interventions [89].

SST programs about healthy relationships can include content on healthy relationships, sexual feelings and behavior, sexual health, boundary setting, mechanics of sex and reproductive health, puberty, and more. The *PEERS*-Decision Making (PEERS-DM) curriculum teaches about peer pressure, relationships, and a four-step strategy for effective decision-making. After implementing the program at a school with students served by the special education system (autistic youth predominating), students who participated in the PEERS-DM curriculum earned better scores on measures of interpersonal decision-making action responses, risk perception, and understanding of peer pressure [92]. Another similar program, the Tackling Teenage Training (TTT) program, is a manualized psychosexual education intervention for youth on the spectrum. TTT is implemented in a one-on-one clinical setting and consists of a series of exercises and homework assignments with content on puberty, appearances, first impressions, physical and emotional development, friendships, love and dating, sexuality, pregnancy, boundary setting, and safe Internet usage [93]. Youth aged 12–18 who participated in TTT reported improved psychosexual knowledge after treatment and received higher parent ratings on understanding boundary setting [90]. These changes in the treatment group were driven by younger adolescents (ages 12–16), indicating that earlier intervention may be more effective. Finally, Supporting Teens with Autism on Relationships (STAR) is a manualized parent-mediated intervention that includes a parent curriculum and interactive computer game for autistic youth, with modules comprising topics such as relationships, puberty, and sexual health [94]. Parents and youth who completed the intervention reported greater knowledge, and parents felt more confident and comfortable talking about sexuality with their children.

Psychoeducational programs on reproductive and sexual health and dating for autistic women would likely benefit from inclusion of several additional topics. Self-care, especially regarding puberty, birth control, and menstruation, all of which have been reported as concerns by parents of autistic girls [19], would be an important topic to include in program content. Given that parents have also highlighted concerns regarding their daughters' potential victimization in sexual exploitation and abuse [19], programs should also spend more time or content on boundary setting and healthy relationships to address these concerns.

9.4.3 Considerations for Future Social Skills Training and Related Programs on Social Skills Training

Given the unique social experiences of autistic girls and women, social skills training curricula should be tailored to address the needs of autistic girls and women. For example, curricula could include discussion of topics such as the ways in which girls are socialized to communicate differently than boys or other topics salient to women, such as sexual health and dating. In addition, since SST programs carry the risk of reinforcing common sex/gender stereotypes regarding the ways individuals should act in a given sociocultural context, the inclusion of sex/gender-sensitive content in these programs (i.e., discussion of gender variance and gender-related social norms and expectations) could help prevent internalization of these gender norms and improve treatment outcomes for autistic women [89]. Finally, because some elements of SST programs teach compensation strategies (defined as alternative ways of acting or thinking to compensate for social-cognitive difficulties associated with ASD), the extent to which these compensation strategies may overlap with camouflaging and masking warrants careful consideration. Dubreucq and Dubreucq highlight the concern that SST programs may actually increase the use of masking and indirectly contribute to increased psychological distress [89]. Thus, it is important for future SST research to examine the distinction between compensation strategies and masking behaviors, as well as their respective effects on treatment outcomes and mental health.

9.4.4 Women's Health Programs in ASD

Other content areas to address include motherhood and parenting for autistic women and the development of support programs for autistic mothers [89]. Given that autistic mothers are at increased risk of perinatal depression and postpartum challenges [95], there is a great need for transparent and accurate information about pregnancy, potential complications, delivery, postpartum care, and improved self-agency and empowerment in such psychological programs for women with ASD [89].

9.5 Peer-Mediated Interventions

Social interaction is one of the main areas of difficulty for individuals with ASD. For school-aged children on the spectrum, deficits in social skills can be particularly challenging. One intervention category aiming to address social interactions is peer-mediated interventions, which utilize the presence of typically developing peers, including classmates, friends, and siblings, as a key component of the intervention [96]. These peer intervention strategies emerged from recognizing the limitations of adult-implemented interventions, including a developed reliance on adult prompting and difficulties generalizing skills to peer interactions [97]. Systematic reviews show that peer-mediated interventions are effective for individuals with ASD. A 2009 review analyzing 42 studies found that 91% of the studies reported positive results, although the studies reported different outcome measures, including joint attention, communication, and social initiation. The participants' ages in the studies ranged from 2 to 13 years, indicating that peer-mediated interventions are effective across a wide age range [98]. Despite these positive findings, Chan et al. noted that treatment fidelity was often limited in the studies assessed. A later review conducted in 2016 found four group design, school-based, peer-mediated interventions with "high" or "adequate" quality [99]. According to Reichow et al.'s framework for evaluating evidence-based practices in ASD, and consistent with Chang and Locke's (2016) findings, peer-mediated interventions have "established evidence-based practice" [99, 100]. Overall, peer-mediated interventions have the highest empirical support of all social interventions for children with autism [96].

Peer initiation training, developed primarily by Strain, Odom, and Goldstein, involves teaching typically developing peers to initiate structured interactions with their peers with ASD through structured training [101]. Modifications have been made to the initial structure of peer initiation training, including enhanced reinforcement and incorporation of peer initiation procedures into daily classroom activities, which led to increased implementation efficacy and higher rates of social interactions [102].

Peer buddy models are another model of peer-mediated interventions. Peer buddy models pair children with autism with a typically developing peer, who serves as a "buddy" throughout the school day. Peer buddy models have been shown to increase the interactions between students with and without disabilities in a classroom context [103]. Furthermore, appropriate social play skills were strengthened when peer buddy programs were implemented, as compared to integrated classroom settings without active buddy assignment [104].

While most peer-mediated interventions utilize classmates and friends as intervention agents, research shows the efficacy of typically developing siblings as peer intervention agents as well. Classroom-based social skills interventions were modified for home-based use, producing significant improvements in sibling interactions [105].

No studies have been conducted assessing the effect of gender in peer-mediated interventions; further research on whether gender plays a role in peer-mediated interventions would be useful.

9.6 Promising Psychosocial Interventions

9.6.1 Mindfulness

Mindfulness-based techniques can be utilized in interventions for individuals with autism, with mindfulness-based interventions often delivered to children with ASD along with their parents. MYmind is one such mindfulness-based intervention consisting of 9 weekly sessions of group mindfulness training for adolescents with ASD and a parallel set of group sessions for their parents. In a 2015 study of MYmind, adolescents with autism indicated no change in mindful awareness or autism spectrum disorder core symptoms following the intervention. However, they displayed an increase in quality of life, a decrease in rumination, and improvements in social responsiveness, social communication, social cognition, preoccupations, and social motivation. The parents participating in the program reported many improvements as well, including in parental mindfulness and general parenting abilities, as well as an increased quality of life [106]. A follow-up study on MYmind with a control group demonstrated similar results [107]. In addition, similar effects were observed when MYmind was delivered to younger children with ASD [108]. Extending the scope of mindfulness interventions, a 2015 pilot study tested an intervention in which mothers of children with autism were trained to teach mindfulness skills to their children. The study found positive results, though limited by the small sample size [109]. Additionally, only mothers were involved in the study. Further research is needed on how the program could extend to fathers, as well as on whether the gender composition of parents and/or children in the program could moderate the program effects.

9.7 Conclusion and Takeaways

There is a great need for more research on treatments for autistic individuals to be sex/gender-balanced and tailored for autistic girls if necessary. In nearly all treatment studies in ASD, participant samples are majority male, and several earlier studies did not report the gender compositions of their samples. A key question concerns whether the response to treatment for individuals with ASD differs or is moderated by sex/gender. However, there is little research on predictors and moderators of treatment in ASD, and of that research, sex/gender is not among the moderators commonly examined [110]. Further, to examine sex/gender as a moderator of treatment, studies need sufficiently large sample sizes of both males and females, and few studies have included such samples. Of the handful of studies that have examined sex/gender as a moderator of treatment, including six multisite randomized controlled trials, findings have not supported sex/gender differences in treatment response [111]. Still, many of these studies include limitations such as heterogeneous sample compositions, which may limit the power to detect effects.

No studies of interventions reviewed in this chapter (except for Girls Night Out) explicitly discuss how the intervention could be tailored to be more useful or effective for autistic girls and women. Females with ASD are the minority of those diagnosed with ASD (~25%) and comprise only 15% of subjects in the ASD research literature [12]. The predominance of men in participant samples in ASD research can lead to sex/gender-related biases in the development of interventions, whereby autism diagnoses and resulting interventions targeting diagnostic symptoms are based on majority-male samples. As such, the unique needs of autistic women can go missed or unaddressed in interventions.

Particular considerations regarding psychosocial treatments for girls on the spectrum, relevant to clinicians and researchers alike, include the following:

Girls on the spectrum are often diagnosed later in life, resulting in poor access to services and interventions, impacting development and mental health. Many of the interventions described in this chapter focus on early intervention and target toddlers and school-age children; however, many females are not diagnosed with autism until adolescence or young adulthood. As such, it is important to consider ways in which the assessment of autism symptoms may be tailored to increase sensitivity to the early signs and symptoms of the disorder in girls. Moreover, continued research on sex/gender differences in the manifestation of autism symptoms is greatly needed, and such research should aim to clarify the extent to which sex/gender differences in symptom presentation warrant changes to current methods of diagnosing ASD in females.

More studies evaluating the efficacy of ASD interventions that include sizable samples of girls and women are needed. Given the preponderance of males in treatment studies for ASD, until larger samples and greater proportions of females are included in these studies, the extent to which the positive effects of these interventions generalize to females remains unknown. Further, in order to systemically examine whether treatment outcomes differ between the sexes, treatment studies with sufficiently large samples of both males and females are needed. Taken together with research examining sex/gender differences in the presentation and experience of females with ASD, the results of such research are likely to further knowledge regarding how to better address the needs of girls and women on the autism spectrum. Consequently, such knowledge is likely to play a key role in the development and refinement of interventions that more precisely align with the needs of females with ASD and/or are delivered in ways that are maximally effective for them.

More research is needed to understand how societal sex/gender expectations for women uniquely impact autistic girls and women. Already faced with pressures to fit into a neurotypical world, societal expectations for women to be communicative and emotionally expressive can add pressure for girls on the spectrum to mask or camouflage their autism symptoms, often leading to heightened stress and anxiety. In addition, the emphasis on closeness, intimacy, and sharing characteristic of female relationships can make it challenging for girls with ASD to navigate friendships, placing them at heightened risk for isolation and loneliness. These pressures, coupled with the elevated risk for girls to develop internalizing symptoms, create a "double whammy" experienced by girls on the spectrum [12]. As such, a better understanding of the pressures faced by autistic girls is important as we strive to develop interventions that not only decrease autism symptomology and increase adaptive functioning, but also promote mental health and general well-being.

Interventions and services for girls and women on the spectrum will be most useful when they address the unique experiences and needs of this population. Research indicates that many topics relevant to females with ASD, including female friendships, impact of societal sex/gender expectations, reproductive and sexual health, puberty and menstruation, and parenting, are largely missing from most psychosocial interventions for girls and women. Parents of autistic girls have also identified other topics of relevance for their daughters, including life skill training, driving lessons, bike riding, social media education, vocational skill preparation, and social networks with typically developing girls. To the extent that these topics and areas for skill building are addressed and promoted in new or existing interventions, females on the autism spectrum are likely to derive more benefit from the services and treatments with which they engage.

However, as we incorporate knowledge about the experiences and needs of females with ASD into intervention development and planning, it is important to remember that much still remains unknown. Continued research on the experiences, interests, challenges, and strengths of females with ASD, as well as on treatment outcomes specific to this population, is greatly needed. In addition, direct feedback and participation from the autistic female community are vital. Only by incorporating the feedback, opinions, and lived experiences of girls and women on the spectrum can we aim to develop interventions that address the complexities and best meet the needs of this population.

References

1. Strang JF, van der Miesen AI, Caplan R, Hughes C, daVanport S, Lai M-C. Both sex-and gender-related factors should be considered in autism research and clinical practice. Autism. 2020;24(3):539–43.
2. Hull L, Petrides K, Mandy W. The female autism phenotype and camouflaging: a narrative review. J Autism Dev Disord. 2020;7:306–17.
3. Lai M-C, Lombardo MV, Auyeung B, Chakrabarti B, Baron-Cohen S. Sex/gender differences and autism: setting the scene for future research. J Am Acad Child Adolesc Psychiatry. 2015;54(1):11–24.

4. Milner V, McIntosh H, Colvert E, Happé F. A qualitative exploration of the female experience of autism spectrum disorder (ASD). J Autism Dev Disord. 2019;49(6):2389–402.
5. Rutherford M, McKenzie K, Johnson T, Catchpole C, O'Hare A, McClure I, et al. Gender ratio in a clinical population sample, age of diagnosis and duration of assessment in children and adults with autism spectrum disorder. Autism. 2016;20(5):628–34.
6. Bargiela S, Steward R, Mandy W. The experiences of late-diagnosed women with autism Spectrum conditions: an investigation of the female autism phenotype. J Autism Dev Disord. 2016;46(10):3281–94.
7. Cage E, Troxell-Whitman Z. Understanding the reasons, contexts and costs of camouflaging for autistic adults. J Autism Dev Disord. 2019;49(5):1899–911.
8. Hull L, Petrides K, Allison C, Smith P, Baron-Cohen S, Lai M-C, et al. "Putting on my best normal": social camouflaging in adults with autism spectrum conditions. J Autism Dev Disord. 2017;47(8):2519–34.
9. Dean M, Kasari C, Shih W, Frankel F, Whitney R, Landa R, et al. The peer relationships of girls with ASD at school: comparison to boys and girls with and without ASD. J Child Psychol Psychiatry. 2014;55(11):1218–25.
10. Jamison TR, Schuttler JO. Examining social competence, self-perception, quality of life, and internalizing and externalizing symptoms in adolescent females with and without autism spectrum disorder: a quantitative design including between-groups and correlational analyses. Mol Autism. 2015;6(1):1–16.
11. Solomon M, Miller M, Taylor SL, Hinshaw SP, Carter CS. Autism symptoms and internalizing psychopathology in girls and boys with autism spectrum disorders. J Autism Dev Disord. 2012;42(1):48–59.
12. Jamison TR, Schuttler JO. Overview and preliminary evidence for a social skills and self-care curriculum for adolescent females with autism: the girls night out model. J Autism Dev Disord. 2017;47(1):110–25.
13. Gesi C, Migliarese G, Torriero S, Capellazzi M, Omboni AC, Cerveri G, et al. Gender differences in misdiagnosis and delayed diagnosis among adults with autism spectrum disorder with no language or intellectual disability. Brain Sci. 2021;11(7):912.
14. Giarelli E, Wiggins LD, Rice CE, Levy SE, Kirby RS, Pinto-Martin J, et al. Sex differences in the evaluation and diagnosis of autism spectrum disorders among children. Disabil Health J. 2010;3(2):107–16.
15. Yianni-Coudurier C, Darrou C, Lenoir P, Verrecchia B, Assouline B, Ledesert B, et al. What clinical characteristics of children with autism influence their inclusion in regular classrooms? J Intellect Disabil Res. 2008;52(10):855–63.
16. May T, Cornish K, Rinehart N. Does gender matter? A one year follow-up of autistic, attention and anxiety symptoms in high-functioning children with autism spectrum disorder. J Autism Dev Disord. 2014;44(5):1077–86.
17. Taylor JL, DaWalt LS. Working toward a better understanding of the life experiences of women on the autism spectrum. Autism. 2020;24(5):1027–30.
18. Halladay AK, Bishop S, Constantino JN, Daniels AM, Koenig K, Palmer K, et al. Sex and gender differences in autism spectrum disorder: summarizing evidence gaps and identifying emerging areas of priority. Mol Autism. 2015;6(1):1–5.
19. Mademtzi M, Singh P, Shic F, Koenig K. Challenges of females with autism: a parental perspective. J Autism Dev Disord. 2018;48(4):1301–10.
20. Taylor JL, Henninger NA, Mailick MR. Longitudinal patterns of employment and postsecondary education for adults with autism and average-range IQ. Autism. 2015;19(7):785–93.
21. Yu Q, Li E, Li L, Liang W. Efficacy of interventions based on applied behavior analysis for autism spectrum disorder: a meta-analysis. Psychiatry Investig. 2020;17(5):432.
22. Carr EG, Dores PA. Patterns of language acquisition following simultaneous communication with autistic children. Anal Interv Dev Disabil. 1981;1(3–4):347–61.
23. Lang R, van der Werff M, Verbeek K, Didden R, Davenport K, Moore M, et al. Comparison of high and low preferred topographies of contingent attention during discrete trial training. Res Autism Spectr Disord. 2014;8(10):1279–86.

24. Lovaas OI. Behavioral treatment and normal educational and intellectual functioning in young autistic children. J Consult Clin Psychol. 1987;55(1):3.
25. Eldevik S, Hastings RP, Jahr E, Hughes JC. Outcomes of behavioral intervention for children with autism in mainstream pre-school settings. J Autism Dev Disord. 2012;42(2):210–20.
26. Lerman DC, Valentino AL, LeBlanc LA. Discrete trial training. Early intervention for young children with autism spectrum disorder: Springer; 2016. p. 47–83.
27. Cariveau T, Shillingsburg MA, Alamoudi A, Thompson T, Bartlett B, Gillespie S, et al. Brief report: feasibility and preliminary efficacy of a behavioral intervention for minimally verbal girls with autism spectrum disorder. J Autism Dev Disord. 2019;49(5):2203–9.
28. Eldevik S, Titlestad KB, Aarlie H, Tønnesen R. Community implementation of early behavioral intervention: higher intensity gives better outcome. Eur J Behav Anal. 2020;21(1):92–109.
29. Reichow B, Barton EE, Boyd BA, Hume K. Early intensive behavioral intervention (EIBI) for young children with autism spectrum disorders (ASD): a systematic review. Campbell Syst Rev. 2014;10(1):1–116.
30. Koegel LK, Koegel RL, Harrower JK, Carter CM. Pivotal response intervention I: overview of approach. J Assoc Pers Sev Handicaps. 1999;24(3):174–85.
31. Koegel RL, O'dell MC, Koegel LK. A natural language teaching paradigm for nonverbal autistic children. J Autism Dev Disord. 1987;17(2):187–200.
32. Bozkus-Genc G, Yucesoy-Ozkan S. Meta-analysis of pivotal response training for children with autism spectrum disorder. Educ Train Autism Dev Disabil. 2016;51(1):13–26.
33. Baker-Ericzén MJ, Stahmer AC, Burns A. Child demographics associated with outcomes in a community-based pivotal response training program. J Posit Behav Interv. 2007;9(1): 52–60.
34. Daniel T, Sukhodolsky D, Ventola P. Sex-based differences of treatment response to PRT for emotional and behavioral symptoms. International Society for Autism Research; 2022.
35. Dawson G, Rogers S, Munson J, Smith M, Winter J, Greenson J, et al. Randomized, controlled trial of an intervention for toddlers with autism: the early start Denver model. Pediatrics. 2010;125(1):e17–23.
36. Sipes M, Matson JL, Worley JA, Kozlowski AM. Gender differences in symptoms of autism spectrum disorders in toddlers. Res Autism Spectr Disord. 2011;5(4):1465–70.
37. Greenspan SI. Intelligence and adaptation: an integration of psychoanalytic and Piagetian developmental psychology. Psychol Issues. 1979;12(3-4):1–408.
38. Wieder S, Greenspan SI. Climbing the symbolic ladder in the DIR model through floor time/ interactive play. Autism. 2003;7(4):425–35.
39. Dionne M, Martini R. Floor time play with a child with autism: a single-subject study. Can J Occup Ther. 2011;78(3):196–203.
40. Mercer J. Examining DIR/Floortime™ as a treatment for children with autism spectrum disorders: a review of research and theory. Res Soc Work Pract. 2017;27(5):625–35.
41. Bruinsma Y, Koegel RL, Koegel LK. Joint attention and children with autism: a review of the literature. Ment Retard Dev Disabil Res Rev. 2004;10(3):169–75.
42. Mundy P. Joint attention and social-emotional approach behavior in children with autism. Dev Psychopathol. 1995;7(1):63–82.
43. Lewy AL, Dawson G. Social stimulation and joint attention in young autistic children. J Abnorm Child Psychol. 1992;20(6):555–66.
44. Kasari C, Freeman SF, Paparella T. Early intervention in autism: joint attention and symbolic play. In: International review of research in mental retardation. 23: Elsevier; 2000. p. 207–37.
45. Whalen C, Schreibman L. Joint attention training for children with autism using behavior modification procedures. J Child Psychol Psychiatry. 2003;44(3):456–68.
46. Rocha ML, Schreibman L, Stahmer AC. Effectiveness of training parents to teach joint attention in children with autism. J Early Interv. 2007;29(2):154–72.
47. Jones EA, Carr EG, Feeley KM. Multiple effects of joint attention intervention for children with autism. Behav Modif. 2006;30(6):782–834.
48. Goods KS, Ishijima E, Chang Y-C, Kasari C. Preschool based JASPER intervention in minimally verbal children with autism: pilot RCT. J Autism Dev Disord. 2013;43(5):1050–6.

49. Shih W, Shire S, Chang YC, Kasari C. Joint engagement is a potential mechanism leading to increased initiations of joint attention and downstream effects on language: JASPER early intervention for children with ASD. J Child Psychol Psychiatry. 2021;62(10):1228–35.
50. Sukhodolsky DG, Bloch MH, Panza KE, Reichow B. Cognitive-behavioral therapy for anxiety in children with high-functioning autism: a meta-analysis. Pediatrics. 2013;132(5):e1341–e50.
51. Wood JJ, Kendall PC, Wood KS, Kerns CM, Seltzer M, Small BJ, et al. Cognitive behavioral treatments for anxiety in children with autism spectrum disorder: a randomized clinical trial. JAMA Psychiatry. 2020;77(5):474–83.
52. Simonoff E, Pickles A, Charman T, Chandler S, Loucas T, Baird G. Psychiatric disorders in children with autism spectrum disorders: prevalence, comorbidity, and associated factors in a population-derived sample. J Am Acad Child Adolesc Psychiatry. 2008;47(8):921–9.
53. White SW, Oswald D, Ollendick T, Scahill L. Anxiety in children and adolescents with autism spectrum disorders. Clin Psychol Rev. 2009;29(3):216–29.
54. Van Steensel F, Bögels S. Cognitive-behavioral therapy for anxiety disorders in children with and without ASD. J Consult Clin Psychol. 2015;83(3):512–23.
55. Olatunji BO, Cisler JM, Deacon BJ. Efficacy of cognitive behavioral therapy for anxiety disorders: a review of meta-analytic findings. Psychiatr Clin. 2010;33(3):557–77.
56. Danial JT, Wood JJ. Cognitive behavioral therapy for children with autism: review and considerations for future research. J Dev Behav Pediatr. 2013;34(9):702–15.
57. Perihan C, Burke M, Bowman-Perrott L, Bicer A, Gallup J, Thompson J, et al. Effects of cognitive behavioral therapy for reducing anxiety in children with high functioning ASD: a systematic review and meta-analysis. J Autism Dev Disord. 2020;50(6):1958–72.
58. Kendall PC, Hedtke KA. Cognitive-behavioral therapy for anxious children: therapist manual. Workbook Publishing; 2006.
59. Barrett PM, Dadds MR, Rapee RM. Family treatment of childhood anxiety: a controlled trial. J Consult Clin Psychol. 1996;64(2):333–42.
60. Fisher PH, Masia-Warner C, Klein RG. Skills for social and academic success: a school-based intervention for social anxiety disorder in adolescents. Clin Child Fam Psychol Rev. 2004;7(4):241–9.
61. Sukhodolsky DGG, Theresa R, Marsh C, L; and Cimino, Kimberly R. Behavioral interventions for irritability in children and adolescents. In: Roy AKB, Melissa A, Leibenluft E, editors. Irritability in pediatric psychopathology. Oxford University Press; 2019. p. 255–75.
62. Riise EN, Wergeland GJH, Njardvik U, Öst L-G. Cognitive behavior therapy for externalizing disorders in children and adolescents in routine clinical care: a systematic review and meta-analysis. Clin Psychol Rev. 2021;83:101954.
63. Sofronoff K, Attwood T, Hinton S, Levin I. A randomized controlled trial of a cognitive behavioural intervention for anger management in children diagnosed with Asperger syndrome. J Autism Dev Disord. 2007;37(7):1203–14.
64. Sukhodolsky DG, Scahill L. Cognitive-behavioral therapy for anger and aggression in children. Guilford Press; 2012.
65. Sukhodolsky DG, Smith SD, McCauley SA, Ibrahim K, Piasecka JB. Behavioral interventions for anger, irritability, and aggression in children and adolescents. J Child Adolesc Psychopharmacol. 2016;26(1):58–64.
66. Demmer DH, Hooley M, Sheen J, McGillivray JA, Lum JA. Sex differences in the prevalence of oppositional defiant disorder during middle childhood: a meta-analysis. J Abnorm Child Psychol. 2017;45(2):313–25.
67. Sedgewick F, Hill V, Yates R, Pickering L, Pellicano E. Gender differences in the social motivation and friendship experiences of autistic and non-autistic adolescents. J Autism Dev Disord. 2016;46(4):1297–306.
68. Henriksen M, Skrove M, Hoftun GB, Sund ER, Lydersen S, Kalvin CB, et al. Exposure to traumatic events poses greater risk for irritability in girls than in boys. J Affect Disord Rep. 2021;6:100204.
69. Burt I, Butler SK. Capoeira as a clinical intervention: addressing adolescent aggression with Brazilian martial arts. J Multicult Couns Dev. 2011;39(1):48–57.

70. Tudor ME, Ibrahim K, Bertschinger E, Piasecka J, Sukhodolsky DG. Cognitive-behavioral therapy for a 9-year-old girl with disruptive mood dysregulation disorder. Clin Case Stud. 2016;15(6):459–75.
71. White SW, Keonig K, Scahill L. Social skills development in children with autism spectrum disorders: a review of the intervention research. J Autism Dev Disord. 2007;37(10):1858–68.
72. Wolstencroft J, Robinson L, Srinivasan R, Kerry E, Mandy W, Skuse D. A systematic review of group social skills interventions, and meta-analysis of outcomes, for children with high functioning ASD. J Autism Dev Disord. 2018;48(7):2293–307.
73. Kasari C, Dean M, Kretzmann M, Shih W, Orlich F, Whitney R, et al. Children with autism spectrum disorder and social skills groups at school: a randomized trial comparing intervention approach and peer composition. J Child Psychol Psychiatry. 2016;57(2):171–9.
74. Gates JA, Kang E, Lerner MD. Efficacy of group social skills interventions for youth with autism spectrum disorder: a systematic review and meta-analysis. Clin Psychol Rev. 2017;52:164–81.
75. Dubreucq J, Haesebaert F, Plasse J, Dubreucq M, Franck N. A systematic review and meta-analysis of social skills training for adults with autism Spectrum disorder. J Autism Dev Disord. 2021;52(4):1598–609.
76. Laugeson EA, Ellingsen R, Sanderson J, Tucci L, Bates S. The ABC's of teaching social skills to adolescents with autism spectrum disorder in the classroom: the UCLA PEERS® program. J Autism Dev Disord. 2014;44(9):2244–56.
77. Laugeson EA, Gantman A, Kapp SK, Orenski K, Ellingsen R. A randomized controlled trial to improve social skills in young adults with autism spectrum disorder: the UCLA PEERS® program. J Autism Dev Disord. 2015;45(12):3978–89.
78. Schohl KA, Van Hecke AV, Carson AM, Dolan B, Karst J, Stevens S. A replication and extension of the PEERS intervention: examining effects on social skills and social anxiety in adolescents with autism spectrum disorders. J Autism Dev Disord. 2014;44(3): 532–45.
79. Gantman A, Kapp SK, Orenski K, Laugeson EA. Social skills training for young adults with high-functioning autism spectrum disorders: a randomized controlled pilot study. J Autism Dev Disord. 2012;42(6):1094–103.
80. Shum KK-M, Cho WK, Lam LMO, Laugeson EA, Wong WS, Law LS. Learning how to make friends for Chinese adolescents with autism spectrum disorder: a randomized controlled trial of the Hong Kong Chinese version of the PEERS® intervention. J Autism Dev Disord. 2019;49(2):527–41.
81. Yamada T, Miura Y, Oi M, Akatsuka N, Tanaka K, Tsukidate N, et al. Examining the treatment efficacy of PEERS in Japan: improving social skills among adolescents with autism Spectrum disorder. J Autism Dev Disord. 2020;50(3):976–97.
82. Yoo HJ, Bahn G, Cho IH, Kim EK, Kim JH, Min JW, et al. A randomized controlled trial of the K orean version of the PEERS® parent-assisted social skills training program for teens with ASD. Autism Res. 2014;7(1):145–61.
83. Laugeson EA, Frankel F, Gantman A, Dillon AR, Mogil C. Evidence-based social skills training for adolescents with autism Spectrum disorders: the UCLA PEERS program. J Autism Dev Disord. 2012;42(6):1025–36.
84. Mandelberg J, Laugeson EA, Cunningham TD, Ellingsen R, Bates S, Frankel F. Long-term treatment outcomes for parent-assisted social skills training for adolescents with autism spectrum disorders: the UCLA PEERS program. J Ment Health Res Intellect Disabil. 2014;7(1):45–73.
85. Laugeson EA, Frankel F. Social skills for teenagers with developmental and autism spectrum disorders: the PEERS treatment manual. Routledge; 2011.
86. Coucouvanis J. Super skills: a social skills group program for children with Asperger syndrome, high-functioning autism and related challenges. AAPC Publishing; 2005.
87. Wolstencroft J, Kerry E, Denyer H, Watkins A, Mandy W, Skuse D. New approaches to social skills training: blended group interventions for girls with social communication difficulties. Autism Res. 2021;14(5):1061–72.

88. McVey AJ, Schiltz H, Haendel A, Dolan BK, Willar KS, Pleiss S, et al. Brief report: does gender matter in intervention for ASD? Examining the impact of the PEERS® social skills intervention on social behavior among females with ASD. J Autism Dev Disord. 2017;47(7):2282–9.
89. Dubreucq M, Dubreucq J. Toward a gender-sensitive approach of psychiatric rehabilitation in autism Spectrum disorder (ASD): a systematic review of women needs in the domains of romantic relationships and reproductive health. Front Psych. 2021;12:456.
90. Visser K, Greaves-Lord K, Tick NT, Verhulst FC, Maras A, van der Vegt EJ. A randomized controlled trial to examine the effects of the tackling teenage psychosexual training program for adolescents with autism spectrum disorder. J Child Psychol Psychiatry. 2017;58(7):840–50.
91. Holmes LG, Ofei LM, Bair-Merritt MH, Palmucci PL, Rothman EF. A systematic review of randomized controlled trials on healthy relationship skills and sexual health for autistic youth. Rev J Autism Dev Disord. 2021;9(4):555–70.
92. Khemka I, Hickson L, Mallory SB. Evaluation of a decision-making curriculum for teaching adolescents with disabilities to resist negative peer pressure. J Autism Dev Disord. 2016;46(7):2372–84.
93. Dekker LP, Van Der Vegt EJ, Visser K, Tick N, Boudesteijn F, Verhulst FC, et al. Improving psychosexual knowledge in adolescents with autism spectrum disorder: pilot of the tackling teenage training program. J Autism Dev Disord. 2015;45(6):1532–40.
94. Pugliese CE, Ratto AB, Granader Y, Dudley KM, Bowen A, Baker C, et al. Feasibility and preliminary efficacy of a parent-mediated sexual education curriculum for youth with autism spectrum disorders. Autism. 2020;24(1):64–79.
95. Pohl A, Crockford S, Blakemore M, Allison C, Baron-Cohen S. A comparative study of autistic and non-autistic women's experience of motherhood. Mol Autism. 2020;11(1):1–12.
96. Bass JD, Mulick JA. Social play skill enhancement of children with autism using peers and siblings as therapists. Psychol Sch. 2007;44(7):727–35.
97. Strain PS, Kohler FW, Goldstein H. Learning experiences... An alternative program: peer-mediated interventions for young children with autism. Psychosocial treatments for child and adolescent disorders: empirically based strategies for clinical practice. American Psychological Association; 1996. p. 573–87.
98. Chan JM, Lang R, Rispoli M, O'Reilly M, Sigafoos J, Cole H. Use of peer-mediated interventions in the treatment of autism spectrum disorders: a systematic review. Res Autism Spectr Disord. 2009;3(4):876–89.
99. Chang Y-C, Locke J. A systematic review of peer-mediated interventions for children with autism spectrum disorder. Res Autism Spectr Disord. 2016;27:1–10.
100. Reichow B, Volkmar FR, Cicchetti DV. Development of the evaluative method for evaluating and determining evidence-based practices in autism. J Autism Dev Disord. 2008;38(7):1311–9.
101. Strain PS, Odom SL. Peer social initiations: effective intervention for social skills development of exceptional children. Except Child. 1986;52(6):543–51.
102. Storey K, Smith DJ, Strain PS. Use of classroom assistants and peer-mediated intervention to increase integration in preschool settings. Exceptionality. 1993;4(1):1–16.
103. English K, Goldstein H, Shafer K, Kaczmarek L. Promoting interactions among preschoolers with and without disabilities: effects of a buddy skills-training program. Except Child. 1997;63(2):229–43.
104. Laushey KM, Heflin LJ. Enhancing social skills of kindergarten children with autism through the training of multiple peers as tutors. J Autism Dev Disord. 2000;30(3):183–93.
105. Strain PS, Danko CD. Caregivers' encouragement of positive interaction between preschoolers with autism and their siblings. J Emot Behav Disord. 1995;3(1):2–12.
106. de Bruin EI, Blom R, Smit FM, van Steensel FJ, Bögels SM. MYmind: mindfulness training for youngsters with autism spectrum disorders and their parents. Autism. 2015;19(8):906–14.
107. Salem-Guirgis S, Albaum C, Tablon P, Riosa PB, Nicholas DB, Drmic IE, et al. MYmind: a concurrent group-based mindfulness intervention for youth with autism and their parents. Mindfulness. 2019;10(9):1730–43.

108. Ridderinkhof A, de Bruin EI, Blom R, Bögels SM. Mindfulness-based program for children with autism spectrum disorder and their parents: direct and long-term improvements. Mindfulness. 2018;9(3):773–91.
109. Hwang Y-S, Kearney P, Klieve H, Lang W, Roberts J. Cultivating mind: mindfulness interventions for children with autism spectrum disorder and problem behaviours, and their mothers. J Child Fam Stud. 2015;24(10):3093–106.
110. Klinger LG, Cook ML, Dudley KM. Predictors and moderators of treatment efficacy in children and adolescents with autism Spectrum disorder. J Clin Child Adolesc Psychol. 2021;50(4):517–24.
111. Cariveau T, McCracken CE, Bradshaw J, Postorino V, Shillingsburg MA, McDougle CJ, et al. Gender differences in treatment-seeking youth with autism Spectrum disorder. J Child Fam Stud. 2021;30(3):784–92.

Pharmacological Interventions and an Emerging Understanding of the Need to Consider Sex Differences in Treatment Planning

10

Annie Fanta, Aniela Bordofsky, Cheyanne Sebolt, and Roger Jou

10.1 Introduction

Currently, there are no FDA-approved medications in the United States for treating the core symptoms of autism spectrum disorder (ASD). While two medications are approved specifically for treating irritability in children with autism, risperidone, and aripiprazole, the research on pharmacological treatments that target core symptoms of autism is limited and still in the stages of investigational clinical trials [1].

As a result, the pharmacological treatment of ASD tends to focus primarily on comorbid disorders, with numerous medications currently being used to treat comorbid diagnoses in the ASD population. However, it is essential to note that most research on pharmacological treatments of autism and comorbid disorders is based on a male population. There are no evidence-based differences between pharmacological treatments for males and females with ASD. This demonstrates a need for future research to investigate the differences in comorbid disorders in females with ASD and how pharmacological treatments might differ for the female ASD population.

Before discussing the various pharmacological treatments used to treat comorbid psychiatric disorders, it is first essential to understand the most common diagnoses in the ASD population. When compared to a psychiatrically referred population of non-ASD adults, it is found that ASD adults experience higher rates of current and lifetime psychiatric comorbidities [2]. In the pediatric population, up to 85% of children with autism have at least one other psychiatric diagnosis, and 35% take at least one medication as treatment [3]. This chapter focuses primarily on the pharmacological treatments of mood disorders, anxiety disorders, and attention-deficit/

A. Fanta · A. Bordofsky · C. Sebolt · R. Jou (✉)
Yale Child Study Center, New Haven, CT, USA
e-mail: Roger.Jou@yale.edu

L. Mazzone et al. (eds.), *Autism Spectrum Disorder: Understanding the Female Phenotype*, https://doi.org/10.1007/978-3-031-62072-0_10

hyperactivity disorder (ADHD), as they are most prevalent in the ASD population [3]. Other comorbidities discussed in this chapter include obsessive-compulsive disorder (OCD) and eating disorders. Sufficient evidence was not found to support how psychotic disorders, tic disorders, and Tourette syndrome should be treated differently when co-occurring with ASD. It is important to note that while many medications are used to treat the symptoms of these comorbid disorders, there is still a strong need for further research on how these medications can specifically target ASD symptoms and how they differ between female and male populations.

10.2 Mood Disorders

Individuals diagnosed with ASD are often diagnosed with a comorbid mood disorder. Symptoms of mood disorders in ASD can include depression, euphoria/mania, and sleep disturbance, often presenting alongside irritability [4]. Existing literature on mood disorders comorbid with ASD reports a wide prevalence range due to different diagnostic measures, age ranges, etc. However, mood disorders are frequently comorbid with ASD.

In a 2008 preliminary study of 44 adolescents and young adults with ASD, 36% of participants had a mood disorder of either major depressive disorder or bipolar disorder [5]. In a more recent 2019 study, depression was seen in 38% of a sample of 255 individuals with ASD [6]. Most research on comorbid depression and ASD has focused on children and adolescents [6]. Maternal ratings for 350 children with autism indicated that 54% of children with low support needs and 42% of children with high support needs had depression [7]. These high percentages reflect how often mood disorders impact individuals with ASD and the need for appropriate and effective pharmacological interventions.

Where an individual falls on the spectrum, the level of support needed appears to affect mood disorder comorbidity levels. This also makes diagnosing more challenging if an individual has an intellectual disability (ID) comorbid with ASD because they cannot elaborate on their personal experience, and one without ID [8]. The same is true for individuals with ASD that have limited expressive language, as these scenarios inevitably rely on caregiver and diagnostician observation for diagnosis [8]. When diagnosing, clinicians must be aware that individuals with ASD can present standard depressive symptoms seen in the neurotypical population, but it is also possible that depressive symptoms might be more specific to ASD, such as changes in repetitive behaviors or an increase in compulsivity or irritability [9]. When discussing mood disorders comorbid with ASD, it is essential to remember that every individual presents differently.

Studies report varying depression rates in adults with ASD with conflicting results. Results from a 30-year longitudinal study in Utah reported that adults with autism and ID are less likely to be identified as having comorbid depression than adults with autism that do not have ID [8]. In contrast, a 2019 Australian study of 255 individuals with ASD, high support needs, and *female gender* predicted an increase in depressive symptoms, with 38% of this sample reporting clinically significant depression [6]. These contradicting results likely highlight the previously mentioned differences across individuals and how they are impacted and the general lack of research on mood disorders in the ASD population. In this review, the latter-mentioned study was one of the few that mentioned female gender as a prediction of depressive symptoms, signaling a clear need for research on female-specific experiences regarding mood disorders and ASD.

Multiple pharmacological medications are used to treat mood disorders in individuals with ASD. Selective serotonin reuptake inhibitors (SSRIs) have been commonly used to treat depression in the ASD population, though evidence for efficacy is limited and conflicting. When treating children and adolescents with SSRIs, clinicians should be especially aware of increased potential side effects such as hyperactivity, aggression, and suicidal thoughts [9]. Research on SSRIs in children and adolescents with ASD has shown potential therapeutic benefits, including decreased ritualistic, stereotyped, and repetitive behaviors [10].

Atypical antipsychotic medications are also used in mood disorder treatment. Most existing studies target symptoms suggestive of a mood disorder (i.e., irritability, self-injury, severe tantrums, and aggression). Still, risperidone and aripiprazole are the only FDA-approved medications for these symptoms in ASD [9]. Risperidone and aripiprazole, antipsychotic medications, have successfully targeted irritability when treating children with ASD [4]. In treating irritability symptoms, risperidone is more effective than a placebo in treating repetitive or aggressive behaviors, irritability, anxiety, and depression [10]. However, the side effects of risperidone can cause the individual to feel more hungry, tired, or dizzy than usual [10]. Also, an antipsychotic, aripiprazole, is commonly prescribed to ASD patients with schizophrenia and bipolar disorder but can also be used in conjunction with other medications to treat depression and irritability [10]. Weight gain has been observed as a side effect of aripiprazole during treatment [10]. If an individual can tolerate or does not experience these side effects, risperidone or aripiprazole could help improve many symptoms of mood disorders comorbid with ASD.

Lithium is a psychotropic medication prescribed to individuals with ASD as a mood stabilizer, specifically for comorbid bipolar disorder. Yet, limited evidence-based research exists for its use, specifically in the ASD population [9]. Before 2014, the authors of the following study were aware of only five individuals with ASD that were ever examined for the efficacy of lithium [4]. In a study of 30 individuals with ASD, researchers determined that 43% of subjects demonstrated improvement when treated with lithium, and 71% of those with two or more pre-treatment mood disorder symptoms improved [4]. In the previously mentioned study, almost half of the sample experienced side effects from lithium, such as vomiting, tremor, fatigue, and irritability [4]. There is cause for concern in the administration of lithium because the rate of side effects observed is higher than most side effect rates of other psychotropic medicines for ASD [4]. Lithium as a treatment for mood disorders in ASD continues to be cautionary but does demonstrate results in some cases.

As discussed, the literature on pharmacological treatment options for females with ASD is limited. This remains consistent when examining comorbid mood disorders and demonstrates a clear need for further research on mood disorder treatment options for the autism community and a focus on female-specific treatment.

10.3 Anxiety Disorders

Anxiety disorders also make up many comorbid diagnoses in the ASD population. While the research shows ranging levels of prevalence for this comorbidity, it has been reported that 40% of children and adolescents with ASD meet the criteria for clinically significant anxiety [6]. This is much higher than non-ASD children and adolescents and children and adolescents with other neurodevelopmental diagnoses [6]. This high prevalence of anxiety is also present in adult ASD populations. It could be even higher, with studies reporting that up to 53.6% of adults with ASD meet the criteria for clinically significant anxiety [6].

These high rates can have a significant impact on individuals with ASD. A comorbid diagnosis of anxiety is associated with increased severity of core ASD symptoms and psychosocial functioning [11]. Additionally, autism severity has been reported to predict anxiety in children and adolescents [7]. Research has also identified risk factors of increasing IQ, age, and autism severity for anxiety in autistic youth and adolescents [7]. Consistent with this is a study that used maternal ratings as a measurement and found that 79% of children with low support needs had anxiety compared to 67% of children with high support needs [7]. While there is limited research on the sex/gender differences of comorbid anxiety, some literature shows that females experience higher levels of affective symptoms of anxiety [6].

Despite the high prevalence, identifying anxiety as a comorbid diagnosis with ASD can be challenging as the core features of ASD and anxiety often overlap. For example, a social avoidance behavior could be categorized as a social communication deficit of autism or a presentation of anxiety [9]. It can also be challenging to distinguish between restrictive and repetitive behaviors, a core component of ASD, and ritualistic behaviors, which manifest anxiety [9].

Once a comorbid diagnosis of anxiety is identified in an individual with autism, pharmacological treatments are often considered. However, it is essential to note that the research on the efficacy of these medications is primarily focused on neurotypical populations, and the data on specifically ASD populations is limited. In the neurotypical adult population, the most common medications used to treat anxiety disorders are selective serotonin reuptake inhibitors (SSRIs) due to their efficacy and relatively minimal adverse effects [9]. Randomized placebo-controlled trials have reported that 40–60% of individuals have improved their anxiety from taking a placebo, while 60–75% have improved results from SSRI medications [12]. SSRIs remain the most common medication for anxiety in typically developing youth populations, with research showing evidence that SSRIs are effective in a pediatric population [13].

Due to the potential anxiolytic effects of SSRIs, they are also the most common medications for children with anxiety and ASD. Some clinical data indicate that SSRIs could effectively treat comorbid ASD and anxiety, especially for children

[11]. However, because of a lack of large-scale randomized controlled trials on the efficacy of SSRIs in treating children with anxiety and ASD, there is no evidence to support the widespread prescribing of SSRIs to this population [14]. Additionally, some studies have reported that the behavioral activation effects of SSRIs in ASD children could present more negatively than in typically developing children, with a potential increase in irritability, aggression, and agitation [11].

Similarly, very few studies have examined the efficacy of SSRIs in treating anxiety in adults with ASD. The results from the few existing studies are mixed, with some reporting evidence of the effectiveness of SSRIs on anxiety within the ASD population and others reporting no change in anxiety symptoms [9]. While there is currently no evidence of an association between serotonin activity and ASD symptoms, SSRIs are hypothesized to regulate the abnormal serotonin activity in ASD individuals that experience anxiety and compulsive behaviors [11]. This supports a strong need for further research on the efficacy of SSRIs in treating anxiety within an ASD population.

Benzodiazepines are also commonly used to treat generalized anxiety disorder as they are known to be efficacious and fast acting. Following SSRIs, benzodiazepines are the second-most widely used medication to treat youth with anxiety [13]. However, they can also have limitations to treatment and adverse side effects, such as minimal efficacy in treating comorbid depression symptoms, drowsiness, memory impairment, dependence, impaired psychomotor function, and withdrawal symptoms [15]. Due to these issues, benzodiazepines are typically prescribed for specific scenarios, such as short-term treatment for anxiety or for patients who have exhausted other options.

10.4 Attention-Deficit/Hyperactivity Disorder

Attention-deficit/hyperactivity disorder (ADHD) is another neurodevelopmental disorder commonly comorbid with ASD. Gender differences in individuals diagnosed with both ASD and ADHD have not been widely studied to date. However, a few conclusions regarding this subject have been made as secondary findings in various studies. Due to the lack of research in this area, ADHD is treated similarly in males and females with ASD and in neurotypical populations. Before the release of the DSM-5 in 2013, clinicians were discouraged from making comorbid ADHD and ASD diagnoses due to some of the overlap between the disorders [16]. After this restriction was lifted, more research began to be carried out on the overlap between ASD and ADHD, a field of research that will presumably only continue to grow.

While the sex/gender differences in individuals diagnosed with ASD and ADHD have not been widely studied, one study found that ASD females with low support needs have higher levels of inattention than ASD males with low support needs [17]. Typically developing (TD) populations are often characterized by males having higher rates of ADHD than females [17].

While few studies have examined sex/gender differences in individuals with ASD and ADHD, others have been conducted to compare differing age groups living with these disorders. In children, ADHD and ASD have a high rate of comorbidity, with 40–70% of children with ASD also having an ADHD diagnosis [16]. Due to the high proportion of children diagnosed with both ADHD and ASD, many parents consider pharmacological treatments. Regarding adults with ASD, ADHD occurs at similar rates as in childhood, with one study finding that 39% of adults in the sample had both diagnoses [2]. This finding signifies that while ADHD is often a childhood-onset disorder, it persists into adulthood, impacting individuals throughout their lifespan [2]. Many effective pharmacological treatments have been developed to treat ADHD, and thus it is hopeful that individuals with ADHD and ASD can benefit from these treatments.

Multiple pharmacological treatments have shown effectiveness in treating individuals with ASD and ADHD and some of their overlapping symptomatology. Social impairment is one of these overlapping symptoms that individuals with ASD and ADHD often struggle with. For individuals with ADHD, this can manifest through impulsivity or disruptive behaviors. In contrast, in individuals with ASD, this lack of social competence is often due to an absence of socially adaptive behaviors such as eye contact [16]. Researchers have found that prescribing medications to treat ADHD in individuals with ADHD and ASD can help with these social competency issues by targeting other behaviors. One study found that 86% of youth with comorbid ASD and ADHD have been prescribed medication for ADHD symptoms to target aggression and hyperactive-impulsive behaviors [16]. This type of treatment targets the symptoms characteristic of ADHD, such as impulsivity, but can also have positive impacts on children's social capabilities.

According to the American Academy of Pediatrics [18], there are two forms of stimulants approved to treat attention deficits and hyperactivity disorders: immediate-release (short-acting) medications and extended-release (intermediate-acting and long-acting) medications. In the ASD population, stimulants are the most commonly prescribed medications for treating comorbid ADHD. However, some studies have found adverse side effects in ASD populations. The results of a meta-analysis of methylphenidate, a stimulant frequently used to treat ADHD, showed lower effect sizes in individuals with ASD and ADHD than for individuals with only ADHD [16]. It was also reported that methylphenidate could result in more severe side effects, such as depression, social withdrawal, and irritability when used in an ASD population [16]. Some parents or independent adults with ASD and ADHD may not want to risk developing these side effects for a potentially less effective treatment. Nevertheless, stimulants like methylphenidate continue to be the most commonly prescribed medication for individuals with comorbid disorders of ASD and ADHD.

Other medications have been tested in treating ADHD in populations with ASD in recent studies. Drugs such as atomoxetine (an SSRI) and guanfacine (an alpha agonist) can treat ADHD in ASD. One study showed that atomoxetine reduced ADHD symptoms in 43% of children with ASD and an intellectual disability [16]. An 8-week clinical trial of guanfacine in youth with ASD and ADHD reported significant reductions in parent-reported oppositional behaviors but no differences in parent-reported anxiety and sleep issues [16]. While these treatments are prescribed less often than stimulants, parents may want other options based on their primary behavioral concerns. Additionally, some families may opt for more nontraditional therapies for ADHD to avoid some possible side effects when taking stimulants.

With ADHD being one of the most commonly occurring comorbid disorders with ASD, families need to be aware of the different pharmacological treatment options for individuals with these diagnoses. It would be beneficial for more research to be conducted in this area, especially surrounding how males and females respond to different treatment options.

10.5 Obsessive-Compulsive Disorder

Obsessive-compulsive disorder (OCD) is another disorder that often occurs alongside ASD and has overlapping symptomatology. Similar to other comorbid disorders discussed in this chapter, little research has been conducted on females with ASD and OCD. Based on the lack of differentiation between genders in this study, females and males with OCD and ASD are treated using a similar pharmacological approach.

Due to the high similarities between ASD and OCD, making a comorbid diagnosis can be difficult; nevertheless, studies demonstrate that OCD often occurs with ASD [8]. Some of the overlapping symptoms of ASD and OCD can be differentiated by clinicians based on the intricacies of each disorder. In children and adolescents with ASD, rates of OCD have been reported at varying speeds, from 2.6 to 37.2% [19]. In one 2006 study that surveyed over 100 children, 37% qualified for an OCD diagnosis [20]. While these comorbidity rates vary, it is apparent that OCD commonly occurs with ASD in children and adolescents. Regarding adults with ASD, one study found that 22% of the sample met the lifetime criteria for an OCD diagnosis, despite researchers removing the OCD item that coincides with an ASD criterion [8]. By removing this item, the OCD diagnosis gains accuracy as the chance of overlap between ASD and OCD decreases in this instance.

Some common compulsions are found among those diagnosed with ASD and OCD. The most common compulsion found in a study of children with ASD and OCD was a ritual that involves other people, such as having their parents complete certain daily routines in a specific way [20]. This compulsion is often unique to those who have also been diagnosed with ASD and can inform clinicians' diagnostic process.

The use of pharmacological treatments for OCD in the general population has been widely studied, and many individuals find that these medications alleviate some of the unwanted symptoms of OCD. However, there is a lack of research conducted on using these medications for individuals with OCD and ASD diagnoses. Selective serotonin reuptake inhibitors (SSRIs) and serotonin-norepinephrine reuptake inhibitors (SNRIs) are the most commonly prescribed medications used to treat OCD in the general population. However, there is insufficient evidence available on the usage of these medications in the ASD population [19]. Furthermore, some evidence points toward individuals with ASD being more sensitive to the negative side effects of these medications, some of which are impulsivity and insomnia [19]. This finding may concern some individuals being treated for ASD and OCD.

One common SSRI, fluoxetine, has been studied in a few randomized control trials to determine its ability to reduce ASD symptoms and compulsive and repetitive behaviors in children [11]. While one study did see a decrease in repetitive behaviors in the treatment group, more extensive studies of fluoxetine in individuals with ASD saw no change in repetitive behaviors [11]. In another study which consisted of six adults with ASD, no decreases in ASD symptoms were seen, and overall reductions in anxiety and repetitive behaviors were found among participants [11]. The highly variable results of these studies indicate inconsistencies in the knowledge surrounding how individuals with both ASD and OCD respond to this medication.

In addition to the fluoxetine studies in adults and children with ASD and OCD, a few other studies have been conducted to examine the potential benefits of other SSRIs and SNRIs, with mixed results. Due to the lack of ample research, the pharmacological treatment of comorbid ASD and OCD should be handled cautiously.

More research in this field would benefit individuals diagnosed with ASD and OCD, as this is a significant part of the population. Furthermore, studies examining the sex/gender differences in individuals with ASD and OCD would help determine effective treatment methods for both groups.

10.6 Eating Disorders

It has been observed that more males are diagnosed with ASD, yet females with ASD are disproportionately represented in the adult eating disorder population [21]. In a 2013 systematic review of eight studies published between 1992 and 2011 in Sweden [13] or the UK [16], in which all eight studies screened for both eating disorders and ASD, a 22.9% prevalence rate of ASD was discovered [22]. This highlights a clear overrepresentation of ASD in these eating disorder samples [22]. While the review did not assess sex/gender differences and the impact of eating disorders in the female ASD population, others emphasized females. For example, a 2017 clinical audit study evaluating the effects of ASD traits on treatment outcomes of restrictive eating disorders found that ASD traits were higher than expected in the general population but did not affect treatment outcomes [21].

While the highest rates of ASD and eating disorders are within the adult population, it should be noted that treatment guidelines suggest that medication should not be used as the primary treatment of children and adolescents with anorexia nervosa; family-based psychological therapies should be used instead as they are the most evidence-based treatment option for anorexia nervosa [12]. There is also a wide range of eating disorder presentations in those with ASD, and it is therefore recommended to facilitate a trait-based approach, which may increase success in treatment [23].

There has been cautionary success with antidepressant medication treatment for those with ASD and anorexia nervosa due to some having significant side effects and a general lack of research [12]. Studies that assess fluoxetine to treat anorexia nervosa often have high dropout rates or show no considerable success [12]. However, in the treatment of adults with bulimia nervosa, fluoxetine allows both binging and purging to decrease significantly [12]. An article published in 2007 noted that a few case reports suggested that the atypical antipsychotic olanzapine may help treat anorexia nervosa. However, this proved successful in those with low body weights [12]. To date, there has not been any research that studies how effective olanzapine is in the treatment of eating disorders comorbid with ASD. Other antipsychotics, such as risperidone, have even less research to support their usage. The same goes for tricyclic antidepressants, which have been studied in controlled trials with no increase in weight gain for hospitalized patients [12].

Most existing research on eating disorder treatment pertains to the general population, with few studies assessing treatment options for individuals with ASD, especially females. Ideally, in the future, more treatment options will be trait-specific to the individual with ASD, and medication will be prescribed on a case-by-case basis.

10.7 Conclusion

With no medications currently approved to treat the core symptoms of autism, pharmacological treatments for individuals with autism are primarily used to treat comorbid diagnoses. As this chapter discusses, the most prevalent comorbid diagnoses in individuals with ASD include mood disorders, anxiety disorders, ADHD, OCD, and eating disorders. Therefore, the most common medications used in the ASD population are prescribed for these comorbid conditions. However, it is essential to note that many other comorbid diagnoses occur within the autism population.

With a lack of research on sex/gender differences in comorbid diagnoses within ASD and their respective pharmacological treatments, comorbid diagnoses are treated similarly in males and females with ASD. This demonstrates a strong need for future research to investigate the differences in comorbid disorders in females with ASD and how pharmacological treatments might differ for the female ASD population.

Key Points

- Currently, in the United States, there are no FDA-approved medications for treating the core symptoms of autism spectrum disorder (ASD), and therefore the pharmacological therapies for individuals with ASD focus on treating comorbid conditions.
- The most common comorbid diagnoses in the ASD population are mood disorders, anxiety disorders, attention-deficit/hyperactivity disorder (ADHD), obsessive-compulsive disorder (OCD), and eating disorders. Medications for these comorbid diagnoses, among the most frequently prescribed within the ASD population, are SSRIs, benzodiazepines, stimulants, antipsychotics, lithium, and guanfacine.

- Most research on pharmacological treatments of autism and comorbid disorders is based on the male population. There are no evidence-based differences between pharmacological treatments for males and females with ASD. This demonstrates a need for future research to investigate the differences in comorbid disorders in females with ASD and how pharmacological treatments might differ for the female ASD population.
- Additionally, there is a need for future research to investigate pharmacological treatments that target the core symptoms of ASD and how therapy might differ between males and females.

References

1. LeClerc S, Easley D. Pharmacological therapies for autism spectrum disorder: a review. P & T. 2015;40(6):389–97.
2. Joshi G, Wozniak J, Petty C, Martelon MK, Fried R, Bolfek A, et al. Psychiatric comorbidity and functioning in a clinically referred population of adults with autism spectrum disorders: a comparative study. J Autism Dev Disord. 2012;43(6):1314–25. https://doi.org/10.1007/s10803-012-1679-5.
3. Bennett A. Autism's clinical companions: frequent comorbidities with ASD. Children's Hospital of Philadelphia; 2017. https://www.chop.edu/news/autism-s-clinical-companions-frequent-comorbidities-asd#:~:text=Psychiatric%20comorbidities,1%20psychotropic%20medication%20as%20treatment. Accessed 1 Jun 2021.
4. Siegel M, Beresford CA, Bunker M, Verdi M, Vishnevetsky D, Karlsson C, et al. Preliminary investigation of lithium for mood disorder symptoms in children and adolescents with autism spectrum disorder. J Child Adolesc Psychopharmacol. 2014;24(7):399–402. https://doi.org/10.1089/cap.2014.0019.
5. Munesue T, Ono Y, Mutoh K, Shimoda K, Nakatani H, Kikuchi M. High prevalence of bipolar disorder comorbidity in adolescents and young adults with high-functioning autism spectrum disorder: a preliminary study of 44 outpatients. J Affect Disord. 2008;111(2–3):170–5. https://doi.org/10.1016/j.jad.2008.02.015.
6. Uljarević M, Hedley D, Rose-Foley K, Magiati I, Cai RY, Dissanayake C, et al. Anxiety and depression from adolescence to old age in autism spectrum disorder. J Autism Dev Disord. 2019;50(9):3155–65. https://doi.org/10.1007/s10803-019-04084-z.
7. Mayes SD, Calhoun SL, Murray MJ, Zahid J. Variables associated with anxiety and depression in children with autism. J Dev Phys Disabil. 2011;23(4):325–37. https://doi.org/10.1007/s10882-011-9231-7.
8. Buck T, Viskochil J, Farley M, Coon H, McMahon W, Morgan J, Bilder D. Psychiatric comorbidity and medication use in adults with autism spectrum disorder. J Autism Dev Disord. 2014;44:3063–71. https://doi.org/10.1007/s10803-014-2170-2.
9. Mazzone L, Vitiello B. Anxiety in autism spectrum disorder. In: Psychiatric symptoms and comorbidities in autism Spectrum disorder. Springer International Publishing; 2016. p. 21–32.
10. Eissa N, Al-Houqani M, Sadeq A, Ojha SK, Sasse A, Sadek B. Current enlightenment about etiology and pharmacological treatment of autism spectrum disorder. Front Neurosci. 2018;12:304. https://doi.org/10.3389/fnins.2018.00304.
11. Nadeau J, Sulkowski ML, Ung D, Wood JJ, Lewin AB, Murphy TK, et al. Treatment of comorbid anxiety and autism spectrum disorders. Neuropsychiatry (London). 2011;1(6):567–78. https://doi.org/10.2217/npy.11.62.
12. Couturier J, Lock J. A review of medication use for children and adolescents with eating disorders. J Can Acad Child Adolesc Psychiatry. 2007;16(4):173–6. https://www.ncbi.nlm.nih.gov/pmc/articles/PMC2247460/pdf/ccap16_4p173.pdf.

13. Bushnell GA, Compton SN, Dusetzina SB, Gaynes BN, Brookhart MA, Walkup JT, et al. Treating pediatric anxiety: initial use of SSRIs and other antianxiety prescription medications. J Clin Psychiatry. 2018;79(1):16m11415. https://doi.org/10.4088/JCP.16m11415.
14. Vasa RA, Carroll LM, Nozzolillo AA, Mahajan R, Mazurek MO, Bennett AE, et al. A systematic review of treatments for anxiety in youth with autism spectrum disorders. J Autism Dev Disord. 2014;44(12):3215–29. https://doi.org/10.1007/s10803-014-2184-9.
15. Baldwin D, Waldman S, Allgulander C. Evidence-based pharmacological treatment of generalized anxiety disorder. Int J Neuropsychopharmacol. 2011;14(5):697–710. https://doi.org/10.1017/S1461145710001434.
16. Antshel KM, Russo N. Autism spectrum disorders and ADHD: overlapping phenomenology, diagnostic issues, and treatment considerations. Curr Psychiatry Rep. 2019;21(34):1–11. https://doi.org/10.1007/s11920-019-1020-5.
17. Worley JA, Matson JL. Psychiatric symptoms in children diagnosed with an autism spectrum disorder: examining gender differences. Res Autism Spectr Disord. 2011;5(3):1086–91. https://doi.org/10.1016/j.rasd.2010.12.002.
18. Common ADHD medications & treatments for children. American Academy of Pediatrics. 2019. https://www.healthychildren.org/English/health-issues/conditions/adhd/Pages/Determining-ADHD-Medication-Treatments.aspx. Accessed 1 Jun 2021.
19. Postorino V, Kerns C, Vivanti G, Bradshaw J, Siracusano M, Mazzone L. Anxiety disorders and obsessive-compulsive disorder in individuals with autism spectrum disorder. Curr Psychiatry Rep. 2017;19(92):1–8. https://doi.org/10.1007/s11920-017-0846-y.
20. Leyfer O, Folstein S, Bacalman S, Davis N, Dinh E, Morgan J, et al. Comorbid psychiatric disorders in children with autism: interview development and rates of disorders. J Autism Dev Disord. 2006;36:849–61. https://doi.org/10.1007/s10803-006-0123-0.
21. Stewart CS, McEwen FS, Konstantellou A, Eisler I, Simic M. Impact of ASD traits on treatment outcomes of eating disorders in girls. Eur Eat Disord Rev. 2017;25(2):123–8. https://doi.org/10.1002/erv.2497.
22. Huke V, Turk J, Saeidi S, Kent A, Morgan JF. Autism spectrum disorders in eating disorder populations: a systematic review. Eur Eat Disord Rev. 2013;21(5):345–51. https://doi.org/10.1002/erv.2244.
23. Treasure J. Coherence and other autistic spectrum traits and eating disorders: building from mechanism to treatment. The Birgit Olsson lecture. Nord J Psychiatry. 2012;67(1):38–42. https://doi.org/10.3109/08039488.2012.674554.

Part V

Quality of Life for Transition Age Youth

Autism and Gender and Sexuality Diversity

11

Jeroen Dewinter, Zosia Zaks, Nikki Brörmann, Ivan Henczyk, Elizabeth K. Graham, and John F. Strang

11.1 Introduction and Terminology

Over the past decade, there has been increasing interest in the diverse genders and sexualities of autistic people [1–4]. Previously, sexuality in autism was largely ignored, or approached as a reason for concern [5] with a focus on knowledge and behaviors [6, 7]. Only recently has research focused on self-report and the lived experience of sexuality and gender in autistic individuals [8, 9]. Outside of clinical research, the growing autistic self-advocacy movement—which emphasizes the perspectives and needs of autistic communities—has pointed out the broad experiences of gender and sexuality among autistic people [10]

J. Dewinter
Clinical psychologist at the Unit for Children and Adolescents at GGzE, Eindhoven, The Netherlands and senior researcher at Tranzo, the scientific center for care and wellbeing, Tilburg School of Social and Behavioral Sciences, Tilburg University, Tilburg, The Netherlands
e-mail: Jeroen.dewinter@ggze.nl

Z. Zaks
Zaks Autism Consulting, Baltimore, MD, USA

N. Brörmann · I. Henczyk
Autiroze, The Netherlands

E. K. Graham
The Arc of Prince George's County, Largo, MD, USA

J. F. Strang (✉)
Children's National Hospital, Washington, DC, USA
e-mail: JStrang@childrensnational.org

L. Mazzone et al. (eds.), *Autism Spectrum Disorder: Understanding the Female Phenotype*, https://doi.org/10.1007/978-3-031-62072-0_11

Situated within a book examining autism in girls and women, this chapter presents intersections with female designated sex *and* female gender, and thereby challenges commonly held by sex-difference frameworks [11]. The intersections of LGBTQ+ identities (further explained below) with the *female* gender- and/or designated sex-related focus of the larger book have an obvious link for transgender people of female gender identity, cisgender female individuals who are not heterosexual, and any LGBTQ+ individual designated female sex at birth. Only a few subgroups within the broad LGBTQ+ would be omitted for lack of clear intersection with female-designated sex/gender (e.g., gay and bisexual cisgender males), but even within these subgroups, there may be the presence—for some individuals—of more "femme" expressions and/or a range of interests common in girls and women [12]. Therefore, in order to appropriately cover the topic of the intersection of LGBTQ+ identities and autism, we will take the literary liberty of including the full LGBTQ+ spectrum in our review and discussion.

A proportional overrepresentation (i.e., as compared to the general population) of gender and sexuality diversity in autistic people is often reported in research (e.g., [2, 4, 13–15]) and is also featured in autistic testimonials and writings (e.g., [16, 17]). Autistic self-advocates have emphasized the importance of listening to and including the voices and perspectives of autistic individuals regarding their experience in their gender and sexuality [11, 18], yet the majority of available research on gender and sexuality diversity in autism has not included autistic co-researchers', nor autistic community's, perspectives. Therefore, to counterbalance potential neuronormative, cisnormative, and/or heteronormative biases within the available literature (i.e., a literature written primarily by non-autistic cisgender individuals, many of whom are also heterosexual), the authors of this chapter have joined together as an intentionally representative group of autistic and non-autistic, gender-diverse and cisgender, and gay, lesbian, and bisexual contributors. In this chapter, the existing research on gender and sexuality in autism is discussed through a double lens: (1) from the perspective of non-autistic researchers in the field [JD; JS] and, concurrently, (2) from the perspectives of research partners with lived experience of being autistic and gender and/or sexuality diverse [NB; EG; IH; ZZ]. Through this diverse author partnership, we seek to provide an overview of the present research pertaining to the intersection of autism and gender, sexual attraction and identity diversity, as well as autistic perspectives regarding directions in which researchers might next focus their work.

The terms employed in this chapter may require definition and explanation. Importantly, terminology in the field of gender and sexuality diversity, as well as in autism, is in flux, and so some of the vocabulary employed here may not stand the test of time. Because many of the terms used describe the personal experience and identities of individuals, we would like to proactively apologize to any readers who find our language problematic, now or in the future. Our team worked to employ language that we understood, based on standards from current gender and sexuality diversity advocacy initiatives [19], to be the most affirming and respectful available. In a parallel manner, to refer to autism and neurodivergence, we have endeavored to employ language that is contemporary and affirmative of autistic experiences and identities [20, 21]. However, it must be acknowledged that there is variation in preferred autism-related language among autistic people; for example, there is no overall consensus regarding identity-first (i.e., autism-first language; an "autistic person") versus person-first language (a person "with autism"; [21, 22]). Further, the characterization of autism as a disorder, disability, identity, strength, challenge, and/or diagnosis remains an ongoing discussion [23].

In terms of language and concepts, we differentiate designated sex and gender. Designated sex refers to primary physiological components of a person, which often includes sex-related chromosomes [24]. Readers will note that in this chapter, we always add the word "designated" before the word "sex" to remind readers that the "designated sex" may be very different from a person's gender identity; in the context of the contemporary gender-affirming movement, the word "sex" alone is insufficient and should be preceded by "designated" or "assigned." In this way, a transgender woman might have a "designated sex at birth" that is male, but her gender identity (or just "gender") is female [25]. It is important to acknowledge that sex is more complex than a binary construct; even outside of variations in sex development (e.g., differences of sex development; intersex identities), components of sex can be multi-categorized [26]. Gender identity (or "gender") refers to the core gender that a person experiences themselves as (e.g., male, female, non-binary, agender, fluid). The word "gender" is complex as it can refer to gender identity, but also relates to multiple aspects of the gender experience beyond identity, such as societal components and expectations of gender roles, societal conventions and individual gender expressions, and gender-related interests [27].

The term "gender diversity" has been claimed by communities of providers and researchers working with transgender, non-binary, and other people whose gender identities differ from their designated sex at birth [28]. In this chapter, "gender diversity" will refer to the gender experience of that broad group of people who experience variation in gender identity from the designated sex at birth as well as people with gender expressions that differ from the expressions associated with the designated sex at birth or gender role in a specific time and culture. We acknowledge that the term gender diversity is used in contrasting ways for other contexts (e.g., to describe inclusion of women in the workplace), but these broader definitions of the term are not employed within this chapter. The term "transgender" refers to people who experience gender identity diversity. In this way, transgender is very similar to gender diversity, though it does not include people who experience gender expression diversity, without diversity in gender identity. Non-binary refers to genders that are not male or female, specifically. This can include genders that are neither male nor female or genders that have components of more than one gender. Agender refers to no experience of gender. Finally, cisgender describes the experience of a gender congruent with the designated sex at birth.

In terms of sexuality, lesbian refers to a person whose gender is female and who is attracted to women. Gay men have male gender and are attracted to men. Bisexual people are of any gender and experience attraction to two genders. Pansexual people are people of any gender and experience attraction to multiple genders. Asexuality is the absence of sexual desire for other people, and the asexual spectrum refers to diversity within asexuality (e.g., gray- or demi-asexual; [29]). Taken together, the identities and experiences of gender diversity and sexual orientation diversity are often expressed with the descriptor, LGBTQ+, where "L" refers to lesbian, "G" to gay (presumably gay male), "B" to bisexual, "T" to transgender, and "Q" to questioning (as in still exploring or concerned with applying a specific label) or queer (queer being an umbrella term referring to the entire LGBTQ+ spectrum and its intersections); "+" refers to all other gender and sexuality identities. Some also add an "I" (for intersex people) and an "A" for agender and/or asexual. We will use "straight" and "heterosexual" to describe people who are attracted to the other binary gender, alone. We do not use the word "homosexual" because within some LGBTQ+ communities, the term is experienced as less affirming [30]. We provide this level of terminology review to assist researchers and clinicians in knowing key components of experience and appropriate types of language when working with the gender-diverse and/or sexuality-diverse autistic communities.

11.2 Overview of the Importance of Understanding the LGBTQ+/Autism Intersection

As noted above, a series of studies have reported a significant (proportional) overrepresentation of gender diversity and sexual orientation diversity in autism [3, 31–33]. Independently, studies of gender-diverse populations have reported a significant proportional overrepresentation of autism (at the level of diagnosis and traits) in gender-diverse samples [1, 4, 34, 35]. Finally, a link between autistic traits and gender diversity has been reported in the nonclinical general population [13].

These apparent proportional overrepresentations have implications in terms of research, ethics, rights, and clinical practice. We briefly discuss some of these. For example, in research, ignoring the gender and sexuality dimensions of autistic people may result in a loss of critical information. For instance, some aspects of autistic experience, including components of mental health, may be better understood and measured by variations in gender, beyond designated sex [36]. Yet, the vast majority of autism research fails to model gender beyond designated sex. Also, our insight into the needs of gender- and sexuality-diverse individuals is still limited, although we know that this group experiences more mental health problems [37]. In clinical practice, attention to the needs of gender and sexual diversity in autistic individuals is important to provide attuned care. There is a history of doubting autistic people's experiences of sexual and/or gender identities and related needs [38]. This led to major US advocacy organizations joining together to develop a declaration of the rights of autistic gender-diverse individuals following the death of Kayden Clark, an autistic transgender man who died following what he described as a long history of being denied gender-affirming medical care due to his autism status [39]. There have been apparent improvements in the climate of affirmation and acceptance for autistic LGBTQ+ people, but profound disparities in access to supports still exist above and beyond disparities associated with being autistic or LGBTQ+ independently [40].

Broader research on autism and sexual and gender diversity is needed, as well as attention to this diversity in clinical practice. Within the field of research on LGBTQ+ intersection with autism, there are notable emerging disparities. First, samples within studies tend to be fairly monocultural and focused on primarily White individuals; the majority of studies lack race and ethnicity diversity (for an exception, see [41]). Also, research studies on the intersection of autism and gender diversity (especially in youth) profoundly outnumber studies of sexuality diversity in ASD. Yet, the measurement and modeling of sexual orientation may be to some degree explanatory in brain-related studies, and perhaps especially as a control variable in studies of sex and gender [42]. Further, gender expression and gender-related interests may be more expansive for LGB individuals than for straight individuals [43]. The way we examine play in children and for autism diagnosis is primarily based on heterosexual cisgender male models of play. The focus on cisgender male play in regard to the diagnosis of autism has been critiqued for its reduced relevance in cisgender girls, who may have less obvious characteristics of autism in social interaction and interests [44, 45]. Given the common variations in play interests and other gender characteristics in LGB youth, and LGBTQ+ youth more broadly, it is possible that some play for autistic LGBTQ+ youth may not fit within typical gender-related patterns. Therefore, both gender *and* sexuality variation in autism may be important additional factors to consider in the presentation of autism characteristics (also known as "symptoms"). Yet, we have no acceptable vocabulary to even begin this investigation, as terms such as the "female autism phenotype" or the "female presentations of autism" are inappropriate for people who have genders other than female (e.g., transgender males, non-binary individuals, femme gay boys). Therefore, the authors of this chapter, along with other advocates in the field, call upon sex-difference researchers in autism to engage in dialogue with LGBTQ+ autistic communities to improve the current language employed to describe variations in autism by sex, so as to include the full range of genders and sexualities in the terminology [11].

11.3 Gender Diversity and Autism

The intersection of gender diversity and autism was first identified in gender clinic-based studies, which reported high rates of both autism spectrum disorder (ASD, i.e., diagnosis) and autistic traits more broadly in gender-referred samples [1, 46, 47]. Methodologically, some of these studies suffered from the lack of specificity provided by ASD screening tools; critiques noted that elevations on ASD measures among gender-diverse individuals might well be due to anxiety and depression, and not ASD symptoms specifically [48]. However, even among several of the studies that employed autism screening tools, rates of clinical ASD were reported, with rates of ASD showing large effect size proportional overrepresentation, even when compared with the most inclusive base rates for ASD in the general population [34]. In the largest study to date ($N = 641{,}860$), the odds of being autistic among gender-diverse individuals was ~6.4 that of being autistic among cisgender individuals [4].

In the largest study to date of children and adolescents, specifically ($N = 292{,}572$), the odds ratio of a child meeting the criteria for gender dysphoria (the DSM-5 classification for distress related to gender incongruence) was ~4.4 if they were autistic as compared to non-autistic [31]. A significant overrepresentation of neurodiversity (beyond autism) in gender-diverse populations has also been reported in some studies, including broad neurodevelopmental diversity [4], ADHD specifically [36], and executive functioning differences [49, 50]. Finally, the intersection of autism and gender diversity has been reported at a trait level in a nonclinical community-based sample [13].

Some have commented on the nature of the autism and gender diversity co-occurrence from the perspective of etiology. For example, some have suggested that the over-occurrence could be the result of the culturally unanticipated and strong interests common in autism [51]. However, self-report descriptions from youth themselves do not concord with such descriptions, and instead speak to a deep-felt experience of gender dysphoria and gender identity diversity by many autistic transgender young people [14]. It has also been suggested that a deeper biological link (e.g., sex hormone) might drive sex/gender variation in autism [52]. Finally, some autistic commentators have described that autistic people may be less likely to abide by—or be aware of—social restrictions against gender diversity, and therefore may be more likely to express gender variation (J. F [53].).

There have also been messages by autistic commentators discouraging an over-focus on etiology, and instead focusing research efforts on strategies to understand and support gender-diverse autistic individuals [53]. This position against focusing research on etiology of the over-occurrence accords with larger concerns expressed within the transgender community regarding probes of biological determinants of gender identity, for fear of how these findings could be used to gatekeep services (e.g., for those who do not show the expected biological indicators) or for attempts to biologically suppress gender diversity itself [54].

Initial work examining experiences and needs of autistic gender-diverse individuals have identified an increased risk for mental health challenges, above and beyond mental health risks associated with autism or gender minority stress independently [36, 37, 55, 56]; no studies to date have accounted for potential additional disparities related to other intersecting minoritized statuses or identities. Qualitative work with autistic gender-diverse adolescents has identified intersectional mechanisms such as the need for time to discover one's identities, competing challenges related to being autistic and gender diverse, and intersectional stressors that may in part drive greater mental health burden: autistic transgender teens described the challenges of being autistic (with associated executive function and social differences) on gender affirmation processes, such as problems accessing gender care, managing the routines required for gender transition, and advocating for gender-related needs [14]. These experiences were translated into a self-report measure, the Gender-diversity-related Barriers Questionnaire (GBQ; [57]), which was administered to cohorts of autistic transgender and non-autistic transgender youth. As predicted, autistic transgender youth reported many more gender transition-related barriers related to executive function differences than non-autistic transgender youth, and executive function-related gender barriers predicted both internalizing problems and suicidality [36]. Of importance, these executive function-related gender barriers were more predictive of suicidality among transgender youth than experiences of LGBT-related stigma.

Preliminary work has been done on specific clinical supports for gender-diverse autistic people. Importantly, the DSM-5 mentions autism as a common co-occurring experience with gender dysphoria [58], and the upcoming Standards of Care 8 through the World Professional Association for Transgender Health (WPATH) provide specific references to and guidance for supporting autistic transgender children and adolescents. Further, the Global Education Initiative through WPATH, the primary certification program for gender care providers internationally, includes didactics specifically dedicated to the intersection of gender diversity and neurodiversity. In terms of research, a set of initial clinical guidelines for the care of autistic gender-diverse adolescents were developed through a consensus study with expert providers and researchers in the co-occurrence (J. F [59].). Primary recommendations included (1) the importance of screening for autism among gender-diverse youth, (2) slower timelines (typically) for moving forward with potentially irreversible gender-affirming medical interventions in autistic youth due to communication and processing speed differences, and (3) in spite of slower timelines, the importance of providing gender-affirming supports (including medical gender-affirming treatments) for autistic youth when the need is clear over time. A second clinical study took a different approach, turning to neurodivergent gender-diverse adolescents, their parents, and a diverse team of self-advocates and community experts to develop a support group model for neurodiverse gender-diverse youth [60]. The model developed included several features: supports of autism-related differences to reduce the impact of executive function, social, and sensory differences on gender-related needs; enrichment of the program with visits from divergent "role models" with lived experience of various gender journeys to help the young people more concretely learn about various options and outcomes related to gender (i.e., "concrete exemplars" of gender); and importance of facilitating interpersonal connections between neurodivergent gender-diverse youth, which can support positive self-identification, hopefulness, and social connectedness.

The continuity or discontinuity of gender diversity experiences in autistic people has only begun to be explored in the literature, and interpretation of the findings is complex. This is also because no study to date has compared continuity/discontinuity of gender diversity between autistic and non-autistic gender-diverse people, and therefore no conclusions can be made regarding whether autistic people are less, more, or equally likely to show shifts in gender diversity-related experiences, identities, and needs over time compared to their non-autistic gender-diverse counterparts. Two studies have reported that a subset of autistic gender-diverse youth move away from these experiences and identities over time [1, 14]. A study of detransitioned adults (i.e., those who previously were transgender and then "detransitioned" and now are cisgender) reported that approximately 20% of detransitioned respondents indicated that they were autistic [61]. Importantly, detransition and fluctuation of gender identity and gender-related needs are also reported in non-autistic gender-diverse populations, so this should not be understood as an autism-specific phenomenon.

11.4 Sexual Diversity and Autism

Attention to sexual attraction and the diversity in sexual identities of autistic adults has increased over the last decade, yet has been mostly focused on identifying the prevalence of sexual diversity in autistic individuals rather than understanding lived experiences, challenges, or needs of autistic people who are diverse in sexual orientation. Bennett and Goodall [18] argued for more attention to and research on the experiences and well-being of autistic people who identify as LGBT+, given that little is known about the unique issues facing autistic LGBT+ adults, such as coming out and mental health while autistic. Autistic LGB+ individuals (i.e., autistic individuals with non-heterosexual sexual orientations) may be at great risk for mental health issues compared to heterosexual peers [37], but mental health professionals have almost no guidance to inform their practice. Before 2016, studies had already revealed that autistic individuals scored lower on measures of heterosexuality and higher on measures of homo-, bi-, and a-sexuality compared to non-autistic controls and that this difference was larger in autistic women compared to men. The finding that more autistic adults, especially women, report sexual attraction to someone of the same binary gender or to both binary genders, compared to general population peers, was corroborated by several studies [2, 62, 63]. In a large Swedish cohort, 7.5% of participants scored high on an autism screening questionnaire, and only 77% of this subset reported heterosexual orientation, compared to 89.5% in the remaining of the sample [62]. In other larger samples of autistic adults, relatively high levels of sexual diversity were found; Strunz and colleagues reported that 69% of their sample (n = 229) self-identified as heterosexual, 7% as homosexual, and 10% as bisexual [63]. In a sample of Dutch autistic adults (n = 659), 56.6% of women and 81.6% of men reported feeling attraction only to someone of the other assigned sex [2]. In a recent large study, 63% of autistic adolescents and adults identified as heterosexual, compared to 83% of the non-autistic group in this study [15].

The higher prevalence of nonheterosexual interests and identities is less pronounced in studies with adolescent participants, specifically in boys [64, 65]. However, the proportional over-occurrence of sexuality diversity is reported in girls [66]. It is possible that some of these young men were still figuring out their sexual attraction and identity or they did not experience sexual attraction at younger ages [65]. Adolescent autistic boys did report higher levels of acceptance towards homosexuality compared to general population peers [64].

In several of the sexual orientation studies, a notable subset of participants indicated that they did not identify as hetero-, bi-, or gay or did not experience attraction to or sexual interest in the other, same, or both assigned sexes: i.e., about 15% of the female participants in a Dutch sample [2], 19% in a Swedish study [62], 14% in

Strunz and colleagues' study [63], and 15% in Weir and colleagues' study [15]. This finding requires further research to parse whether this group includes individuals who are still figuring out their sexual attraction, who experience their attraction as fluid, who question existing LGBTQ identity categories, who did not wish to answer these questions, or who did not experience or recognize sexual attraction. In a group of autistic adults who identified as female or more fluid non-male, about a third of participants (36%) identified on the asexuality spectrum, and only a minority (8%) identified as heterosexual [29]. Those who identified on the asexuality spectrum reported fewer lifetime sexual experiences, were less likely to have a current sexual partner, and experienced less desire for solo and partnered sexual activity. However, identifying on the asexuality spectrum did not exclude the reported need for love or romantic relationships. In Weir et al. [15], 10% of the autistic participants identified as asexual.

Some initial qualitative work has been conducted with autistic LGB+ individuals. These studies provide some information on how autistic individuals may experience LGB+ identities [67–69]. Autistic adults described how autism delayed or complicated the understanding of their sexual feelings, attraction, and identity, while they did not experience a direct influence of their autism on their sexual orientation [69]. Participants in this study described how it took time to define and accept their identities (e.g., autistic identity, LGB+ or asexual identity, romantic identity) and that they experienced that others, including others in LGB+ communities, found it difficult to understand their perspectives. Across several studies, with heterosexual and LGBT+ identifying participants, autistic individuals described difficulties enjoying their sexuality (e.g., related to sensory issues, overstimulation), communicating with a partner about their wishes and desires, and finding a partner and a satisfying relationship [67–69]. Flirting and dating were experienced as challenging by some, related to challenges understanding nonverbal and subtle, indirect verbal communication, including online; problems with flirting and dating sometimes resulted in loneliness. Sex education was often experienced as inadequate and not accounting for autism-related issues such as sensory dysregulation or communication needs; sex education was also critiqued for failing to adequately discuss diversity in sexual desires. Autistic men in same-sex relationships described insufficient professional support and concerns for being misunderstood by healthcare professionals [68]. Yet, strategies for success related to sexuality and relationships have also begun to be identified such as allowing downtime, open communication about needs and desires, and experimenting with alternative sexual techniques [67].

The relationship between sexual identity or identifying as LGB+ and mental health has also been studied since the call from Bennett and Goodall [18] on the importance of such research. George and Stokes [37] found that all minority groups (i.e., autistic, nonheterosexual, gender-dysphoric) in an online study of intersecting autism, sexual orientation diversity, and gender diversity reported reduced mental health and lower levels of well-being. Mental health burden increased when individuals had more than one minoritized group membership. George and Stokes hypothesized that belonging to a minority within a minority might increase the stress people experience, although their findings did not support theory related to sexual orientation, specifically. In addition to mental health issues, Hall and colleagues report that autistic LGB+ adults report more physical health issues and inappropriate healthcare (e.g., due to a lack of knowledge by healthcare professionals regarding autism and sexuality, a lack of insurance coverage; [40]).

There is no current understanding of why sexual orientation diversity is common in autistic populations. Some have criticized theoretical attempts to explain the proportional over-occurrence for taking non-autistic individuals as the "norm," for heteronormativity, and for assuming autism as an explanation for the sexual and/or gender diversity [70]. Early research on the lived experience of autistic individuals with sexual orientation diversity has shed some light on issues related to identity formation, well-being, and mental health in this population. Yet, a multitude of questions remain, as identified in the work by autistic adults and stakeholders [71]. Specifically, autistic adults and stakeholders prioritized future research efforts to study sexual and relationship well-being, sexual identity development (e.g., development of sexual identity and its intersectionality with autism), and experiences and needs of LGBT+ identifying autistic individuals. Regarding the latter, autistic adults and stakeholders emphasized research addressing how autistic LGBTQ+ individuals conceal or divulge multiple identities, the experience of living under "double rainbows," relatedness with the broad LGB+ community, managing societal reactions to LGBTQ+ autistic individuals, and the importance of a sense of belonging.

11.5 Conclusion: Reflections from the Autistic LGBTQ+ Co-Authors

These above components of the chapter were conceptualized and developed through a collaborative effort between the autistic and non-autistic authors. This conclusion section was primarily crafted by the autistic LGBT+ co-authors, specifically, to center their voices and perspectives. We believe that this is critical, given the limited opportunities autistic LGBTQ+ individuals have been afforded to drive and interpret research that pertains to their own lives.

While homosexuality was removed from the Diagnostic and Statistical Manual since its third edition in 1980, autism is still mostly viewed as a medical issue: a disorder people suffer from and for which they are pathologized as such. The emancipation of autism from a conceptualization rooted in pathology to perspectives that focus on the abilities and identities of autistic people—abilities and identities that may be neurodivergent—still has a long way to go. In that sense, the autistic movement can learn from the LGBTI+ movement about emancipation, depathologization, and importance of safe spaces for identity-based communities. The rapid development of AutiRoze (a Dutch national organization by and for autistic LGBTQ+ individuals) since its creation in 2015, and the expansion of the Autism Women's Network to intentionally embrace gender-diverse autistic people (e.g., as reflected in their new name, the Autistic Women and Nonbinary Network), signals the increasing need for the development of safe spaces at the intersection between sexuality diversity, gender diversity, and autism.

Access to quality (mental) healthcare that meets the specific needs of autistic people with questions and/or diversity related to their gender and/or sexuality is lacking too often, even in places with wide acceptance of LGBTQ+ individuals. Autistic people who are not cisgender or not heterosexual face the obstacles faced by gender and sexual minority populations in general, but little is known about how the intersection of autism with LGBTQ+-related disparities functions. Additional insight in the challenges autistic LGBTQ+ individuals experience is needed to develop ways to support them or to question and challenge societal constraints.

We worry especially about autistic LGBTQ+ persons in the countries with (de facto) provisions criminalizing consensual same-gender conduct [72] or gender identity diversity. Even in the countries that offer legal protection, there are still many cases of violence, hatred, discrimination, and exclusion based on (perceived) sexual orientation and/or gender diversity, especially for people with intersectional identity such as (dis)ability, religion, race, ethnicity, or class. This reality poses barriers for autistic people to access and receive the healthcare they need, to find the support they need in realizing their sexuality and/or gender as well as their ability to freely express their sexuality and gender, and to establish meaningful relationships. These experiences are often missing from research and statistics and may render the needs of the autistic LGBTQ+ communities largely invisible and excluded.

Discovering and freely expressing one's autism along with gender and sexuality can be challenging, especially for neurodivergent kids and adults who struggle to know and understand their feelings in general. We do not yet understand how the environment that autistic children experience, which tells them for example daily that heterosexuality or being cisgender is normal or, even worse, that being gay and/or gender diversity is bad and should be punished, impacts their development of a sense of self. Autistic LGBTQ+ people must deal with several sets of stigmas (autism, gender diversity, and/or sexual diversity) and often daily confrontations with a *double coming out*, which is difficult to navigate. When autistic people are met with acceptance and care providers knowledgeable of sexual and gender diversity, this can ease the fear and challenges that we face in our sexual and gender development. Future research on the intersections between autism, gender, and sexuality is needed to give visibility to the needs of these intersections and to better understand and meet them. While the autistic movement can learn from the LGBTQ+ movement, further understanding of the intersection between autism, gender, and sexuality can strengthen both movements to be more inclusive and better advocate for gender, sexual, and neurodiversity and equal rights and treatment.

References

1. de Vries ALC, Noens ILJ, Cohen-Kettenis PT, van Berckelaer-Onnes IA, Doreleijers TA. Autism spectrum disorders in gender dysphoric children and adolescents. J Autism Dev Disord. 2010;40(8):930–6. https://doi.org/10.1007/s10803-010-0935-9.
2. Dewinter J, De Graaf H, Begeer S. Sexual orientation, gender identity, and romantic relationships in adolescents and adults with autism Spectrum disorder. J Autism Dev Disord. 2017;47(9):2927–34. https://doi.org/10.1007/s10803-017-3199-9.

3. George R, Stokes MA. Gender identity and sexual orientation in autism spectrum disorder. Autism. 2018a;22(8):970–82.
4. Warrier V, Greenberg DM, Weir E, Buckingham C, Smith P, Lai M-C, Baron-Cohen S. Elevated rates of autism, other neurodevelopmental and psychiatric diagnoses, and autistic traits in transgender and gender-diverse individuals. Nat Commun. 2020;11(1):1–12.
5. Rosqvist HB. Becoming an 'autistic couple': narratives of sexuality and couplehood within the Swedish autistic self-advocacy movement. Sex Disabil. 2014;32(3):351–63.
6. Stokes M, Newton N, Kaur A. Stalking, and social and romantic functioning among adolescents and adults with autism spectrum disorder. J Autism Dev Disord. 2007;37(10):1969–86. https://doi.org/10.1007/s10803-006-0344-2.
7. Stokes MA, Kaur A. High-functioning autism and sexuality: a parental perspective. Autism. 2005;9(3):266–89. https://doi.org/10.1177/1362361305053258.
8. Øien RA, Cicchetti DV, Nordahl-Hansen A. Gender dysphoria, sexuality and autism Spectrum disorders: a systematic map review. J Autism Dev Disord. 2018;48(12):4028–37. https://doi.org/10.1007/s10803-018-3686-7.
9. Sala G, Pecora L, Hooley M, Stokes MA. As diverse as the Spectrum itself: trends in sexuality, gender and autism. Curr Dev Disord Rep. 2020;7(2):59–68.
10. Alison, C. (2019). Autistic Women & Nonbinary Network (AWN). https://awnnetwork.org/autistic-women-non-binary-network-awn/.
11. Strang JF, van der Miesen AIR, Caplan R, Hughes C, daVanport S, Lai MC. Both sex- and gender-related factors should be considered in autism research and clinical practice. Autism. 2020b;24(3):539–43. https://doi.org/10.1177/1362361320913192.
12. Skidmore WC, Linsenmeier JA, Bailey JM. Gender nonconformity and psychological distress in lesbians and gay men. Arch Sex Behav. 2006;35(6):685–97.
13. Nabbijohn AN, van der Miesen AIR, Santarossa A, Peragine D, de Vries AL, Popma A, VanderLaan DP. Gender variance and the autism spectrum: an examination of children ages 6–12 years. J Autism Dev Disord. 2019;49(4):1570–85.
14. Strang JF, Powers MD, Knauss M, Sibarium E, Leibowitz SF, Kenworthy L, Anthony LG. "they thought it was an obsession": trajectories and perspectives of autistic transgender and gender-diverse adolescents. J Autism Dev Disord. 2018b;48(12):4039–55. https://doi.org/10.1007/s10803-018-3723-6.
15. Weir E, Allison C, Baron-Cohen S. The sexual health, orientation, and activity of autistic adolescents and adults. Autism Research; 2021.
16. Lawson WB, Lawson BM. Transitioning together: one Couple's journey of gender and identity discovery. Jessica Kingsley Publishers; 2017.
17. Mendes EA, Harris BT. Gender identity, sexuality and autism: voices from across the spectrum. Jessica Kingsley Publishers; 2019.
18. Bennett M, Goodall E. Towards an agenda for research for lesbian, gay, bisexual, transgendered and/or intersexed people with an autism Spectrum diagnosis. J Autism Dev Disord. 2016;46(9):3190–2. https://doi.org/10.1007/s10803-016-2844-z.
19. Bouman WP, Schwend AS, Motmans J, Smiley A, Safer JD, Deutsch MB, Winter S. Language and trans health. In: Taylor & Francis; 2017.
20. Bottema-Beutel K, Kapp SK, Lester JN, Sasson NJ, Hand BN. Avoiding ableist language: suggestions for autism researchers. Autism in Adulthood. 2021;3(1):18–29.
21. Kenny L, Hattersley C, Molins B, Buckley C, Povey C, Pellicano E. Which terms should be used to describe autism? Perspectives from the UK autism community. Autism. 2016;20(4):442–62.
22. Sequenzia, A. (2017). The failings of person first language.
23. Insel T. The four kingdoms of autism. In: Director Post Series; 2013. https://www.nimh.nih.gov/about/directors/thomas-insel/blog/2013/the-four-kingdoms-of-autism.
24. van Anders SM, Schudson ZC, Abed EC, Beischel WJ, Dibble ER, Gunther OD, Silver ER. Biological sex, gender, and public policy. Policy Insights Behav Brain Sci. 2017;4(2):194–201.
25. Hyde JS, Bigler RS, Joel D, Tate CC, van Anders SM. The future of sex and gender in psychology: five challenges to the gender binary. Am Psychol. 2019;74(2):171.

26. Joel D, Mccarthy MM. Incorporating sex as a biological variable in neuropsychiatric research: where are we now and where should we be? Neuropsychopharmacology. 2017;42(2):379–85.
27. World Health Organization. (2021). Gender and Health. https://www.who.int/health-topics/gender#tab=tab_1.
28. Thorne N, Yip AK-T, Bouman WP, Marshall E, Arcelus J. The terminology of identities between, outside and beyond the gender binary–a systematic review. Int J Transgend. 2019;20(2–3):138–54.
29. Bush HH, Williams LW, Mendes E. Brief report: asexuality and young women on the autism Spectrum. J Autism Dev Disord. 2021;51(2):725–33.
30. GLAAD. (2021). Terms to Avoid. https://www.glaad.org/reference/offensive.
31. Hisle-Gorman E, Landis CA, Susi A, Schvey NA, Gorman GH, Nylund CM, Klein DA. Gender dysphoria in children with autism spectrum disorder. LGBT Health. 2019;6(3):95–100. https://doi.org/10.1089/lgbt.2018.0252.
32. van der Miesen AIR, Hurley H, de Vries ALC. Gender dysphoria and autism spectrum disorder: a narrative review. Int Rev Psychiatry. 2016;28(1):70–80. https://doi.org/10.3109/09540261.2015.1111199.
33. Walsh RJ, Krabbendam L, Dewinter J, Begeer S. Brief report: gender identity differences in autistic adults: associations with perceptual and socio-cognitive profiles. J Autism Dev Disord. 2018;48(12):4070–8. https://doi.org/10.1007/s10803-018-3702-y.
34. Strang JF, Janssen A, Tishelman A, Leibowitz SF, Kenworthy L, McGuire JK, Anthony LG. Revisiting the link: evidence of the rates of autism in studies of gender diverse individuals. J Am Acad Child Adolesc Psychiatry. 2018a;57(11):885–7. https://doi.org/10.1016/j.jaac.2018.04.023.
35. Strauss P, Cook A, Winter S, Watson V, Wright Toussaint D, Lin A. Trans pathways: the mental health experiences and care pathways of trans young people. Perth, Australia; 2017.
36. Strang JF, Anthony LG, Song A, Lai MC, Knauss M, Sadikova E, Kenworthy L. In addition to stigma: cognitive and autism-related predictors of mental health in transgender adolescents. J Clin Child Adolesc Psychol. 2021a;53:1–18. https://doi.org/10.1080/15374416.2021.1916940.
37. George R, Stokes MA. A quantitative analysis of mental health among sexual and gender minority groups in ASD. J Autism Dev Disord. 2018b;48(6):2052–63. https://doi.org/10.1007/s10803-018-3469-1.
38. ASAN. (2016). Joint Statement on the Death of Kayden Clark. https://autisticadvocacy.org/2016/02/asan-joint-statement-death-of-kayden-clarke/.
39. Autistic Self Advocacy Network, National Center for Transgender Equality, & LGBTQ Task Force. Autistic self advocacy network, National Center for transgender equality, and LGBTQ task force joint statement on the rights of transgender and gender non-conforming autistic people. Washington, DC; 2016.
40. Hall JP, Batza K, Streed CG Jr, Boyd BA, Kurth NK. Health disparities among sexual and gender minorities with autism spectrum disorder. J Autism Dev Disord. 2020;50(8):3071–7. https://doi.org/10.1007/s10803-020-04399-2.
41. Chang JC, Lai MC, Tai YM, Gau SS. Mental health correlates and potential childhood predictors for the wish to be of the opposite sex in young autistic adults. Autism. 2021;26(1):146–59. https://doi.org/10.1177/13623613211024098.
42. Burke SM, Manzouri AH, Savic I. Structural connections in the brain in relation to gender identity and sexual orientation. Sci Rep. 2017;7(1):17954. https://doi.org/10.1038/s41598-017-17352-8.
43. D'augelli AR, Grossman AH, Starks MT. Gender atypicality and sexual orientation development among lesbian, gay, and bisexual youth: prevalence, sex differences, and parental responses. J Gay Lesbian Ment Health. 2008;12(1–2):121–43.
44. Carpenter, B., Happé, F., & Egerton, J. (2019). *Girls and autism: educational, family and personal perspectives*: Routledge.
45. Duvekot J, van der Ende J, Verhulst FC, Slappendel G, van Daalen E, Maras A, Greaves-Lord K. Factors influencing the probability of a diagnosis of autism spectrum disorder in girls versus boys. Autism. 2017;21(6):646–58. https://doi.org/10.1177/1362361316672178.

46. Shumer DE, Reisner SL, Edwards-Leeper L, Tishelman A. Evaluation of Asperger syndrome in youth presenting to a gender dysphoria clinic. LGBT health. 2016;3(5):387–90. https://doi.org/10.1089/lgbt.2015.0070.
47. van der Miesen AIR, de Vries AL, Steensma TD, Hartman CA. Autistic symptoms in children and adolescents with gender dysphoria. J Autism Dev Disord. 2018;48(5):1537–48.
48. Turban JL, van Schalkwyk GI. "gender dysphoria" and autism Spectrum disorder: is the link real? J Am Acad Child Adolesc Psychiatry. 2018;57(1):8–9.e2. https://doi.org/10.1016/j.jaac.2017.08.017.
49. Akgül GY, Ayaz AB, Yildirim B, Fis NP. Autistic traits and executive functions in children and adolescents with gender dysphoria. J Sex Marital Ther. 2018;44(7):619–26. https://doi.org/10.1080/0092623x.2018.1437489.
50. Strang JF, Chen D, Nelson E, Leibowitz SF, Nahata L, Anthony LG, Kenworthy L. Transgender youth executive functioning: relationships with anxiety symptoms, autism Spectrum disorder, and gender-affirming medical treatment status. Child Psychiatry Hum Dev. 2021b;53(6):1252–65. https://doi.org/10.1007/s10578-021-01195-6.
51. VanderLaan DP, Postema L, Wood H, Singh D, Fantus S, Hyun J, Zucker KJ. Do children with gender dysphoria have intense/obsessional interests? J Sex Res. 2015;52(2):213–9. https://doi.org/10.1080/00224499.2013.860073.
52. Bejerot S, Eriksson JM, Bonde S, Carlström K, Humble MB, Eriksson E. The extreme male brain revisited: gender coherence in adults with autism spectrum disorder. Br J Psychiatry J Ment Sci. 2012;201:116–23. https://doi.org/10.1192/bjp.bp.111.097899.
53. Strang JF, Klomp SE, Caplan R, Griffin AD, Anthony LG, Harris MC, van der Miesen AIR. Community-based participatory design for research that impacts the lives of transgender and/or gender-diverse autistic and/or neurodiverse people. Clin Pract Pediatr Psychol. 2019;7(4):396.
54. Llaveria Caselles E. Epistemic injustice in brain studies of (trans) gender identity. Front Sociol. 2021;6:63.
55. Mahfouda S, Panos C, Whitehouse AJO, Thomas CS, Maybery M, Strauss P, Lin A. Mental health correlates of autism spectrum disorder in gender diverse young people: evidence from a specialised child and adolescent gender clinic in Australia. J Clin Med. 2019;8(10):1503. https://doi.org/10.3390/jcm8101503.
56. Strauss P, Cook A, Watson V, Winter S, Whitehouse A, Albrecht N, Lin A. Mental health difficulties among trans and gender diverse young people with an autism spectrum disorder (ASD): findings from trans pathways. J Psychiatr Res. 2021;137:360–7. https://doi.org/10.1016/j.jpsychires.2021.03.005.
57. Strang JF, Sadikova E. Gender-diversity-related barriers questionnaire (GBQ): a self-report of gender diverse/transgender adolescent and young adult barriers achieving gender diversity-related needs and goals. Washington, DC: Children's National Hospital; 2017.
58. American Psychiatric Association. *Diagnostic and statistical manual of mental disorders*. 5th ed. Washington, D.C: American Psychiatric Association; 2013.
59. Strang JF, Meagher H, Kenworthy L, de Vries ALC, Menvielle E, Leibowitz S, Anthony LG. Initial clinical guidelines for co-occurring autism spectrum disorder and gender dysphoria or incongruence in adolescents. J Clin Child Adolesc Psychol. 2016;47(1):1–11. https://doi.org/10.1080/15374416.2016.1228462.
60. Strang JF, Knauss M, van der Miesen AIR, McGuire JK, Kenworthy L, Caplan R, Anthony LG. A clinical program for transgender and gender-diverse neurodiverse/autistic adolescents developed through community-based participatory design. J Clin Child Adolesc Psychol. 2020a;50(6):730–45. https://doi.org/10.1080/15374416.2020.1731817.
61. Vandenbussche E. Detransition-related needs and support: a cross-sectional online survey. J Homosex. 2021;69(9):1602–20.
62. Rudolph CES, Lundin A, Åhs JW, Dalman C, Kosidou K. Brief report: sexual orientation in individuals with autistic traits: population based study of 47,000 adults in Stockholm County. J Autism Dev Disord. 2018;48(2):619–24. https://doi.org/10.1007/s10803-017-3369-9.

63. Strunz S, Schermuck C, Ballerstein S, Ahlers CJ, Dziobek I, Roepke S. Romantic relationships and relationship satisfaction among adults with Asperger syndrome and high-functioning autism. J Clin Psychol. 2017;73(1):113–25.
64. Dewinter J, Vermeiren R, Vanwesenbeeck I, Van Nieuwenhuizen C. Adolescent boys with autism spectrum disorder growing up: follow-up of self-reported sexual experience. Eur Child Adolesc Psychiatry. 2016;25(9):969–78. https://doi.org/10.1007/s00787-016-0816-7.
65. Hartmann K, Urbano MR, Raffaele CT, Qualls LR, Williams TV, Warren C, Deutsch SI. Sexuality in the autism Spectrum study (SASS): reports from young adults and parents. J Autism Dev Disord. 2019;49(9):3638–55. https://doi.org/10.1007/s10803-019-04077-y.
66. May T, Pang KC, Williams K. Brief report: sexual attraction and relationships in adolescents with autism. J Autism Dev Disord. 2017;47(6):1910–6. https://doi.org/10.1007/s10803-017-3092-6.
67. Barnett JP, Maticka-Tyndale E. Qualitative exploration of sexual experiences among adults on the autism Spectrum: implications for sex education. Perspect Sex Reprod Health. 2015;47(4):171–9. https://doi.org/10.1363/47e5715.
68. Hogan MS, Micucci JA. Same-sex relationships of men with autism spectrum disorder in middle adulthood: an interpretative phenomenological study. Psychol Sex Orientat Gend Divers. 2020;7(2):176–85. https://doi.org/10.1037/sgd0000372.
69. Lewis LF, Ward C, Jarvis N, Cawley E. "Straight sex is complicated enough!": the lived experiences of autistics who are gay, lesbian, bisexual, asexual, or other sexual orientations. J Autism Dev Disord. 2021;51(7):2324–37. https://doi.org/10.1007/s10803-020-04696-w.
70. Jackson-Perry D. The autistic art of failure? Unknowing imperfect systems of sexuality and gender. Scand J Disabil Res. 2020;22(1):221–9.
71. Dewinter J, van der Miesen AIR, Holmes LG. INSAR special interest group report: stakeholder perspectives on priorities for future research on autism, sexuality, and intimate relationships. Autism Res. 2020;13(8):1248–57. https://doi.org/10.1002/aur.2340.
72. Mendos LBK, Carrano Lelis R, de la Peña EL, Savelev I, Tan D. State-sponsored homophobia 2020: global legislation overview update. ILGA World; 2020.

Evaluation of Sexual and Socio-Emotional Well-Being in Persons Affected by ASD: Are We Ready?

12

Erika Limoncin, Giacomo Ciocca, Tommaso B. Jannini, Martina Siracusano, Luigi Mazzone, and Emmanuele A. Jannini

12.1 ASD and Unconventional-Paraphilic Interests, Hypersexuality, Sexual Victimization

12.1.1 Introduction

Why is it so important to speak about sexuality within people with autism spectrum disorder (ASD)? And why this topic appears still controversial, and so difficult to manage? A possible explanation may be related to the general difficulty the society has in accepting that sexual needs are needs also for people with every kind of disability. When it comes to sexuality, there seems to be a great public debate on

E. Limoncin (✉) · G. Ciocca
Department of Dynamic, Clinical Psychology and Health Studies, Sapienza University of Rome, Rome, Italy
e-mail: erika.limoncin@uniroma1.it; giacomo.ciocca@uniroma1.it

T. B. Jannini · E. A. Jannini
Department of Systems Medicine, University of Rome Tor Vergata, Rome, Italy

M. Siracusano
Child Neurology and Psychiatry Unit, Department of Neurosciences, Policlinico Tor Vergata Hospital, Rome, Italy

Biomedicine and Prevention Department, University of Rome Tor Vergata, Rome, Italy

L. Mazzone
Department of Systems Medicine, University of Rome Tor Vergata, Rome, Italy

Child Neurology and Psychiatry Unit, Department of Neurosciences, Policlinico Tor Vergata Hospital, Rome, Italy

L. Mazzone et al. (eds.), *Autism Spectrum Disorder: Understanding the Female Phenotype*, https://doi.org/10.1007/978-3-031-62072-0_12

victimization, abuse, inappropriate behaviour, and deviance. Sexuality may, in other words, imperil people with disabilities for several traumas, both auto-experienced and auto-committed [1]. Hence, the tendency is to eliminate risk factors inducing persons with disabilities to distract themselves from sexuality and sexual needs. This supposition is supported by the evidence of a scarce scientific literature on this topic. Literature data are still represented by qualitative studies, or by case reports or case series, which limit the scientific understanding of sexuality and sexual programmes for clinical population. Recent evidence points out how people with ASD show a wide array of sexual behaviours and a true interest in sexuality as well as intimate relationships [2, 3]. Nevertheless, core symptoms of autism, such as impairments in social cognition and communication, could prevent them to properly experience sexuality. In addition, a consistent number of people with ASD do not have access to an appropriate sexual education [4]. As a result, this may lead to naïve inappropriate sexual conducts, ranging across public masturbations, frottage, stalking, and hypersexuality [5].

The aim of this chapter is to provide readers with scientific evidence—even if limited—regarding the issue of legal consequences deriving from unconventional sexual behaviours which could damage public privacy. In addition, the assessment of sexual functioning in ASD population—supported by psychometric measurements—will be presented/addressed.

The road is still uphill, but scientists must be aware of the necessity to talk about it, to study, and to understand the way people with ASD live in terms of sexuality and intimacy. It is also important to find adequate measures for the evaluation of sexual behaviours and to promote sexual education and programmes able to give to persons the instruments for understanding associated risk factors, rather than simply denying their sexual life.

12.2 ASD as a Risk Factor for Coming into Contact with Criminal Justice System

What does it happen when we travel in another country, where we do not perfectly know the social rules and habits and maybe we do not perfectly know the spoken language? It is possible that for someone with this misunderstanding may bring some problems with the law. It is reasonable to suppose that the same happens to some persons with ASD, who do not really understand social situations, the others' intentions, or the way in which it is socially accepted to manifest sexual interest or desire towards another person. To this end, literature presents a broader number of scientific studies documenting how people with ASD tend to have a higher risk to be imprisoned. Among the different causes, also the adoption of inappropriate sexual behaviours (i.e. masturbating in public areas, trying to kiss a stranger, considering a stranger as a stable partner, touching the genitalia in public areas) is considered a frequent motivation [6, 7].

An emerging cause of encountering the criminal justice system is, unfortunately, viewing films and images of child exploitation. A recent systematic review explains how unemployment or underemployment may, in fact, produce a consistent amount of spare time that is frequently spent online [5].

For what concerns the psychiatric diagnoses prevalent among imprisoned people, a recent study evidenced a significantly higher prevalence of attention deficit hyperactivity disorder (ADHD), post-traumatic stress disorder (PTSD), and autistic traits with significantly lower verbal IQ [8] compared to individuals without a history of imprisonment. Because of the difficulty in understanding social rules, a higher risk was also documented for some ASD persons to become sexually violent [9, 10].

It is important to highlight, however, that although specific features of ASD were found in individuals who committed crimes, maybe due to some problems with Theory of Mind (ToM) [11], or due to the relational inexperience [10], this risk seems to be the same as for individuals without ASD. In addition, given the specific focus of this book on female ASD phenotype, it is also important to note that literature regarding inappropriate sexual behaviours or sexual violence within ASD is strictly related to male sex/gender. Probably, the gendered nature of the law brings to a firm consideration of the perpetrator as a male, and of the victim as a female. Another consideration that must be made is related to the fact that other variables may determine this sex/gender discrepancy. The most significant is probably the female ability to better understand what is correct and legitimate, and vice versa what is legally wrong. This ability permits females with a diagnosis of ASD to understand that some sexual needs necessitate to be postponed or not manifested in public areas [12]. Nevertheless, it is necessary to consider the vulnerability of ASD individuals to engage in inappropriate sexual behaviours and to prevent problems with justice implementing sexual education.

12.3 ASD and Unconventional-Paraphilic Interests, Hypersexuality, Sexual Victimization, and Gender Identity

Problems with sociability, restricted interests, and sensorial sensitivity are all connected with the possible development of the interest towards unconventional sexuality or the adoption of paraphilic behaviours. Unfortunately, also for this topic, scientific evidence is scarce. In most cases, case reports showed that ASD individuals presented excessive masturbation because of the pharmacological treatment [13–17], exhibitionism [18], paedophilic fantasies and/or behaviours [19, 20], fetishism [21, 22], sadomasochism [17], or other paraphilias [23]. However, the most important limitation of these case studies is the description of exclusively males, with important IQ limitations. Hence, it is reasonable to suppose that unconventional sexual behaviour is a manifestation of underlying cognitive difficulties (low IQ) and/or clinical features characteristic of ASD—among which the most probable ones are the restricted interests and the obsessive behaviours [24].

To the best of our knowledge, Schottle and colleagues' study is the only research evaluating within ASD the prevalence of hypersexuality and of paraphilic behaviours in both males and females without intellectual impairment [25]. As regards hypersexuality, ASD males obtained higher scores than male controls at the Hypersexual Behaviour Inventory (HBI), and a significantly higher number of ASD males ranged above the proposed cut-off. Such differences did not emerge between ASD females and female controls. Similarly, paraphilic fantasies and/or behaviours were significantly more prevalent among ASD males than among male controls. Within female samples, instead, no statistically significant differences were found for the prevalence of paraphilic interests/fantasies/behaviours, except for the frequency of masochistic behaviours, which were more prevalent among female controls. A possible explanation for this interesting finding could be the limitations in the comprehension and the acceptance, during childhood, of the social role which considers the female gender in a subordinate position in respect to the male. Hence, ASD females, due to the inability to adhere to this social script, might not adopt the masochistic behaviour as the female controls.

Based on these limited data, we can preliminarily conclude that ASD females with low level of support needs do not frequently manifest unconventional sexual behaviours, or paraphilic interests/fantasies/behaviours. In addition, for what concerns in general the population of subjects with low support needs, the manifestation of such behaviours should be interpreted, diagnosed, and treated as the result of other comorbid conditions, such as the IQ, and the autistic features.

Core symptoms of autism, such as an impaired ToM, problems in social understanding, and lack of communication skills, are probably the main cause for an increased risk of sexual victimization [26]. Young people with ASD have a sad primacy for sexual abuse (16.6%) compared to general population [5]. From a gender perspective, female individuals with ASD have an increased risk in sexual victimization compared to males [27]. A scarce sexual knowledge is one of the main reasons for this phenomenon. A lack of sexual education may, in fact, lead to ingenuous promiscuities, which are often misunderstood by abusive partners [5]. Interestingly, recent evidence has shown how female homosexual individuals with ASD tend to be more vulnerable to sexual harassments compared to ASD heterosexual females [28].

This may be explained by the fact that in general, both non-ASD homosexual females and female ASD individuals tend more easily to experience affective and mood disturbances, such as anxiety and depression [29].

12.4 Psychometric Evaluation of Sexual and Socio-Emotional Well-Being in Persons Affected by ASD: Are We Ready?

Maybe the most realistic response to the question if we are ready for a standardized evaluation of the sexual functioning in people affected by ASD is "no". Several are in fact the possible reasons for this scientific gap. First, the study of sexuality in this population has been subjected to a retard due to the social stigma, which considered people with intellectual disabilities as asexual persons [30]. However, it is also important to highlight some methodological issues related to the difficulty in structuring questionnaires adequate to the autistic subjects' IQ, or questionnaires overpassing the problem related to the ability to understand verbal messages, by using pictures [31]. A second problem may be represented by the limited sexual experience ASD individuals may have in a relational context [18]. In fact, the most frequent criterion necessary for the fulfilment of tools measuring sexual functioning is the presence of a sexual intercourse (i.e. vaginal penetration) in a specific period anterior to the evaluation. Improvements have been made in recent years in the field of the measurement of solitary sexual activity [32]. However, we are still far from the same measurement in the case of people affected by disabilities. Last, but not least, there is the difficulty in building a questionnaire able to measure sexual functioning in a population with a heterogeneous clinical phenotype.

What is nowadays available for clinicians and researchers are tools, which have been originally developed for the evaluation of sexual functioning in a general population and have been then modified, adequate, and in some cases validated for the evaluation of sexuality of ASD persons (Table 12.1). Among these, there is the Knowledge of Sexual Health Questionnaire [33], which has not been developed for the measurement of sexual functioning within autistic persons, but it has been used in this population. In addition, we can find other qualitative instruments, such as interviews for ASD persons or for caregivers, as well as non-validated tools, which try to describe—directly or indirectly—the sexual functioning, grade of sexual knowledge, sexual cognitions, or sexual satisfaction. An example of a qualitative measure is the self-report written questionnaire completed by caregivers [34], which was developed for an indirect evaluation of sexual functioning.

Table 12.1 describes the questionnaires mostly used in research, hoping to give to the reader an indication about its scientific solidity and its application [33, 35–42]. So much must be made to have adequate tools for the measurement of sexuality in ASD people. However, the attention towards this aspect in the ASD population represents a starting point. Now the objective is to continue to broaden the knowledge, first for the ASD features, and second for the way these features modulate sexuality. We can affirm that the study of sexual functioning may be considered a good explanatory model showing the persons' relational abilities. The final effort will be represented, not only for ASD people but also for the general population, by the necessity to think about a sexual intervention considering gender. As previously stated, in fact, also in the case of ASD males and females, gender plays a role in the way people live with sexual needs and sexual experiences.

Table 12.1 Questionnaires for the measurement of sexuality and sexual knowledge in the ASD population

Questionnaire's name, authors, year of publication	Outcome	Number of items	Validation/ standardization	Development for evaluation in ASD context
Knowledge of sexual health questionnaire, revised (Joseph J.M., Sawyer R., Desmond S., 1995)	Susceptibility to STDs and pregnancy; sexual behaviour; method of contraception used; reasons why condoms were not used; preventive health behaviours; sources of health information; sexual knowledge	76	No	No
Sexual experiences survey-victimization (SES-V) (Testa, M., VanZile-Tamsen, C., Livingston, J. A., & Koss, M. P., 2004)	Measure of sexual victimization	10	Yes	No
Global measure of sexual satisfaction (GMSEX; Lawrance K. et al., 2011)	Measure of sexual satisfaction	5	Yes	No
Hurlbert Index of Sexual Assertiveness (Hurlbert DF, 1991)	Assessment of the frequency of sexual activities related to assertive behaviour in sexual situations	25	Yes	No
Sexual Arousability and Sexual Anxiety Inventory (Hoon EF et al., 1976)	Evaluation of specific sexual situations	14	Yes	No
Sexual Desire Inventory (Spector IP et al., 1998)	Measure of the frequency and intensity of sexual desire in different situations	14	Yes	No
Sexual functioning questionnaire (MacNeil S. And byers ES., 1997)	Evaluation of specific sexual problems	9	No	No
Sexual Cognitions Checklist (SCC; Renaud CA and Byers ES, 2011)	Evaluation of sexual cognitions	57	Yes	No
Global Measure of Relationship Satisfaction (Lawrence K, Byers ES, 2011)	Evaluation of the quality of relationship	5 scales	Yes	No

12.5 Conclusion

A recent burst in clinical research has more focused on sexuality and on sexual unusual interests among people with ASD. In addition, new pieces of evidence reported more accurate findings on sexual behaviour among ASD females [27].

However, although a broader knowledge has been reached in the last few years, there is still an urgent need of quantitative studies to further deepen our understanding of ASD sexual functioning, and specifically of the functioning of ASD females. For instance, a still open question would be the reasons of the higher rate of sexual victimization among ASD females, which requires to immediately take an action on this argument, building programs or services that are specifically tailored for them. These would indeed encourage self-awareness enhancing positive social interactions and reducing negative sexual experiences.

Key Points

- The evaluation of sexuality and of sexual functioning in the field of ASD persons is subjected to several methodological problems: the enrolment of ASD persons not representative of the general ASD population and evaluation of sexual functioning through the interviews with caregivers.
- ASD represents a risk factor for problems with justice exclusively in male population.
- The adoption of unconventional sexual behaviours or paraphilic behaviours seems to be more prevalent in male ASD persons.
- Standardized psychometric tools evaluating sexuality and sexual functioning are lacking.

References

1. Baarsma ME, et al. Sexuality and autistic-like symptoms in juvenile sex offenders: a follow-up after 8 years. J Autism Dev Disord. 2016;46(8):2679–91.
2. Dewinter J, et al. Sexual orientation, gender identity, and romantic relationships in adolescents and adults with autism Spectrum disorder. J Autism Dev Disord. 2017 Sep;47(9):2927–34.
3. Dewinter J, et al. Autism and normative sexual development: a narrative review. J Clin Nurs. 2013 Dec;22(23–24):3467–83.
4. Mackin ML, et al. Parent perceptions of sexual education needs for their children with autism. J Pediatr Nurs. 2016;31(6):608–18.
5. Pecora LA, et al. Sexuality and gender issues in individuals with autism Spectrum disorder. Child Adolesc Psychiatr Clin N Am. 2020;29(3):543–56.
6. Green J, et al. Social and psychiatric functioning in adolescents with Asperger's syndrome compared with conduct disorder. J Autism Dev Disord. 2000;30:279–93.
7. Katz N, et al. Criminal responsibility in Asperger's syndrome. Isr J Psychiatry Relat Sci. 2006;43:166–73.
8. Bebbington PE, et al. The mental health of ex-prisoners: analysis of the 2014 English National Survey of psychiatric morbidity. Soc Psychiatry Psychiatr Epidemiol. 2021;56(11):2083–93.
9. Fujikawa Y, et al. Sexual crimes committed by adolescents with Asperger's disorder: problems of management by the viewpoint of probation officers at a family court. Japanese Journal of Child and Adolescent Psychiatry. 2002;43:280–9.

10. Murrie DC, et al. Asperger's syndrome in forensic settings. Int J Forensic Ment Health. 2002;1(1):59–70.
11. Goldberg BR, et al. Predictors of aggression on the psychiatric inpatient service: self-esteem, narcissism, and theory of mind deficits. J Nerv Ment Dis. 2007;195(5):436–42.
12. Sturrock A, et al. A subtle profile with a significant impact: language and communication difficulties for autistic females without intellectual disability. Front Psychol. 2021 Aug;9(12):621742.
13. Hergüner S, et al. Combination of risperidone and paroxetine for inappropriate sexual behaviors in an adolescent with autism and mental retardation. Arch Neuropsychiatry. 2012;49:311–3.
14. Shahani L. Use of lithium for sexual obsessions in Asperger's disorder. J Neuropsychiatry Clin Neurosci. 2012;24(4):E17.
15. Nguyen M, et al. Mirtazapine for excessive masturbation in an adolescent with autism. J Am Acad Child Adolesc Psychiatry. 2001;40(8):868–9.
16. Deepmala AM. Use of propranolol for hypersexual behavior in an adolescent with autism. Ann Pharmacother. 2014;48(10):1385–8.
17. Müller JL. Are sadomasochism and hypersexuality in autism linked to amygdalohippocampal lesion? J Sex Med. 2011;8(11):3241–9.
18. Coshway L, et al. Medical therapy for inappropriate sexual behaviors in a teen with autism spectrum disorder. Pediatrics. 2016;137(4):e20154366.
19. Realmuto GM, et al. Sexual behaviors in autism: problems of definition and management. J Autism Dev Disord. 1999;29(2):121–7.
20. Fosdick C, et al. Case report: resolution of severe sexual aggression in a developmentally disabled adolescent during leuprolide acetate use. J Autism Dev Disord. 2016;46(6):2267–9.
21. Dozier CL, et al. Assessment and treatment of foot-shoe fetish displayed by a man with autism. J Appl Behav Anal. 2011;44(1):133–7.
22. Early MC, et al. Case report: 16-year-old male with autistic disorder with preoccupation with female feet. J Autism Dev Disord. 2012;42(6):1133–7.
23. Silva JA, et al. Paraphilic psychopathology in a case of autism spectrum disorder. Am J Forensic Psychiatry. 2003;24(3):5–20.
24. Haskins BG, et al. Asperger's disorder and criminal behavior: forensic psychiatric considerations. J Am Acad Psychiatry Law. 2006;34(3):374–84.
25. Schottle D, et al. Sexuality in autism: hypersexual and paraphilic behavior in women and men with high-functioning autism spectrum disorder. Dialogues Clin Neurosci. 2017;19(4)
26. Goldberg Edelson M. Sexual abuse of children with autism: factors that increase risk and interfere with recognition of abuse. Disabil Stud Quart. 2010;30(1)
27. Pecora LA, et al. Characterising the sexuality and sexual experiences of autistic females. J Autism Dev Disord. 2019;49(12):4834–46.
28. Pecora LA, et al. Gender identity, sexual orientation and adverse sexual experiences in autistic females. Mol Autism. 2020;11(1):57.
29. Collier KL, et al. Sexual orientation and gender identity/expression related peer victimization in adolescence: a systematic review of associated psychosocial and health outcomes. J Sex Res. 2013;50(3–4):299–317.
30. Esmail S, et al. Attitudes and perceptions towards disability and sexuality. Disabil Rehabil. 2010;32(14):1148–55.
31. Johnson CN, et al. Cognitive correlates of autism spectrum disorder symptoms. Autism Res. 2021;14(11):2405–11.
32. Limoncin E, et al. The masturbation erection index (MEI): validation of a new psychometric tool, derived from the six-item version of the international index of erectile function (IIEF-6) and from the erection hardness score (EHS), for measuring erectile function during masturbation. BJU Int. 2019 Mar;123(3):530–7.
33. Sawyer RG, et al. A comparison of sexual knowledge, behavior, and sources of health information between deaf and hearing university students. J Health Education. 1996;27(3):144–55.
34. Haracopos D, et al. Sexuality and autism: Danish report. United Kingdom: Society for the Autistically Handicapped; 1992.

35. Testa M, et al. (sexual experiences survey, victimization version). Assessing women's experiences of sexual aggression using the sexual experiences survey: evidence for validity and implications for research. Psychol Women Q. 2004;28(3):256–65.
36. Lawrance K, et al. (Global measure of sexual satisfaction). Sexual satisfaction in long-term heterosexual relationship: the interpersonal exchange model of sexual satisfaction. Pers Relat. 1995;2:267–85.
37. Hurlbert DF. (Hurlbert index of sexual assertiveness). The role of assertiveness in female sexuality: a comparative study between sexually assertive and sexually nonassertive women. J Sex Marital Ther. 1991;17:183–90.
38. Hoon EF, et al. (Sexual Arousability and sexual anxiety inventory). An inventory for the measurement of female sexual arousability: the SAI. Arch Sex Behav. 1971;5:291–300.
39. Spector IP, et al. (Sexual desire inventory). Sexual desire inventory. In: Davis C, Yarber WL, Bauserman R, Schreer G, Davis S, editors. Handbook of sexuality-related measures. Thousand Oaks, CA: Sage; 1998. p. 174–6.
40. MacNeil S, et al. (Sexual functioning questionnaire). The relationships between sexual problems, communication, and sexual satisfaction. Can J Hum Sex. 1997;6:277–83. Sexual Arousability and Sexual Anxiety Inventory (modified version)
41. Renaud CA, et al. Sexual cognitions checklist (SCC; positive and negative sexual cognitions: subjective experience and relationships to sexual adjustment). J Sex Res. 2001;38(3):252–62.
42. Lawrance K, et al. Global measure of relationship satisfaction interpersonal exchange model of sexual satisfaction questionnaire. In: Fisher TD, Davis CM, Yarber WL, Davis S, editors. Handbook of sexuality-related measures. 2nd ed. New York: Routledge; 2011. p. 525–30.

Independent Living and Employment Options

13

Laura Maria Fatta, Martina Siracusano, and Luigi Mazzone

13.1 ASD and Work: Which Are Female Needs?

Work is a crucial aspect of a person's quality of life, representing an opportunity for social inclusion and contributing to independent living [1, 2]. Given the growth in ASD prevalence rates [3], it is estimated that approximately half a million autistic youth will become adults worldwide [4, 5]. Considering the well-known male-to-female ratio (4:1) [3], it is plausible that there will be a lot of autistic women in the coming decades with the desire to work and have an independent life.

Therefore, identifying the work needs of autistic women and promoting independent living represent key topics. Most of the knowledge concerning job expectations of autistic women comes from studies including samples of autistic individuals without intellectual disability (ID), and most of the information derives from their caregivers (without reflecting the needs of the whole autism spectrum). A better understanding of the female phenotype could provide a better definition of "sex/gender-targeted treatment" [6].

L. M. Fatta (✉)
Research Coordination and Support Service, Istituto Superiore di Sanità, Rome, Italy
e-mail: laura.fatta@iss.it

M. Siracusano
Department of Biomedicine and Prevention, University of Rome Tor Vergata, Rome, Italy

Child Neurology and Psychiatry Unit, Department of Wellbeing of Mental and Neurological, Dental and Sensory Organ Health, Policlinico Tor Vergata Hospital, Rome, Italy

L. Mazzone
Child Neurology and Psychiatry Unit, Department of Wellbeing of Mental and Neurological, Dental and Sensory Organ Health, Policlinico Tor Vergata Hospital, Rome, Italy

Systems Medicine Department, University of Rome Tor Vergata, Rome, Italy
e-mail: luigi.mazzone@uniroma2.it

L. Mazzone et al. (eds.), *Autism Spectrum Disorder: Understanding the Female Phenotype*, https://doi.org/10.1007/978-3-031-62072-0_13

13.1.1 Employment Challenges

For some decades, employment in ASD has represented a clinical and scientific topic of interest. Before defining the challenges usually addressed by autistic adults, it is necessary to distinguish between competitive work and supported work—distinctive conditions in the disability framework. Within *competitive work*, the individual is not supported by a job coach or a work team. The autistic person can be initially assisted to detect a more suitable job for him/her and to enhance the suitable skills to join the workplace. However, colleagues may not be aware of the diagnosis (and of what a condition of ASD implies in terms of social difficulties and atypical behaviors), and the environment may present additional barriers related to ASD *core* features (i.e., sensory over-responsivity, lack of routines, and scheduled activities). Vice versa, in *supported employment*, which primarily addresses autistic individuals with substantial support needs, the central role of the job coach is to provide full supervision [7]. Considering all these issues, autistic individuals have to face several challenges strictly connected to their features (i.e., the cognitive profile, the impact of autism-related characteristics) and the type of support their work community offers.

Autistic people have different professional needs in the workplace than individuals with other disabilities or with typical development [7, 8]. Specifically, social and communicative skills impairment influences job recruitment and the working relationship with colleagues. Likewise, repetitive and restricted interests could result in pedantic behaviors misinterpreted as a braggart attitude. Finally, sensory needs might not be adequately considered in the work context (i.e., noise, light, smell).

Regarding the professional needs of autistic women, the actual knowledge is limited. The main job-related challenges that autistic adults experience are unemployment, underemployment, and difficulties in maintaining employment, regardless of sex/gender [1, 2, 9–11].

Worldwide *employment rates* within the autistic population are very low, ranging from 4.1 to 11.8%—regardless of cognitive profile [12]—although autistic individuals with a higher IQ level are generally characterized by more remarkable employment outcomes [13]. ASD employment rates are also lower than other disabilities [4, 14, 15]. Rates of employment within ASD vary across studies depending on the cognitive and adaptive functioning of individuals examined and the type of employment considered (full-time vs. part-time and supported vs. mainstream job employment). An extensive survey study estimated that among graduated autistic individuals, only 34% have a job [14]. Among autistic adults with a salaried job, 80% have part-time jobs [4, 5, 16]. This phenomenon affects autistic people across all countries [17].

Concerning sex/gender, autistic women present lower employment levels than both autistic men [18, 19] and employed neurotypical women [14]. Taylor and Mailick (2014) examined 10-year trajectories of vocational and educational activities in autistic adults and highlighted the declines in the level of independence over time, especially for autistic women.

The *underemployment* includes low wages [12, 20], obstacles to getting a career [13], and downgrading. Underemployment affects autistic individuals' quality of life, sense of self-efficacy [15], and mental and physical well-being, regardless of sex/gender [2, 11]. Autistic women, similar to neurotypical women, aspire to have full-time employment that aligns with their interests and skills, considering this aspiration a fundamental need [2, 21].

Maintaining a job position is another big challenge in autism. Among autistic adults with a salaried job, only 20–25% are estimated to maintain a job position over time [22]. Difficulties in social skills impact negatively 90% of cases about keeping the job [1, 2, 8, 9, 14, 15]. Social impairment represents the main challenge to be faced in the job environment for both males and females (60%) [23]. Conversational skills are related to verbal and nonverbal comprehension abilities [2], which imply understanding language's implicit and explicit meanings [1, 2]. Not surprisingly, job-related interpersonal interactions, such as contacting clients, meeting customers, and understanding the social context's nuances, are highly challenging and overwhelming for autistic individuals of both sex/gender [23].

Sensory hyper/hypo-responsivity related to job environment may represent a crucial factor influencing the work performance of autistic individuals of both sexes/genders [1, 9, 10]. Most of the women report sensory overload as an element that they perceive as relevant in their workplace; however, a minor percentage (29%) declares that their job place supports these sensory needs [23]. Overall, studies highlight that lack of sensory needs' tolerance may negatively influence the work productivity of autistic individuals.

Finally, underemployment and unemployment impact autistic women's economic independence [11], leading to a sense of frustration, reduced self-esteem, anxiety, and depression [1, 10, 14, 23].

As a whole, all the information above discussed comes from studies with methodological limitations such as small and not representative samples of females, lack of a control group of individuals with typical development [15, 23–27], scarce employment of quantitative measures to investigate the needs, and job expectations [8, 15].

13.1.2 Female Social Work-Related Skill Barriers

The main social difficulties—related to job environment—which characterize autistic females, consist of holding conversations with colleagues and responding to phone calls. However, work-related skills do not exactly overlap with social skills but rather focus on social etiquette in work relationships. These abilities also include assertive communication, maintaining a positive attitude, ability to cooperate and work in a team, respecting the authority of supervisors, and social rules [8]. Regarding working relationships, although autistic females have a strong desire to connect with female peers, they often report a better feeling when engaging with autistic males [23, 25, 28]. As a matter of fact, both autistic girls/women (11–40+ years old) described difficulty in making and keeping friends and, joining the conversation on gender clichés– i.e., make-up and shopping [25, 27].

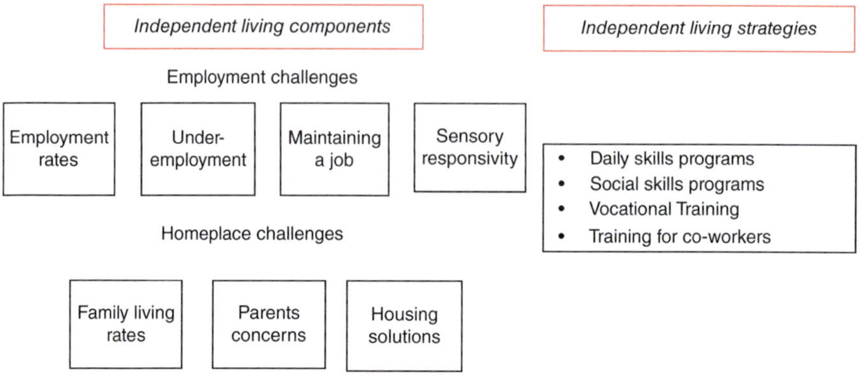

Fig. 13.1 Independent living components and strategies

13.1.3 Employment Options

Employment is one of the components of independent living. With autistic individuals having less work experience than neurotypical peers, they have been exposed to fewer job opportunities with subsequent difficulties in understanding to which profession they are more prone.

Autistic people are often involved in information technology (IT) programs [29]. These areas fit in with a range of skills (task structuring, attention to detail, error detection, systems thinking, visualization, efficiency, honesty, precision, low absenteeism) characteristic of autistic cognitive style [9, 29]. While there is a common belief that autistic people are prone to performing calculations and rather gifted at engineering and computer science [30], some autistic individuals have a talent for performative arts [24] or natural sciences [15]. Autistic women express interest in creative arts, mainly writing, performing, and visual arts [23]. It is not fully understood if these attitudes are driven by gender norms and/or consequences of camouflage efforts.

Among types of professions in which autistic females are employed, there are community and personal service jobs (24%), clerical and administrative jobs (24%), professional jobs (i.e., doctor, teacher, lawyer, author) (22%), technicians, and trade jobs (12%) [7, 23]. Figure 13.1 summarizes independent living components and strategies discussed in the following sections.

13.2 ASD and Transition for Independent Living: Are There Female Needs?

The transition period between adolescence and adulthood is crucial for an autistic person to create the basis for an independent life, including a satisfying job and suitable housing. The transition to independent living raises new challenges for the autistic individual and his/her family. The transition age is experienced as "falling off a cliff"; during this period, school support is not provided anymore, and there is a lack of health services addressed to autistic young adults [5, 22]. This lack of support corresponds to a great desire of independent living. Most autistic women complain of not being "understood" from school years until adulthood included [23], and their needs remain unheard.

13.2.1 Accommodation Arrangement Challenges

Evidence indicates that autistic individuals without ID have more independence in both work and residential contexts than those with ASD and ID [17]. Compared to other developmental disabilities, autistic adults show lower degrees of independent living [31]. Austic adults have in fact high rates of "living in the family," mainly if they have co-occurring ID [24]. Few studies indicate the *ratio by gender* about accommodation, however highlighting both sex/genders' unmet needs [32].

Many parents of autistic individuals report concerns about their child's independent living. To let a child go away from home represents a physiological step in the family life cycle. From one side, this process is postponed for families with a family member with a disability implying a strong emotional impact which includes a sense of guilt [28]. From the other side, independent living implicates advantages for the whole family (raising an autistic child is considered as a "24-h" task) [28]. Concerning sex/gender, females are less likely to live with their parents and more likely to live alone compared to males [23, 33]. In contrast, other studies report a trend inversion [28]. Often, however, the *concerns of autistic females' parents*—regardless of the level of support needs—are related to daily living skills (e.g., taking care of the house, doing laundry, hygiene, etc.), safety [26], and risk of abuse [28].

Independent living in the context of structured programs and *housing solutions* is related to a better outcome and greater self-confidence in autistic individuals [28, 34]; however, it generally represents a hard decision for a family. As a matter of fact, the family should be involved in all the process, from the residence choice to the individualized activities. The *Treatment and Education of Autistic and Communication Handicapped Children* (TEACCH) is an example of a program that can be applied in residential setting [34].

Clinicians and service providers have a responsibility to promote competence in these areas to enable autistic females to pursue independent living opportunities.

13.3 Which Strategies Can Promote Independent Living in ASD Women?

In recent decades, programs and training to support the independent living trajectories of autistic people have multiplied. As a matter of fact, having a job leads to greater chances to live independently. The studies agreed on attending behavioral and social interventions to promote employment and independent life in autistic youth; however, evidence for gender-oriented programs is currently limited to low-quality evidence on social skills training.

Most of these programs indirectly increase the probability of success in recruiting a job. Several programs have been developed to support autistic individuals during transition age (from school to work; from young age to adulthood). Among these, there is a recent online program named TrASDition training aiming to evaluate the impact of parental training (focused on specific topics related to this critical age) on parental well-being [35]. Moreover, the BOOST-A™ is a manageable and flexible online program focused on self-determination and managing work planning, and involving the community to promote personal inclusion [36].

Despite the undoubted usefulness of these programs, sex/gender differences are not usually taken into account, maybe due to a scarce representation of females within their samples [35, 36]. A recent meta-analysis, including transition programs, addressed youth with neurodevelopmental disorders (not just autism) and psychiatric disorders [37] finding that the reduction of caregivers' depressive symptoms represented the main outcome. However, even this meta-analysis did not consider sex/gender effects.

13.3.1 Daily Skills Programs

Adaptive skills are crucial for independence, family release, and employment. In order to live outside the household, adaptive skills have a crucial role, but only a few training programs are specifically focused on these domains. Supporting adaptive skills also implies economic benefits for the healthcare system [16]. Daily skills often represent a target domain of more comprehensive programs [33, 38]; therefore, efficacy in daily skills programs is difficult to define.

A meta-analysis that selected 52 studies (majority single-case studies) with 133 autistic adults [39] found large to moderate effect sizes on functional life skill-based interventions. The finding indicates high levels of responsiveness in adults in learning functional life skills. The high rate of improvement in adaptive skills is more significant for those interventions that are based on cognitive-behavioral intervention strategies (CBT) (particularly visual cues) and applied behavior analysis methodology (ABA) (modeling, prompting, reinforcement, and fading). These results also encompass autistic individuals with co-occurring ID [39].

13.3.2 Social Skills Training

Women social skills impairment is perceived as a barrier to independent living [23] and negatively impacts the job productivity of autistic females. However, few studies on social skills training (SST) addressed sex/gender differences, mainly depicting a male-biased gender perspective and giving only a few suggestions concerning females' needs.

SST is an intervention based on learning theory and CBT. Usually, its aimed to implement conversational skills, perspective-taking, social problem-solving, and emotion recognition [40]. Several evidence-based models have focused on enhancing social skills in autistic adults. In a recent meta-analysis, Dubreucq et al. (2021) identified 18 studies, including 5 RCTs (145 participants), which showed a large effect size in the global social skills outcomes. However, these results should be interpreted with caution due to the paucity and quality of the studies [41]. Most of these studies predominantly involved males and young-aged individuals (aged <25 years; 60%). Nevertheless, results on children and adolescents detect moderate [42] and large [43] effect sizes of SST in autism. Given that SST studies have primarily included individuals with an IQ >70, the evidence of SST in ASD with ID is limited (e.g., Rose et al., 2021) [44]. However, findings about efficacy of evidence-based models, such as the *Program for the Education and Enrichment of Relational Skills* (*PEERS*®) has been deeply investigated and has been exported for use with autistic adults in a variety of cultural contexts [46, 47].

The specific difficulties described by mothers and autistic girls/women [25, 27] assume that there may be different responses to treatment based on gender. A study tested this hypothesis in a sample of adolescents, but no results emerged by sex/gender [45].

In 2017, Jamison and Schuttler developed a promising SST and self-care program specifically for autistic female adolescents and young women: *the Girls Night Out Model (GNO)*. However, to the best of our knowledge, evidence is limited to a study that tested the efficacy of GNO with a restricted sample size (34 subjects). The limited sample size and the lack of a comparison control group or waiting list, limit the generalizability of the findings [38].

13.3.3 Vocational Training

Interventions designed to provide strategies to support employment have grown in recent years [20]. The need to develop strategies for dealing with work challenges is self-reported by autistic women [23], but no available evidence supports sex/gender differences in vocational interventions. In line with the lack of evidence, there is a paucity and insufficient quality of research providing female-oriented information on policy and practice developments [11].

Although protocols on social and adaptive skills include modules on work-related abilities [33, 48], vocational training is more focused on job interviews [49] or directed on job-related social skills [50]. Vocational training addresses autistic adults without ID bringing together several ingredients, such as social skills training, group therapy, CBT, and psychoeducation [33, 50]. It is noteworthy that some studies on vocational training have divided the samples based on job goals and attitudes rather than the autism characteristics or support needs or age [48]. Considering women's poor interest in joining the conversation on mainstream topics, having shared goals and preferences with colleagues could be useful for supporting social motivation, self-confidence, and work-related social skills.

Taking into account the recent impact of COVID-19 on work organizations and sensory overload—common in autistic people, including females—evidence pointed out the advantages of smart working in terms of reduced travel time and work flexibility [51]. These findings should be tested on autistic women to evaluate the impact of isolation on emotional issues and difficulty in considering home and work totally separated.

However, autistic adults with significant support needs can benefit from more structured and concrete job-related programs, such as *Project SEARCH plus Autism* [20] based on common CBT strategies as well as ABA methodology. Findings are unsuccessful to infer gender-specific information about autistic women with ID. Therefore, the employment options and needs of women with ID are salient features for future research.

The challenges and barriers faced by autistic individuals should not solely be a concern for families and autistic people themselves.

13.3.4 Strategies for Co-Workers

Workplace organization is based on executive structures, sociocultural norms, and expectations derived from the attitudes of neurotypical people [52]. However, the companies' assumption of a perspective of neurodiversity workers is a crucial point to be promoted for enhancing the social inclusion of autistic people, including women.

Research, albeit with limitations, is addressing the need to validate interventions for autistic people to support them in the work environment by developing vocational, social, and daily training. However, the organizational needs able to fit with the successful employment of autistic people and develop mutual inclusiveness with colleagues have been poorly explored. There is a research gap that needs to be addressed to identify coping strategies for employers and colleagues with the aim to better support autistic individuals [1, 4] and to ensure that work environments do not represent a barrier [53]. In this area, knowledge is limited, and sex/gender differences are not considered.

Nonetheless, autistic women report that they would also like to receive help from organizations (in 29% of cases), such as more flexibility in work schedules and tasks [19]. Unfortunately, most workplaces and employers do not currently appear to have adequate levels of awareness to improve work access and experiences for autistic employees [2, 24]. Neurotypical colleagues may be unable to correctly interpret both the attitudes and facial expressions of autistic people [54], reflecting what is referred to as Milton's (2012) "double empathy" problem, where neurotypical people do not behave empathetically toward autistic people as they would toward other neurotypicals [24].

Some research reports that employers are less likely to hire people with disabilities even when the disability does not negatively affect performance (stigma) but at the same time disclosure of the diagnosis can lead to experiencing 26% less chance of being hired by the employer [55]. Other studies show that managers report that autism awareness training positively influences the entire cultural context of work and allows them to gain a high-quality employment brand that helps them attract and retain top talent [24]. In this framework, recruiting autistic people is helpful both for the inclusive culture society and for organizational benefits.

13.4 Conclusion and Research Priority

Evidence about female needs suggests a different vocational profile compared to men, but no specific supports are addressed. However, literature on sex/gender differences in independent life needs is scarce, and other studies should be conducted to correctly identify women's profiles. In particular, studies about employment in autistic women are limited. Therefore, evidence is based on autobiographical or caregiver-reported narratives and qualitative tools, study samples were often mixed (males and females), and statistical analyses of gender differences are rarely performed.

The investigation of sex/gender differences in housing needs is at the very beginning, and it is inconsistent to provide clear interpretations. In line with the findings of INSAR's Special Interest Group (SIG) in 2014 [13], although research on gender in ASD has advanced in recent years, there are still many aspects of employment and independent living that remain to be investigated and understood, especially in adulthood.

It is known that the prevalence of ASD disadvantages the opportunity to design studies with suitable numbers for achieving solid results in women. However, it would be helpful to conduct multiple rigorous studies in several countries, using the RCT model design and including moderators' variables (e.g., age, IQ, geographical area, type of services available, health system, and coverage). A solid methodological approach is needed to evaluate the needs in the "real world" and the efficacy of the interventions according to gender.

In addition, interventions should be based on explicit constructs with a clear theoretical framework to assess whether the intervention ingredients have a specific effect on outcomes. Interventions could be addressed to cover needs identified in women and rephrased in modular proposals on social skills, adaptive skills, self-determination skills, self-efficacy and self-perception skills, soft skills, job-specific skills, training toward co-workers, and home skills. In addition, co-workers and organizations should receive information to sustain the inclusion and work needs of autistic people, specifically women.

In conclusion, further research is indispensable to verify the impact of the primary outcomes and quality of life on autistic women in the workplace and housing.

Key Points

- Autistic females show different work and independent living needs than men.
- The planning of intervention for autistic females in transition to adulthood needs to be focused on social skills, adaptive skills, home skills, and self-perception and self-efficacy skills.
- Improving corporate sustainability and enhancing neurodiversity culture are crucial for organizations and communities.
- Needs and support for residential arrangements should be better investigated in autistic women adults.

References

1. Hurlbutt K, Chalmers L. Employment and adults with Asperger syndrome. Focus autism dev disabil. 2004;19:215–22. https://doi.org/10.1177/10883576040190040301.
2. Müller E, Schuler AL, Burton B, Yates G. Meeting the vocational support needs of individuals with Asperger syndrome and other autism spectrum disabilities. J. Vocat. Rehabil. 2003;18:163–75.
3. Maenner MJ, Warren Z, Williams AR, Amoakohene E, Bakian AV, Bilder DA, et al. Prevalence and characteristics of autism Spectrum disorder among children aged 8 years - autism and developmental disabilities monitoring network, 11 sites, United States, 2020. MMWR Surveill Summ. 2023;72(2):1–14. https://doi.org/10.15585/mmwr.ss7202a1.
4. Roux AM, Shattuck PT, Cooper BP, Anderson KA, Wagner M, Narendorf SC. Postsecondary employment experiences among young adults with an autism spectrum disorder. J Am Acad Child Adolesc Psychiatry. 2013;52(9):931–9. https://doi.org/10.1016/j.jaac.2013.05.019.
5. Shattuck PT, Narendorf SC, Cooper B, Sterzing PR, Wagner M, Taylor JL. Postsecondary education and employment among youth with an autism spectrum disorder. Pediatrics. 2012;129(6):1042–9. https://doi.org/10.1542/peds.2011-2864.
6. Kirkovski M, Enticott PG, Fitzgerald PB. A review of the role of female gender in autism spectrum disorders. J Autism Dev Disord. 2013;43(11):2584–603. https://doi.org/10.1007/s10803-013-1811-1.
7. Khalifa G, Sharif Z, Sultan M, Di Rezze B. Workplace accommodations for adults with autism spectrum disorder: a scoping review. Disabil Rehabil. 2020;42(9):1316–31. https://doi.org/10.1080/09638288.2018.1527952.
8. Gal E, Landes E, Katz N. Work performance skills in adults with and without high functioning autism spectrum disorders (HFASD). Res Autism Spectr Disord. 2015;10:71–7. https://doi.org/10.1016/j.rasd.2014.10.011.
9. Baldwin S, Costley D, Warren A. Employment activities and experiences of adults with high-functioning autism and Asperger's disorder. J Autism Dev Disord. 2014;44(10):2440–9. https://doi.org/10.1007/s10803-014-2112-z.
10. Griffith GM, Totsika V, Nash S, Hastings RP. I just don't fit anywhere': support experiences and future support needs of individuals with Asperger syndrome in middle adulthood. Autism. 2012;16(5):532–46. https://doi.org/10.1177/1362361311405223.
11. Hayward SM, McVilly KR, Stokes MA. Challenges for females with high functioning autism in the workplace: a systematic review. Disabil Rehabil. 2018;40(3):249–58.
12. Taylor JL, Seltzer MM. Employment and post-secondary educational activities for young adults with autism spectrum disorders during the transition to adulthood. J Autism Dev Disord. 2011;41(5):566–74. https://doi.org/10.1080/09638288.2016.1254284.

13. Nicholas DB, Hodgetts S, Zwaigenbaum L, Smith LE, Shattuck P, Parr JR, et al. Research needs and priorities for transition and employment in autism: considerations reflected in a "special interest group" at the international meeting for autism research. Autism Res. 2017;10(1):15–24. https://doi.org/10.1002/aur.1683.
14. Autism Spectrum Australia Aspect. We belong: the experiences, aspirations and needs of adults with Asperger's disorder and high functioning autism. 2013.
15. Lorenz T, Heinitz K. Aspergers--different, not less: occupational strengths and job interests of individuals with Asperger's Syndrome. PLoS One. 2014;9(6):e100358. https://doi.org/10.1371/journal.pone.0100358.
16. Hendricks D. Employment and adults with autism spectrum disorders: challenges and strategies for success. J. Vocat. Rehabil. 2010;32:125–34. https://doi.org/10.3233/JVR-2010-0502.
17. Howlin P, Goode S, Hutton J, Rutter M. Adult outcome for children with autism. J Child Psychol Psychiatry. 2004;45(2):212–29. https://doi.org/10.1111/j.1469-7610.2004.00215.x.
18. Howlin P, Moss P, Savage S, Rutter M. Social outcomes in mid- to later adulthood among individuals diagnosed with autism and average nonverbal IQ as children. J Am Acad Child Adolesc Psychiatry. 2013;52(6):572–81.e1. https://doi.org/10.1016/j.jaac.2013.02.017.
19. Taylor JL, Mailick MR. A longitudinal examination of 10-year change in vocational and educational activities for adults with autism spectrum disorders. Dev Psychol. 2014;50(3):699–708. https://doi.org/10.1037/a0034297.
20. Wehman P, Schall CM, McDonough J, Graham C, Brooke V, Riehle JE, et al. Effects of an employer-based intervention on employment outcomes for youth with significant support needs due to autism. Autism. 2017;21(3):276–90. https://doi.org/10.1177/1362361316635826.
21. Hayward S, McVilly K, Stokes M. "I would love to just be myself": what autistic women want at work. Autism Adulthood. 2019;1:297–305. https://doi.org/10.1089/aut.2019.0020.
22. Howlin P, Alcock J, Burkin C. An 8 year follow-up of a specialist supported employment service for high-ability adults with autism or Asperger syndrome. Autism. 2005;9(5):533–49. https://doi.org/10.1177/1362361305057871.
23. Baldwin S, Costley D. The experiences and needs of female adults with high-functioning autism spectrum disorder. Autism. 2016;20(4):483–95. https://doi.org/10.1177/1362361315590805.
24. Buckley E, Pellicano E, Remington A. "the real thing I struggle with is other People's perceptions": the experiences of autistic performing arts professionals and attitudes of performing arts employers in the UK. J Autism Dev Disord. 2021;51(1):45–59. https://doi.org/10.1007/s10803-020-04517-0.
25. Cridland EK, Jones SC, Caputi P, Magee CA. Being a girl in a boys' world: investigating the experiences of girls with autism spectrum disorders during adolescence. J Autism Dev Disord. 2014;44(6):1261–74. https://doi.org/10.1007/s10803-013-1985-6.
26. Mademtzi M, Singh P, Shic F, Koenig K. Challenges of females with autism: a parental perspective. J Autism Dev Disord. 2018;48(4):1301–10. https://doi.org/10.1007/s10803-017-3341-8.
27. Milner V, McIntosh H, Colvert E, Happé F. A qualitative exploration of the female experience of autism Spectrum disorder (ASD). J Autism Dev Disord. 2019;49(6):2389–402. https://doi.org/10.1007/s10803-019-03906-4.
28. Krauss MW, Seltzer MM, Jacobson HT. Adults with autism living at home or in non-family settings: positive and negative aspects of residential status. J Intellect Disabil Res. 2005;49(Pt 2):111–24. https://doi.org/10.1111/j.1365-2788.2004.00599.x.
29. Morris MR, Begel A, Wiedermann B. Understanding the challenges faced by Neurodiverse software engineering employees: towards a more inclusive and productive technical workforce. In: Proceedings of the 17th international ACM SIGACCESS conference on computers & accessibility; 2015. p. 173–84. https://doi.org/10.1145/2700648.2809841.
30. Annabi H, Locke J. A theoretical framework for investigating the context for creating employment success in information technology for individuals with autism. J Manag Organ. 2019;25(4):499–515. https://doi.org/10.1017/jmo.2018.79.
31. Howlin P. Outcome in adult life for more able individuals with autism or Asperger syndrome. Autism. 2000;4(1):63–83. https://doi.org/10.1177/1362361300004001005.

32. Dudley KM, Klinger MR, Meyer A, Powell P, Klinger LG. Understanding service usage and needs for adults with ASD: the importance of living situation. J Autism Dev Disord. 2019;49(2):556–68. https://doi.org/10.1007/s10803-018-3729-0.
33. Oswald TM, Winder-Patel B, Ruder S, Xing G, Stahmer A, Solomon M. A pilot randomized controlled trial of the ACCESS program: a group intervention to improve social, adaptive functioning, stress coping, and self-determination outcomes in young adults with autism Spectrum disorder. J Autism Dev Disord. 2018;48(5):1742–60. https://doi.org/10.1007/s10803-017-3421-9.
34. Galli-Carminati G, Gerber F, Baud MA, Baud O. Evaluating the effects of a structured program for adults with autism spectrum disorders and intellectual disabilities. Res Autism Spectr Disord. 2007;1(3):256–65. https://doi.org/10.1016/j.rasd.2006.11.001.
35. Siracusano M, Calsolaro J, Riccioni A, Gialloreti LE, Benvenuto A, Giovagnoli G, et al. TrASDition training: an online parental training for transition-age youth with autism spectrum disorder. Psychiatry Res. 2021;300:113930. https://doi.org/10.1016/j.psychres.2021.113930.
36. Hatfield M, Falkmer M, Falkmer T, Ciccarelli M. Effectiveness of the BOOST-A™ online transition planning program for adolescents on the autism spectrum: a quasi-randomized controlled trial. Child Adolesc Psychiatry Ment Health. 2017;11:54. https://doi.org/10.1186/s13034-017-0191-2.
37. Hothi H, Bedard C, Ceccacci A, DiRezze B, Kwan MYW. Evaluated interventions addressing developmental transitions for youth with mental health disorders: a meta-analysis. Disabil Rehabil. 2022;44(21):6155–65. https://doi.org/10.1080/09638288.2021.1960440.
38. Jamison TR, Schuttler JO. Overview and preliminary evidence for a social skills and self-care curriculum for adolescent females with autism: the girls night out model. J Autism Dev Disord. 2017;47(1):110–25. https://doi.org/10.1007/s10803-016-2939-6.
39. Ninci J, Leslie C, Neely LC, Hong ER, Boles MG, Gilliland WD, et al. Meta-analysis of single-case research on teaching functional living skills to individuals with ASD. Rev J Autism Dev Disord. 2015;2:184–98. https://doi.org/10.1007/s40489-014-0046-1.
40. Moody CT, Laugeson EA. Social skills training in autism Spectrum disorder across the lifespan. Child Adolesc Psychiatr Clin N Am. 2020;29(2):359–71. https://doi.org/10.1016/j.chc.2019.11.001.
41. Dubreucq J, Haesebaert F, Plasse J, Dubreucq M, Franck N. A systematic review and meta-analysis of social skills training for adults with autism Spectrum disorder. J Autism Dev Disord. 2022;52(4):1598–609. https://doi.org/10.1007/s10803-021-05058-w.
42. Reichow B, Steiner AM, Volkmar F. Cochrane review: social skills groups for people aged 6 to 21 with autism spectrum disorders (ASD). Evid Based Child Health. 2013;8(2):266–315. https://doi.org/10.1002/ebch.1903.
43. Wolstencroft J, Robinson L, Srinivasan R, Kerry E, Mandy W, Skuse D. A systematic review of group social skills interventions, and meta-analysis of outcomes, for children with high functioning ASD. J Autism Dev Disord. 2018;48(7):2293–307. https://doi.org/10.1007/s10803-018-3485-1.
44. Rose AJ, Kelley KR, Raxter A. Effects of PEERS(®) social skills training on young adults with intellectual and developmental disabilities during college. Behav Modif. 2021;45(2):297–323. https://doi.org/10.1177/0145445520987146.
45. McVey AJ, Schiltz H, Haendel A, Dolan BK, Willar KS, Pleiss S, et al. Brief report: does gender matter in intervention for ASD? Examining the impact of the PEERS(®) social skills intervention on social behavior among females with ASD. J Autism Dev Disord. 2017;47(7):2282–9. https://doi.org/10.1007/s10803-017-3121-5.
46. Laugeson EA, Gantman A, Kapp SK, Orenski K, Ellingsen R. A randomized controlled trial to improve social skills in young adults with autism Spectrum disorder: the UCLA PEERS(®) program. J Autism Dev Disord. 2015;45(12):3978–89. https://doi.org/10.1007/s10803-015-2504-8.
47. Chien YL, Tsai WC, Chen WH, Yang CL, Gau SS, Soong WT, et al. Effectiveness, durability, and clinical correlates of the PEERS social skills intervention in young adults

with autism spectrum disorder: the first evidence outside North America. Psychol Med. 2021;53(3):966–76. https://doi.org/10.1017/S0033291721002385.
48. Connor A, Sung C, Strain A, Zeng S, Fabrizi S. Building skills, confidence, and wellness: psychosocial effects of soft skills training for young adults with autism. J Autism Dev Disord. 2020;50(6):2064–76. https://doi.org/10.1007/s10803-019-03962-w.
49. Morgan L, Leatzow A, Clark S, Siller M. Interview skills for adults with autism spectrum disorder: a pilot randomized controlled trial. J Autism Dev Disord. 2014;44(9):2290–300. https://doi.org/10.1007/s10803-014-2100-3.
50. Gorenstein M, Giserman-Kiss I, Feldman E, Isenstein EL, Donnelly L, Wang AT, et al. Brief report: a job-based social skills program (JOBSS) for adults with autism Spectrum disorder: a pilot randomized controlled trial. J Autism Dev Disord. 2020;50(12):4527–34. https://doi.org/10.1007/s10803-020-04482-8.
51. McNaughton D, Rackensperger T, Dorn D, Wilson N. "home is at work and work is at home": telework and individuals who use augmentative and alternative communication. Work. 2014;48(1):117–26. https://doi.org/10.3233/WOR-141860.
52. Maroto M, Pettinicchio D. Twenty-five years after the ADA: situating disability in America's system of stratification. Disability Studies Quarterly. 2015;35:1–34. https://doi.org/10.18061/dsq.v35i3.4927.
53. Whetzel M. Interviewing tips for applicants with autism spectrum disorder (ASD). J. Vocat. Rehabil. 2014;40:155–9. https://doi.org/10.3233/JVR-140668.
54. Sheppard E, Pillai D, Wong GT, Ropar D, Mitchell P. How easy is it to read the minds of people with autism Spectrum disorder? J Autism Dev Disord. 2016;46(4):1247–54. https://doi.org/10.1007/s10803-015-2662-8.
55. Johnson TD, Joshi A. Dark clouds or silver linings? A stigma threat perspective on the implications of an autism diagnosis for workplace Well-being. J Appl Psychol. 2016;101(3):430–49. https://doi.org/10.1037/apl0000058.

Part VI

Case Reports

Clinical Case Reports

14

Assia Riccioni, Martina Siracusano, and Luigi Mazzone

In this chapter, we provide two case reports suggestive of the clinical pictures which more frequently occur within females with ASD.

Case 1 (Sarah) illustrates a traditional onset of autism symptoms in a girl with low cognitive skills and high level of support needs. Case 2 (Elisa) depicts parental understanding of their daughter's atypical behaviors after years of worries. Sarah and Elisa are imaginary names.

A. Riccioni (✉)
Child Neurology and Psychiatry Unit, Department of Wellbeing of Mental and Neurological, Dental and Sensory Organ Health, Policlinico Tor Vergata Hospital, Rome, Italy

M. Siracusano
Child Neurology and Psychiatry Unit, Department of Wellbeing of Mental and Neurological, Dental and Sensory Organ Health, Policlinico Tor Vergata Hospital, Rome, Italy

Department of Biomedicine and Prevention, University of Rome Tor Vergata, Rome, Italy

L. Mazzone
Child Neurology and Psychiatry Unit, Department of Wellbeing of Mental and Neurological, Dental and Sensory Organ Health, Policlinico Tor Vergata Hospital, Rome, Italy

Department of System Medicine, University of Rome Tor Vergata, Rome, Italy
e-mail: luigi.mazzone@uniroma2.it

L. Mazzone et al. (eds.), *Autism Spectrum Disorder: Understanding the Female Phenotype*, https://doi.org/10.1007/978-3-031-62072-0_14

Case 1: "She doesn't Seem to Be Interested in Others, she doesn't Speak. Sometimes I Have the Feeling she Is Deaf": The Case of Sarah, a 2-Year-Old Autistic Female

Sarah is a 24-month baby girl. Her parents are concerned about a language and communication delay: some vocalizations are just coming out, however hardly ever used for communicative and socio-relational purposes. Sarah primarily makes requests by using her parent's arm, reaching and placing the hand on the desired object. By contrast, she has achieved all the motor milestones.

At the age of 20 months, she started the nursery school: educators reported in Sarah the fear related to unfamiliar people, lack of eye contact, and reduced use of gestures (i.e., pointing). A poor range of spontaneous play was also noticed in the scholar context.

As time goes by, atypical behaviors occur and become pervasive: lights are an irresistible attraction for Sarah, and unexpected sounds provoke fear and impulsive reactions. She expresses excitement and emotions flapping her hands and arms, running back and forth. Routine adherence and difficulties in managing changes with a tendency to the sameness arise impacting her family's quality of life.

Any modifications in her routine (domestic, scholar), including her look or that one of familiar people (i.e., haircut), determine unexpected, impulsive, negative (aggressive and extreme) reaction in Sarah (crying, hitting herself). Change is synonymous of pressure. Travelling everyday along the same road to reach school turned into a duty for her parents. Given the unusual food habits of Sarah (bread and crunchy food were the only accepted on her plate), going for grocery shopping suddenly became such a stressful moment for them. Specific brand and shape of pasta represented the target of a strenuous search—sometimes disastrous with irreparable implications on daily meals—in most of the supermarkets of the city center.

Hearing impairment was the first parental concern which could have explained all the difficulties of Sarah: calling her repeatedly does not generate any reaction. However, auditory screening was negative, spreading such a different scenario that parents did not expect at all. In this way, Sarah was referred to the child psychiatric unit receiving diagnosis of ASD.

Case 2: "Suddenly the Difficulties of My Daughter Make Sense": The Case of Elisa, a 10-Year-Old Girl

"A wunderkind, tidy and extremely routine girl" is how the mother of Elisa defines their daughter. All these features determine admiration in friends of their parents, whose children are not characterized by such behavioral traits. However, parents of Elisa have some concern about their child even if her development is adequate. She prefers to be involved—too much involved—in her interests rather than interacting with peers. Something does not add up.

Elisa is a cheerful and smart 10-year-old Italian girl. She has always been highly curious, probably excessively curious. Whereupon she is particularly interested about a topic, Elisa becomes overfocused on it, learning as much as possible information. Currently, she is obsessed by the singer Michael Bublè. Biography, recordings (title, year of publication of all his albums, duration in minutes and seconds of the songs), and date of concerts (actually and of the years gone by) of Bublè constitute her main conversational theme at school, at home, wherever. Moreover, she insists in listening Christmas songs even in seasons during which the Christmas atmosphere should be far away. No contradiction is contemplated leading to quarrel with school mates and emargination.

Teachers are bothered about Elisa's area of interest, a topic appropriate for age but nor for intensity.

Elisa has always been described as very smart and precocious. Nevertheless, despite the presence of outstanding skills (reading and recognizing numbers at the age of 2; use of too polished language; great academic performances) since early childhood, social relationships were her weakness. Social exchange and reciprocal conversation were very challenging for Elisa and the interlocutors. This difficulty was mainly due to her tendency to literally interpret conversational topics.

Routine represents a safety zone for Elisa; order and method permeate meals, sleep (bed routine), and games.

When Elisa was finally referred to a child psychiatric unit, receiving diagnosis of ASD, everything acquired sense for her parents. The initial behavioral difficulties when she was admitted at primary school (Elisa refused to talk for at least 6 months) and the poor tolerance for noises including crowded places (even if amusing) were attributed to ASD symptoms.

MIX
Papier aus verantwortungsvollen Quellen
Paper from responsible sources
FSC® C105338

If you have any concerns about our products,
you can contact us on
ProductSafety@springernature.com

In case Publisher is established outside the EU,
the EU authorized representative is:
Springer Nature Customer Service Center GmbH
Europaplatz 3, 69115 Heidelberg, Germany

Printed by Libri Plureos GmbH
in Hamburg, Germany